BREAST CANCER IN THE POST-GENOMIC ERA

CURRENT CLINICAL ONCOLOGY

Maurie Markman, MD, SERIES EDITOR

For other titles published in this series, go to
www.springer.com/series/7631

BREAST CANCER IN THE POST-GENOMIC ERA

Edited by

ANTONIO GIORDANO

Sbarro Institute for Cancer Research and Molecular Medicine, Center for Biotechnology College of Science and Technology, Temple University, Philadelphia, PA, USA

NICOLA NORMANNO

Cell Biology and Biotherapy Unit, INT-Fondazione Pascale, Via Mariano Semmola, 80131 Naples, Italy

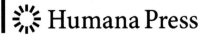

Editors

Antonio Giordano
Sbarro Institute for Cancer Research
  and Molecular Medicine
Center for Biotechnology College
  of Science and Technology
Temple University
Philadelphia, PA 19122
USA
and
Department of Human Pathology and Oncology
University of Siena
53100 Siena
Italy

Nicola Normanno
Cell Biology and Biotherapy Unit
INT-Fondazione Pascale
Via Mariano Semmola
80131 Naples
Italy

ISBN: 978-1-60327-944-4   e-ISBN: 978-1-60327-945-1
DOI: 10.1007/978-1-60327-945-1
Springer Dordrecht Heidelberg London New York

Library of Congress Control Number: 2009920073

© Humana Press, a part of Springer Science+Business Media, LLC 2009
All rights reserved. This work may not be translated or copied in whole or in part without the written permission of the publisher (Humana Press, c/o Springer Science+Business Media, LLC, 233 Spring Street, New York, NY 10013, USA), except for brief excerpts in connection with reviews or scholarly analysis. Use in connection with any form of information storage and retrieval, electronic adaptation, computer software, or by similar or dissimilar methodology now known or hereafter developed is forbidden.
The use in this publication of trade names, trademarks, service marks, and similar terms, even if they are not identified as such, is not to be taken as an expression of opinion as to whether or not they are subject to proprietary rights.
While the advice and information in this book are believed to be true and accurate at the date of going to press, neither the authors nor the editors nor the publisher can accept any legal responsibility for any errors or omissions that may be made. The publisher makes no warranty, express or implied, with respect to the material contained herein

Cover illustration: The selected image shows a section through a lobule-limited LacZ-positive outgrowth in full-term pregnant host composed entirely of progeny from PI-MEC. The growth comprises both luminal and myoepithelial cells and small-undifferentiated light cells.

Printed on acid-free paper

Springer is part of Springer Science+Business Media (www.springer.com)

Preface

Breast cancer is the most common tumour in women and it is the second leading cause of cancer deaths worldwide. Important advances have been made in breast cancer research that might allow for a significant improvement in breast cancer patient outcome over the next few years. The aim of this book is to provide a comprehensive approach to the biology, diagnosis, prevention and treatment of human breast carcinoma.

Specific chapters highlight the most recent findings in different fields of tumour biology. Our knowledge of the pathophysiology of the mammary gland has greatly increased over the last decade. Using high throughput technologies, it has been possible to identify groups of genes that are involved in breast tissue development and differentiation. These genes might also play a major role in breast cancer susceptibility by affecting the ability of mammary epithelial cells to undergo apoptosis, repair DNA defects and/or detoxify xenobiotic substances. The identification of breast cancer susceptibility genes has increased our knowledge of the mechanisms of transformation of mammary epithelial cells and has allowed for the development of counselling programs for high-risk individuals. In addition, the recognition and characterization of putative stem cells of the mammary gland that can give rise to breast cancer will allow for the development of specific drugs that might be useful for breast cancer treatment or prevention.

Different chapters of this book describe the use of gene profiling techniques, which recently made it possible to classify breast carcinomas in distinct entities with specific molecular, clinical and prognostic features. A number of different prognostic and predictive "gene signatures" have been identified, and clinical trials are ongoing to assess whether this novel approach might improve our ability to select more appropriate treatments for breast cancer patients.

Increasing evidence suggests that epigenetic mechanisms are involved in the pathogenesis of breast cancer as well. The most recent findings in this field are described in various chapters of the book. Changes in DNA methylation that lead to reduced expression of tumour suppressor genes or increased expression of prometastatic genes have been identified in breast cancer. This tumour is also characterized by profound alterations in the expression of cell cycle regulatory genes, as a result of genetic and epigenetic changes and growth factor stimuli. Indeed, several different growth factors synthesized either by tumour cells or by the surrounding stroma have been shown to promote breast cancer progression. In this regard, transgenic mice strains that have been developed for the purpose of modelling breast cancer have proven to be an invaluable tool to investigate genes implicated in the induction and progression of breast cancer, and might represent an important setting in which to test novel therapeutics.

Finally, two chapters are dedicated to novel therapeutic approaches in breast cancer. In fact, the identification of the above-described mechanisms that regulate proliferation and survival of tumour cells is leading to the development of novel agents, directed against specific signalling molecules expressed in tumour cells. Target-based agents such as trastuzumab, lapatinib and bevacizumab have been shown to significantly improve the efficacy of standard chemotherapy-based treatment in breast cancer patients, and have been approved for treatment of these patients. However, these drugs represent rather an exception. In fact, little clinical activity of the majority of signalling inhibitors explored in breast cancer patients has been reported up to now, at least when used as monotherapy.

The novel findings summarized in this book suggest that a broader approach that takes into account the complexity of the disease is definitely required to improve the efficacy of novel therapeutic methods in breast cancer. In this regard, we hope that this book might contribute to significant advances in this field by prompting the scientific community to look at breast cancer pathogenesis, diagnosis and treatment under a more comprehensive light.

Philadelphia, PA   *Antonio Giordano*
Naples, Italy   *Nicola Normanno*

Contents

Preface.. v

Contributors ix

1 The Genomic Basis of Breast Development and Differentiation....... 1
   Jose Russo and Irma H. Russo

2 Mammary Glands, Stem Cells, and Breast Cancer 19
   David L. Mack, Gilbert H. Smith,
   and Brian W. Booth

3 The Genetics of Breast Cancer: Application in Clinical Practice 39
   Antonio Russo, Valentina Agnese, Sergio Rizzo,
   Laura La Paglia, and Viviana Bazan

4 Alterations in Cell Cycle Regulatory Genes in Breast Cancer........... 55
   Annalisa Roberti, Marcella Macaluso,
   and Antonio Giordano

5 Neuregulins in the Nucleus... 79
   Carol M. McClelland and William J. Gullick

6 Role of the EGF-CFC Family in Mammary Gland
   Development and Neoplasia... 87
   Luigi Strizzi, Kazuhide Watanabe, Mario Mancino,
   David S. Salomon, and Caterina Bianco

7 Modeling Human Breast Cancer: The Use of Transgenic Mice........ 103
   Rachelle L. Dillon and William J. Muller

8 Gene Expression Profiling in Breast Cancer:
   Clinical Applications... 123
   Giuseppe Russo and Antonio Giordano

9 TGF-β Signaling: A Novel Target for Treatment
   of Breast Cancer? 137
   Jason D. Lee and Gerard C. Blobe

10 DNA Methylation in Breast Cancer 151
    Moshe Szyf

11 Signal Transduction Inhibitors in the Treatment of
    Breast Cancer 177
    Monica R. Maiello, Antonella De Luca,
    Marianna Gallo, Amelia D'Alessio, Pietro Carotenuto,
    and Nicola Normanno

12 Integration of Target-Based Agents in Current Protocols
    of Breast Cancer Therapy... 203
    Maria Carmela Piccirillo, Fabiano Falasconi,
    Antonia Del Giudice, Gianfranco De Feo, Jane Bryce,
    Mario Iaccarino, Francesco Perrone,
    and Alessandro Morabito

Index 225

Contributors

VALENTINA AGNESE • *Department of Surgery and Oncology, Regional Reference Center for the Biomolecular Characterization and Genetic Screening of Hereditary Tumors, Università di Palermo, Via del Vespro 127, 90127 Palermo, Italy*

VIVIANA BAZAN • *Department of Surgery and Oncology, Regional Reference Center for the Biomolecular Characterization and Genetic Screening of Hereditary Tumors, Università di Palermo, Via del Vespro 127, 90127 Palermo, Italy*

CATERINA BIANCO • *Mammary Biology and Tumorigenesis Laboratory, NCI/NIH, 37 Convent Drive, Bethesda, MD 20892, USA*

GERARD C. BLOBE • *Department of Medicine, Duke University Medical Center, Durham, NC 27710, USA*

BRIAN W. BOOTH • *Mammary Biology and Tumorigenesis Laboratory, Center for Cancer Research, National Cancer Institute, Bethesda, MD 20892, USA*

JANE BRYCE • *Clinical Trials Unit, National Cancer Institute, Via Mariano Semmola, 80131 Naples, Italy*

PIETRO CAROTENUTO • *Pharmacogenomic Laboratory, Centro di Ricerche Oncologiche di Mercogliano, Via Ammiraglio Bianco, 83013 Mercogliano (AV), Italy*

AMELIA D'ALESSIO • *Cell Biology and Biotherapy Unit, INT-Fondazione Pascale, Via Mariano Semmola, 80131 Naples, Italy*

GIANFRANCO DE FEO • *Clinical Trials Unit, National Cancer Institute, Via Mariano Semmola, 80131 Naples, Italy*

ANTONIA DEL GIUDICE • *Clinical Trials Unit, National Cancer Institute, Via Mariano Semmola, 80131 Naples, Italy*

ANTONELLA DE LUCA • *Cell Biology and Biotherapy Unit, INT-Fondazione Pascale, Via Mariano Semmola, 80131 Naples, Italy*

RACHELLE L. DILLON • *Goodman Cancer Centre, Department of Biochemistry, McGill University, Montreal, Quebec, Canada*

FABIANO FALASCONI • *Clinical Trials Unit, National Cancer Institute, Via Mariano Semola, 80131 Naples, Italy*

MARIANNA GALLO • *Cell Biology and Biotherapy Unit, INT-Fondazione Pascale, Via Mariano Semmola, 80131 Naples, Italy*

ANTONIO GIORDANO • *Sbarro Institute for Cancer Research and Molecular Medicine, Center for Biotechnology College of Science and Technology, Temple University, Philadelphia, PA 19122, USA; Department of Human Pathology and Oncology, University of Siena, 53100 Siena, Italy; Centro Ricerche Oncologiche Mercogliano, Via Ammiraglio Bianco, 83013 Mercogliano (AV), Italy*

WILLIAM J. GULLICK • *Cancer Biology Laboratory, University of Kent, Canterbury, Kent CT2 7NJ, UK*

MARIO IACCARINO • *Clinical Trials Unit, National Cancer Institute, Via Mariano Semmola, 80131 Naples, Italy*

LAURA LA PAGLIA • *Department of Surgery and Oncology, Regional Reference Center for the Biomolecular Characterization and Genetic Screening of Hereditary Tumors, Università di Palermo, Via del Vespro 127, 90127 Palermo, Italy*

JASON D. LEE • *Department of Pharmacology and Cancer Biology, Duke University Medical Center, 221B MSRB Research Drive, Durham, NC 27710, USA*

MARCELLA MACALUSO • *Sbarro Institute for Cancer Research and Molecular Medicine, Center for Biotechnology College of Science and Technology, Temple University, Philadelphia, PA 19122, USA; Department of Human Pathology and Oncology, University of Siena, 53100 Siena, Italy*

MONICA R. MACELLO • *Cell Biology and Biotherapy Unit, INT-Fondazione Pascale, Via Mariano Semmola, 80131 Naples, Italy*

DAVID L. MACK • *Mammary Biology and Tumorigenesis Laboratory, Center for Cancer Research, National Cancer Institute, Bethesda, MD 20892, USA*

CAROL M. McCLELLAND • *Cancer Biology Laboratory, University of Kent, Canterbury, Kent CT2 7NJ, UK*

MARIO MANCINO • *Mammary Biology and Tumorigenesis Laboratory, NCI/NIH, 37 Convent Drive, Bethesda, MD 20892, USA*

ALESSANDRO MORABITO • *Clinical Trials Unit, National Cancer Institute, Via Mariano Semmola, 80131 Naples, Italy*

WILLIAM J. MULLER • *Goodman Cancer Centre, Departments of Biochemistry and Medicine, McGill University, Montreal, Quebec, Canada*

NICOLA NORMANNO • *Cell Biology and Biotherapy Unit, INT-Fondazione Pascale, Via Mariano Semmola, 80131 Naples, Italy*

FRANCESCO PERRONE • *Clinical Trials Unit, National Cancer Institute, Via Mariano Semmola, 80131 Naples, Italy*

MARIA CARMELA PICCIRILLO • *Clinical Trials Unit, National Cancer Institute, Via Mariano Semmola, 80131 Naples, Italy*

SERGIO RIZZO • *Department of Surgery and Oncology, Regional Reference Center for the Biomolecular Characterization and Genetic Screening of Hereditary Tumors, Università di Palermo, Via del Vespro 127, 90127 Palermo, Italy*

ANNALISA ROBERTI • *Sbarro Institute for Cancer Research and Molecular Medicine, Center for Biotechnology College of Science and Technology, Temple University, Philadelphia, PA 19122, USA; Department of Human Pathology and Oncology, University of Siena, 53100 Siena, Italy*

ANTONIO RUSSO • *Department of Surgery and Oncology, Regional Reference Center for the Biomolecular Characterization and Genetic Screening of Hereditary Tumors, Università di Palermo, Via del Vespro 127, 90127 Palermo, Italy*

GIUSEPPE RUSSO • *Sbarro Institute for Cancer Research and Molecular Medicine, Center for Biotechnology College of Science and Technology, Temple University, Philadelphia, PA 19122, USA; DISI-Department of Computer and Information Sciences, University of Genova, 16146 Genova, Italy*

IRMA H. RUSSO • *Breast Cancer Research Laboratory, Fox Chase Cancer Center, 333 Cottman Avenue, Philadelphia, PA 19111, USA*

JOSE RUSSO • *Breast Cancer Research Laboratory, Fox Chase Cancer Center, 333 Cottman Avenue, Philadelphia, PA 19111, USA*

DAVID SALOMON • *Mammary Biology and Tumorigenesis Laboratory, NCI/NIH, 37 Convent Drive, Bethesda, MD 20892, USA*

GILBERT H. SMITH • *Mammary Biology and Tumorigenesis Laboratory, Center for Cancer Research, National Cancer Institute, Bethesda, MD 20892, USA*

LUIGI STRIZZI • *Children's Memorial Research Center, Robert H. Lurie Comprehensive Cancer Center, Northwestern University Feinberg School of Medicine, 2300 Children's Plaza, Box 222, Chicago, IL 60614-3394, USA*

MOSHE SZYF • *Department of Pharmacology and Therapeutics, McGill University, 3655 Sir William Osler Promenade, Montreal, QC, Canada H3G 1Y6*

KAZUHIDE WATANABE • *Mammary Biology and Tumorigenesis Laboratory, NCI/NIH, 37 Convent Drive, Bethesda, MD 20892, USA*

1

The Genomic Basis of Breast Development and Differentiation

Jose Russo and Irma H. Russo

SUMMARY

The breast attains its maximum development during pregnancy and lactation. After menopause the breast regresses in both nulliparous and parous women containing lobular structures that have been designated lobules type 1. Despite the similarity in the lobular composition of the breast at menopause, the fact that nulliparous women are at higher risk of developing breast cancer than parous women indicates that lobules type 1 in these two groups of women might be biologically different, or exhibit different susceptibility to carcinogenesis. Based on these observations it was postulated that the lobule type 1 found in the breast of nulliparous women and of parous women with breast cancer never went through the process of differentiation, retaining a high concentration of epithelial cells that are targets for carcinogens and therefore susceptible to undergo neoplastic transformation, whereas lobules type 1 structures found in the breast of early parous postmenopausal women free of mammary pathology, on the other hand, are composed of an epithelial cell population that is refractory to transformation. The degree of differentiation acquired through early pregnancy has changed the *genomic signature* that differentiates the lobule type 1 in the early parous women from that in the nulliparous women, making this the postulated mechanism of protection conferred by early full-term pregnancy.

Key Words: Pregnancy; Breast differentiation; Genomic signature; Breast cancer risk; Nulliparity; Development and differentiation

1. ARCHITECTURE OF THE HUMAN BREAST

The breast progressively develops from infancy to puberty under the main stimuli of pituitary and ovarian hormones. The least differentiated structure identified in the breast of postpubertal nulliparous women is the Lob 1, or TDLU, which is composed of clusters of 6–11 ductules per lobule. Lob 1 progresses to Lob 2, which is composed of more numerous

From: *Current Clinical Oncology: Breast Cancer in the Post-Genomic Era,*
Edited by: A. Giordano and N. Normanno, DOI: 10.1007/978-1-60327-945-1_1,
© Humana Press, a part of Springer Science + Business Media, LLC 2009

ductules per lobule and exhibits a more complex morphology. A fully differentiated condition is reached by the end of a full-term pregnancy, under the stimulus of new endocrine organs, the placenta and the developing fetus. These new hormonal influences induce a profuse branching of the mammary parenchyma leading to the formation of secretory lobular structures. During the first and second trimesters of pregnancy Lob 1 and Lob 2 rapidly progress to Lob 3, which are composed of more numerous and smaller small alveoli per lobule. During the last trimester of pregnancy active milk secretion supervenes, the alveoli become distended, and the lobules acquire the characteristic of the Lob 4, which is present during the lactational period. After weaning, all the secretory units of the breast regress, reverting to Lob 3 and Lob 2 *(1–5)*.

2. CELL PROLIFERATION AND STEROID RECEPTOR CONTENT IN THE NORMAL BREAST

The initial classification of lobules into four categories, primarily based on morphological characteristics of these structures *(1–5)* was complemented by analysis of the rate of cell proliferation, a cellular function essential for normal growth *(6–8)*. Normal growth requires a net increase of cycling cells over two other cell populations, resting cells (arrested in G_0), and dying cells (cells lost through programmed cell death or apoptosis). Proliferating cells express the nuclear protein Ki67, which are detected with a monoclonal antibody against it. The proliferative activity of the mammary epithelium varies as a function of the degree of lobular differentiation. The percentage of Ki67-positive cells (Ki67 or proliferation index) decreases progressively as the lobules mature from Lob 1 to Lob 2, and these to Lob 3 and Lob 4 *(6–8)*. These differences were not abrogated when the proliferation index was corrected for the phase of the menstrual cycle *(7,8)*. Parity, in addition to exerting an important influence in the lobular composition of the breast, profoundly influences the proliferative activity of the breast. Estrogens and progesterone are known to promote proliferation and differentiation in the normal breast. Both steroids act intracellularly through nuclear receptors, which become activated by the binding of their respective ligands. This is the most widely accepted model of action of estrogens for inducing cell proliferation and regulating gene expression *(9–19)*. The use of monoclonal antibodies that specifically recognize estrogen receptor alpha (ERa) since the discovery of the ER-beta *(6–8)* and progesterone receptor (PgR) in normal breast tissue revealed that the proliferative activity and percentage of cells positive for both ER-alpha and PgR are highest in Lob 1, and they progressively decrease in an inverse relationship to the degree of lobular differentiation, providing a mechanistic explanation for the higher susceptibility of these structures to be transformed by chemical carcinogens in vitro *(20,21)*.

3. INFLUENCE OF AGE AND PARITY ON BREAST DEVELOPMENT AND CANCER SUSCEPTIBILITY

Chemically induced carcinogenesis in an experimental animal model has shown that the initiation of the neoplastic process is inversely related to the degree of differentiation of the mammary gland, which in turn is a function of age and reproductive history *(22–25)*. These observations indicated that the protective effect of early first full-term pregnancy in women is the result of the differentiation of the breast *(1,2,20,21)*. The breast of nulliparous women contained almost exclusively Lob 1, and their number remained nearly constant throughout the lifespan of the individual *(2)*.

The breast of early parous women contained predominantly the more differentiated Lob 3, whereas Lob 1 were in a very low percentage until the fourth decade of life, when they started to increase, reaching the same level observed in nulliparous women after menopause. The breast of nulliparous women never reached the degree of differentiation found in women who completed an early pregnancy. Even though during the postmenopausal years the preponderant structure is the Lob 1 in the breast of both parous and nulliparous women, only nulliparous women are at high risk of developing breast cancer, whereas parous women remain protected (1,2).

Since ductal breast cancer originates in Lob 1 (TDLU) (22,23), the epidemiological observation that nulliparous women exhibit a higher incidence of breast cancer than parous women (26,27) indicates that Lob 1 in these two groups of women might be biologically different, or exhibit different susceptibility to carcinogenesis (1,2,21). Even though the Lob 1 is the hallmark of the postmenopausal breast, the degree of differentiation acquired through early pregnancy has caused a *genomic signature* that differentiates the Lob 1 in the early parous women from that in the nulliparous women. The identification of such "molecular phenotypes" has provided evidence for functional differences between cells and tissues that may not be obvious at the morphological level (29–31). This new set of information described in the next section has provided another level of complexity for differentiating the breast of early parous women free of cancer in comparison with that of nulliparous or women with cancer. The genomic mapping has added significance to the observations of lower proliferative activity in the Lob 1 of the parous women's breast, and higher in the Lob 1 of the nulliparous women's breast (7,8). Lob 1 and Lob 2 grow faster, have a higher DNA labeling index, and a shorter doubling time than Lob 3 (28). They also exhibit different susceptibility to carcinogenesis (20,21). Cells obtained from Lob 1 and Lob 2 express in vitro phenotypes indicative of neoplastic transformation when treated with chemical carcinogens, whereas cells obtained from Lob 3 do not manifest those changes (20,21).

4. BREAST DEVELOPMENT AND THE PATHOGENESIS OF BREAST CANCER

The Lob 1, the most undifferentiated structure found in the breast of young nulliparous women, is the site of origin of ductal carcinomas (23,32). The finding that the most undifferentiated structures originated the most aggressive neoplasm supports the hypothesis that the presence of Lob 1 explains the higher breast cancer risk of nulliparous women, since they represent the population with the highest concentration of undifferentiated structures in the breast (2,3). Nontumoral breast tissues from cancer-bearing lumpectomy or mastectomy specimens removed from nulliparous women have an architecture dominated by Lob 1; their overall architecture is similar to that of nulliparous females free of mammary pathology (5,33,34). Although the breast tissues of parous women from the general population contain predominantly Lob 3 and a very low percentage of Lob 1, in those parous women who have developed breast cancer their breast tissues have also the Lob 1 as the predominant structure, appearing in this sense similar to those of nulliparous women (5). It is of interest to note that all the parous breast cancer patients we have studied had a history of late first full-term pregnancy or familial history of breast cancer. The analysis of these samples indicated that the architecture of the breast of parous women with breast cancer differs from that of parous women without cancer. The similarities found between the architecture of the breast of nulliparous women and that of parous women with cancer support the hypothesis that the degree of breast development is of importance in the susceptibility to carcinogenesis, and, furthermore, that parous women who develop breast cancer might exhibit a defective response to the differentiating influence of the hormones of pregnancy *(5)*.

Developmental differences might not only provide an explanation for the protective effect induced by pregnancy, but also a new paradigm to assess other differences between the Lob 1 of parous and nulliparous women, such as their ability to metabolize estrogens, or repair genotoxic damage. Such differences exist, and they have been shown to modulate the response of the rodent mammary gland to chemically induced carcinogenesis. It has been postulated *(34)* that unresponsive lobules that fail to undergo differentiation under the stimulus of pregnancy and lactation are responsible for cancer development despite the parity history; it stands to reason that having more of these lobules increases the risk of breast cancer. In fact, the extent of age-related menopausal involution of the Lob 1 appears to influence the risk of breast cancer, and may modify other breast cancer risk factors, including parity. These postulated and early observations *(2,5,34)* have been confirmed in a recent report *(35)* focused on breast biopsy specimens from 8,736 women with benign breast disease. In this publication, the authors have evaluated not only the Lob 1 or terminal ductal lobular unit but also the atrophic or involuted structures resulting by the normal process of aging in the human breast. The extent of involution of the terminal duct lobular units or Lob 1 was characterized as complete (^{3}75% of the lobules involuted), partial (1–74% involuted), or none (0% involuted). The relative risk of breast cancer was estimated based upon standardized incidence ratios by dividing the observed numbers of incident breast cancers by expected values of population-based incident breast cancers from the Iowa Surveillance, Epidemiology and End Results (SEER) registry. The following findings were noted: (a) Greater degrees of involution were positively associated with advancing age, and inversely associated with parity. (b) Overall, the risk of breast cancer was significantly higher for women with no involution, compared to those with partial or complete involution [relative risks (RRs) 1.88, 1.47, and 0.91, respectively]. This particular finding is of great interest because it confirms the previous observations of Russo et al. *(34)* indicating that the Lob1 is a marker of risk. (c) The degree of involution modified the risk of developing breast cancer in women who had atypia in their breast biopsies (RR 7.79, 4.06, and 1.49 for women with none, partial, and complete involution, respectively) as well as for those with proliferative disease without atypia (RR 2.94 and 1.11 for those with no and complete involution, respectively). (d) There was an interaction with family history as well; women with a weak or no family history of breast cancer who had complete involution had a risk for breast cancer that was fivefold lower than the risk of those with a strong family history and no involution (RR 0.59 vs. 2.77, respectively). This data also confirm the previous observations of Russo et al *(34)*. (5) Among nulliparous women, and those whose age at first birth was over the age of 30, the absence of involution significantly increased the risk of breast cancer (RR 2.41 vs. 2.74, respectively). In contrast; for both groups, there was no excess risk if involution was complete.

Altogether the study of Milanese et al. *(35)* provides a powerful confirmation of the risk of Lob 1 or terminal ductal lobular unit in the breast *(2,5,34)* and provides an additional morphological parameter like atrophic or involution of the Lob1 or terminal ductal lobular unit as an indication of protection. However, this conclusion must be taken with reservation because a recent finding of Harvey et al. *(36)* in which postmenopausal women who have received hormonal replacement therapy have shown an increase in breast density associated with a significant increase in the number of Lob 1 or TDLU indicates that reactivation of the so-called involuted Lob1 or terminal ductal lobular unit can increase the risk of a woman to develop breast cancer.

Chapter 1 / The Genomic Basis of Breast Development and Differentiation   5

5. GENOMIC APPROACH TO UNDERSTAND BREAST CANCER SUSCEPTIBILITY

The advances of the human genome project and the availability of new tools for genomic analysis, such as cDNA microarray, laser capture microdissection (LCM), and bioinformatics techniques have allowed to determine whether there are clusters of genes that are differentially expressed in populations that differ in their breast cancer risk *(29–31)*. Those clusters of genes whose expression may be affected by early pregnancy and that can be proven to be functionally relevant in protecting the breast from cancer development could serve as markers for evaluating cancer risk in large populations. This concept has been proven to be correct in the rat model in which a cluster of genes remain activated after the process of involution postpregnancy takes place, conferring a "special genomic signature" to the gland that is responsible for its refractoriness to chemical carcinogenesis *(37,38)*. Early pregnancy imprints in the breast permanent genomic changes, or a "signature," that reduces the susceptibility of the organ to undergo neoplastic transformation *(2,8,29–31)*.

Early first full-term pregnancy imprints a specific genomic signature in the breast epithelia of postmenopausal women. This signature is significantly different from that of women who have had an early full-term pregnancy but developed cancer, and from those who are nulliparous with or without the disease. The genomic signature is made up 129 upregulated and 103 downregulated genes. The gene ontology categories that were overrepresented in the breast epithelia of the parous control breast are related to apoptosis, DNA repair, response to exogenous agents, and gene transcription/gene transcription-regulation *(29–31)*.

5.1. Apoptosis Is Part Genomic Signature of the Breast Epithelia

There are ten genes that are controlling apoptosis that are differentially expressed in the breast epithelia of the parous women (Table 1). Among them, six are upregulated such as the *BCL2 associate X protein or BAX* that belongs to the BCL2 protein family. *BAX* is a proapoptotic

Table 1
Apoptosis and antiapoptosis genes differentially expressed in the breast epithelium of parous control women

Gene name	Gene ID	Symbol	Adj P	Fold increase/ decrease
BCL2-associated X protein	AI565203	*BAX*	0.0230	2.6500
TIA1 cytotoxic granule-associated RNA binding protein	R82978	*TIA1*	0.0173	1.5600
TNF receptor-associated factor 1	R71691	*TRAF1*	0.017	1.7200
TNFRSF1A-associated via death domain	AA916906	*TRADD*	0.027	1.4200
CASP2 and RIPK1	AA285065	*CRADD*	0.0041	1.8900
Protein phosphatase 1F	AA806330	*PPM1F*	0.0142	1.3500
Programmed cell death	AA416757	*PDCD5*	0.0013	−2.1500
Mdm4	AI310969	*MDM4*	0.0134	−1.2500
Baculoviral IAP repeat-containing 6	H10434	*BIRC6*	0.0136	−1.2600
BCL2-associated athanogene 4	H22928	*BAG4*	0.0267	−1.2700

gene that the active p53 stimulates the transcription of it, including the proapoptotic gene *p21*, a cell cycle regulator *(39,40)*. This protein forms a heterodimer with BCL2, and functions as an apoptotic activator *(41)*. The expression of this gene is regulated by the tumor suppressor P53 and has been shown to be involved in P53-mediated apoptosis *(39,42)*. Other genes related to the apoptosis are *the TIA1 cytotoxic granule associated RNA binding protein* and the *tumor necrosis factor receptor 1 (TNFR1)*. The TIA1 possesses nucleolytic activity against cytotoxic lymphocyte (CTL) target cells inducing DNA fragmentation in the target cells *(43)*. TNFR1 can initiate several cellular responses, including apoptosis, which relies on caspases, necrotic cell death, which depends on receptor-interacting protein kinase 1 (RIP1) *(44,45)*. The TNFR-associated death domain (TRADD) protein has been suggested to be a crucial signal adaptor that mediates all intracellular responses from TNFR1 *(46)*. Another upregulated gene in the parous breast epithelial cells is the *CASP2 and RIPK1 domain containing adaptor with death domain or CRADD*. Death domain (DD)-containing proteins are involved in apoptosis signaling induced by activated death receptors *(47)*. Caspase-2 is one of the earliest identified caspases engaged in the mitochondria-dependent apoptotic pathway by inducing the release of cytochrome *c* (Cyt c) and other mitochondrial apoptogenic factors into the cell cytoplasm *(48)*. The *protein phosphatase gene* encodes a protein that is a member of the PP2C family of Ser/Thr protein phosphatases, and the overexpression of this phosphatase has been shown to mediate caspase-dependent apoptosis *(49)*. T*he programmed cell death 5 or PDCD5-and the Mdm4, transformed 3T3 cell double minute 4 (MDM4)* are downregulated in the parous breast epithelia. The *Mdm4* gene is amplified and overexpressed in a variety of human cancers and encode structurally related oncoproteins that bind to the p53 tumor suppressor protein and inhibit p53 activity *(50–53)*. Mice deleted for Mdm4 die during embryogenesis, and the developmental lethality of either mouse model can be rescued by concomitant deletion of p53 *(54)*. The downregulation of the MDM4 in the breast of parous epithelia may act as a protective mechanism and be part of the program cell death pathway active in these cells.

There is also downregulation of antiapoptotic genes. One of them is the *split hand/foot malformation (ectrodactyly) type 1* that is encoding a protein with a BIR (baculoviral inhibition of apoptosis protein repeat) domain and UBCc (ubiquitin-conjugating enzyme E2, catalytic) domain *(55)*. This protein inhibits apoptosis by facilitating the degradation of apoptotic proteins by ubiquitination. The other antiapoptotic gene is the *BCL2-associated athanogene 4* that is a member of the BAG1-related protein family. BAG1 is an antiapoptotic protein that functions through interactions with a variety of cell apoptosis and growth-related proteins including BCL-2, Raf-protein kinase, steroid hormone receptors, growth factor receptors, and members of the heat shock protein 70-kDa family. This protein was found to be associated with the death domain of tumor necrosis factor receptor type 1 (TNF-R1) and death receptor-3 (DR3), and thereby negatively regulates downstream cell death signaling *(56,57)*.

Altogether this cluster of genes seems to maintain the programmed cell death pathway very active in the parous breast epithelia when compared with the parous breast of women with cancer as well as from the epithelia of the breast from nulliparous with and without cancer. Supporting evidence for this statement comes from data in the experimental model *(58–60)* and in the normal breast tissue from reduction mammoplasty specimens of parous women *(29–31)*, in which genes involved in the pathway of apoptosis are significantly upregulated.

5.2. DNA Repair Genes

Upregulation of DNA repair controlling genes is part of the signature induced by pregnancy. This is supported by data generated in the experimental system in which the parous mammary

Chapter 1 / The Genomic Basis of Breast Development and Differentiation 7

epithelial cells have a higher ability to remove the DNA adduct of 7–12 dimethylbenz (a) anthracene *(61,62)*. The greater ability of the parous mammary epithelial cells to remove the DNA adducts has been the first indication that an improved DNA repair was involved in the protective effect induced by pregnancy. DNA repair is central to the integrity of the human genome, and reduced DNA repair capacity has been linked to genetic susceptibility to cancer *(63,64)*. A reduced DNA repair is associated with risk of breast cancer in women *(65)*. The breast epithelial cells of parous control women present four DNA repair related genes that are upregulated significantly when compared with the expression of same genes in the epithelial cells of nulliparous breast with or without cancer, and more importantly, from those parous women with cancer. *RAD51-like 3* is upregulated in the epithelial cells of the parous breast. The RAD51L3 protein encoded by this gene is a member of the RAD51 protein family highly similar to bacterial RecA and Saccharomyces cerevisiae Rad51, which are known to be involved in the homologous recombination and repair of DNA *(66–68)*. We have also reported that the *X-ray repair complementing defective repair 1 (XRCC4)* is upregulated in the breast epithelial cells of the parous breast *(29–31)*. XRCC4 is a nonhomologous end-joining protein employed in DNA double strand break repair and in V(D)J recombination that act as a caretaker of the mammalian genome, a role required both for normal development and for suppression of tumors *(69–71)*. ERCC8 is aso upregulated in the parous breast *(72)*. Another gene related to the DNA repair process is the *ankyrin repeat domain 17 or ANKRD17* and the *translin or TSN* that encodes a DNA-binding protein, which specifically recognizes conserved target sequences at the break point junction of chromosomal translocations. *The three prime repair exonuclease* is also upregulated in the parous breast. The protein encoded by this gene uses two different open reading frames from which the upstream ORF encodes proteins that interact with the ataxia telangiectasia and Rad3 related protein, a checkpoint kinase. The proteins encoded by this upstream ORF localize to intranuclear foci following DNA damage and are essential components of the DNA damage checkpoint *(73,74)*. These data indicate that the activation of genes involved in the DNA repair process is part of the signature induced in the mammary gland by pregnancy confirming previous findings that, in vivo, the ability of the cells to repair carcinogen-induced damage by unscheduled DNA synthesis and adduct removal is more efficient in the postpregnancy mammary gland *(61,62)*.

5.3. Immunosurveillance and Detoxification of Xenobiotic Substances

A cluster of genes that is upregulated in the parous control group are those related to immunosurveillance and detoxification of xenobiotic substances (Table 2). The concept that an immunological process was involved during pregnancy and responsible for its protective effect in mammary carcinogenesis has been reported *(75,76)*. In breast epithelial cells of parous postmenopausal women we found that the *toll-like receptor* gene is upregulated. This gene belongs to the innate immune system recognizing microbial pathogens through toll-like receptors (TLRs), which identify pathogen-associated molecular patterns *(77)*. The fact that the RNA of the epithelial component of the lobules type 1 was obtained by laser capture microdission indicates that this is an epithelial component and not a contaminant of lymphocytes from the stroma. We have also reported that the breast epithelial cells of the parous breast also have *MHC class I HLA-A24*. Upregulated HLA-A24 binding peptides have the capacity to elicit antitumor cytotoxic T lymphocytes in vitro *(78)*. It has been shown that HLA class I antigen downregulation is associated with worse clinical course of ovarian carcinoma that may reflect the escape of tumor cells from immune recognition and destruction. We have also found *regulatory factor X-associated protein* upregulated, which is part of the

Table 2
Response to exogenous agent genes

Gene name	Gene ID	Symbol	Adj P	Fold increase/ decrease
Retinol dehydrogenase 11 (all-trans/9-cis/11-cis)	H82421	*RDH11*	0.0168	1.6428
Epoxide hydrolase 1, microsomal (xenobiotic)	AA838691	*EPHX1*	0.012	1.7800
Thioredoxin reductase 1	AA464849	*TXNRD1*	0.006	1.9200
Immunoglobulin (CD79A) binding protein 1	AA463498	*IGBP1*	0.005	1.3800
Calcium binding atopy-related autoantigen 1	AA992324	*CBARA1*	0.0135	1.3800
Toll-interleukin 1 receptor	AI279454	*TIRAP*	0.0097	1.3800
Scavenger receptor class A, member 3	R10675	*SCARA3*	0.0250	1.3900
Glutathione S-transferase theta 1	T64869	*GSTT1*	0.0139	1.2400
Epoxide hydrolase 1, microsomal (xenobiotic)	AA838691	*EPHX1*	0.012	1.2500
Chromosome 10 open reading frame 59	AI093491	*C10orf59*	0.0130	1.9300
N-acetyltransferase 2 (arylamine *N*-acetyltransferase)	AI460128	*NAT2*	0.0095	1.5000

major histocompatibility (MHC) class II molecules *(79)*. These are transmembrane proteins that have a central role in development and control of the immune system. These data allow us to postulate that the increased immune-surveillance mechanism has been imprinted during the differentiation cycle induced by pregnancy and could be one of the protective factors induced by the cells against neoplastic initiation or progression.

In addition to the increase in the immune surveillance mechanism in the epithelia of the parous breast, there are genes significantly upregulated and involved in the metabolism of xenobiotic substances and oxidative stress. Among them are the *Epoxide hydrolase or EPHX1* that plays an important role in both the activation and detoxification of exogenous chemicals such as polycyclic aromatic hydrocarbons and the *thioredoxin reductase 1 or TXNRD1* that encodes a member of pyridine nucleotide family of oxidoreductases. TXNRD1 protein reduces thioredoxins as well as other substrates, and plays a role in selenium metabolism and protection against oxidative stress *(80)*. Thioredoxin reductase 1 (TR1) is one of the major antioxidant and redox regulators in mammals that supports p53 function and other tumor suppressor activities *(81–83)*. *Glutathione S-transferase (GST) theta 1 (GSTT1)* is a member of a superfamily of proteins that catalyze the conjugation of reduced glutathione to a variety of electrophilic and hydrophobic compounds and is upregulated in the epithelia of the parous breast. Another gene that is also overexpressed is the *N-acetyltransferase 2 [arylamine N-acetyltransferase (NAT2)]* involved in the metabolism of different xenobiotics, including potential carcinogens. The upregulation of these genes is interpreted as an activated system of defense that makes the parous breast cells less vulnerable to genotoxic substances. This contention is supported by data indicating that in primary culture, breast epithelial cells from parous women treated in vitro with chemical carcinogens do not express phenotypes of cell transformation, whereas those from nulliparous women do *(20,21)*.

5.4. Transcription Factors

There are 21 gene encoding proteins controlling gene transcription/gene transcription-regulation that are significantly upregulated in parous breast epithelia and 13 that are downregulated (Table 3) This indicates that during pregnancy transcription modifications are important components of the genomic signature induced by this physiological process. *The Bromodomain PHD finger transcription factor or BPTF* is upregulated in the epithelia of the parous breast. *BPTF* expression is lost or significantly reduced in human lung, prostate,

Table 3
Transcription factor genes

Gene name	Gene ID	Symbol	Adj P	
Bromodomain PHD finger transcription factor	AA704421	*BPTF*	0.066	2.000
Suppressor of Ty 5 homolog (*S. cerevisiae*)	R21511	*SUPT5H*	0.043	2.150
SRY (sex determining region Y)-box 10	AA976578	*SOX10*	0.0281	1.9300
p300/CBP-associated factor	N74637	*PCAF*	0.0500	1.2500
Forkhead box K2	AA136472	*FOXK2*	0.0142	1.2550
Kv channel interacting protein 3, calsenilin	H39123	*KCNIP3*	0.0247	1.3000
Protein inhibitor of activated STAT, 1	N91175	*PIAS1*	0.0280	1.3100
Regulatory factor X-associated protein	AI365571	*RFXAP*	0.0139	1.2400
Zinc finger protein 16	H17016	*ZNF16*	0.012	1.2340
Inhibitor of DNA binding 4	AA464856	*ID4*	0.978	2.100
General transcription factor IIB	H23978	*GTF2B*	0.009	1.53859
Zinc finger protein 26	R97944	*ZNF26*	0.017	1.53388
Zinc finger protein 498	W94267	*ZNF498*	0.0051	2.0074
Zinc finger protein 544	AA885065	*ZNF544*	0.0102	1.2500
Zinc finger protein 710	AI025842	*ZNF710*	0.0054	1.9023
Bromodomain adjacent to zinc finger domain, 2A	AA699460	*BAZ2A*	0.015	1.2450
Homeobox D1	W68537	*HOXD1*	0.0321	1.2600
HIR histone cell cycle regulation defective homolog A	AA609365	*HIRA*	0.0220	1.2600
Transducin-like enhancer of split 3 E(sp1) homolog	AI216623	*TLE3*	0.0131	1.2500
Zinc finger protein 268	AI277336	*ZNF268*	0.0142	1.5000
Zinc finger protein 275	AA406125	*ZNF275*	0.032	1.2800
Histone deacetylase 8	AI053481	*HDAC8*	0.0027	−2.2000

(continued)

Table 3
(continued)

Gene name	Gene ID	Symbol	Adj P	
Zinc finger protein 425	H20279	*ZNF425*	0.0054	−1.6200
PBX/knotted 1 homeobox 2	AI024125	*PKNOX2*	0.0040	−1.6400
Methyl-CpG binding domain protein 3	AI017865	*MBD3*	0.0027	−3.1705
General transcription factor IIIC	AI184450	*GTF3C4*	0.0027	−1.8700
Ring finger protein 12	AA598809	*RNF12*	0.0079	−1.2500
D4, zinc and double PHD fingers family 2	AA496782	*DPF2*	0.016	−1.690
SRY (sex determining region Y)-box 3	AI359981	*SOX3*	0.00476	−2.1142
POU domain, class 6, transcription factor 1	AI123130	*POU6F1*	0.0082	−1.3700
Myeloid/lymphoid or mixed-lineage leukemia	AI197974	*MLLT6*	0.0097	−1.4100
RAR-related orphan receptor A	AI022327	*RORA*	0.0116	−1.4000
GATA zinc finger domain containing 2A	AA458840	*GATAD2A*	0.0224	−1.9700
Zinc finger protein 320	AI025436	*ZNF320*	0.0124	−1.5000

colon, pancreas, and ovarian carcinomas as well as in cell lines established from different human carcinomas. It is speculated that the gene may play a role in suppression of tumors originating from epithelial tissue *(84)*. We have already reported that the *LIM domain binding 2 and SOX 2* are significantly upregulated in the epithelial cells of the parous breast *(29–31)*. SOX-2 is a transcription factor that is expressed by self-renewing and multipotent stem cells of the embryonic neuroepithelium *(85–87)*. SOX 2 is also considered a stem cell marker and it could well represent the marker of the differentiated stem cell 2 previously postulated *(8,39–41)*. Furthermore, genes of the Sox family encode evolutionarily conserved HMG box containing transcription factors, which play key roles in various events of cell determination/differentiation during development *(88–91)*. The *SOX 30 or sex determination region Y (SRY)* is also significantly upregulated in the parous breast epithelial cells. Sox 30 family proteins are characterized by a unique DNA-binding domain, a HMG box which shows at least 50% sequence similarity with mouse Sry, the sex-determining factor. The *SRY (sex determining region Y) box 10 or SOX 10* is also upregulated in the breast of parous women. The SOX group E transcription factors play an integral role in the specification and differentiation of astrocytes and oligodendrocytes *(92)*. *Sox10* may influence transcription of terminal differentiation *(93,94,95,96)*, and therefore the overexpression in the parous breast epithelial cells could be an indication of a more differentiated phenotype acquired by these cells under influence of the physiological process of pregnancy. In contrast, *SOX10*, the *SRY-SOX3* are downregulated in the parous breast, involved in the regulation of embryonic development and in the determination of cell fate *(97,98)*. The final molecular mechanism by which these transcription factors regulate the differentiation properties of the parous breast epithelia still needs more investigation.

Another group of genes whose function is associated to coactivators and chromatin remodeling seem to play an important role on the genomic signature induced by pregnancy

Chapter 1 / The Genomic Basis of Breast Development and Differentiation   **11**

in breast epithelial cells. One of them is the *p300/CBP-associated factor (PCAF)* that is significantly upregulated in the epithelial cells of the parous breast tissue *(66–68)*. p300/CBP-associated factor (PCAF) is a coactivator of the tumor suppressor, p53. PCAF participates in p53's transactivation of target genes through acetylation of both bound p53 and histones within p53 target promoters *(99)*. Interestingly enough, various kinds of cofactors, such as steroid receptor coactivator-1 (SRC-1), transcription intermediary factor 2 (TIF2), and amplified in breast cancer 1 (AIB1), have also been reported to interact with nuclear receptors in a ligand-dependent manner and enhance transcriptional activation by the receptor via histone acetylation/methylation and recruitment of additional coactivator, such as CREB binding protein (CBP)/p300 *(100)*. The role of p300/CBP-associated factor in the differentiated breast epithelial cells of parous women could be similar to the effect of transretinoic acid (ATRA) treatment of metastatic breast cancer cells that by increasing the protein levels of the histone acetyl transferases p300 and CBP suppress the level of histone deacetylase and increase the level of acetylated histone H4. ATRA also has been shown to decrease Bcl-2 and increase BAX and decrease VEGF *(101)*. BAX is upregulated in the parous breast epithelial cells. Real-time PCR confirmed the upregulation of the p300/CBP-associated factor as well as BAX found in the array. The p300/CBP-associated factor (PCAF) has been considered part of the genomic signature of the stem cell 2 *(29–31)*.

ID4 or inhibitor of DNA binding 4, is a member of the ID family of proteins (Id1-Id4), which function as dominant-negative regulators of basic helix-loop-helix transcription factors and are involved in numerous cell processes, including cell proliferation and differentiation *(102)*. Id4 is constitutively expressed in the normal human mammary epithelium but is suppressed in ER-positive breast carcinomas and preneoplastic lesions supporting a possible role of Id4 as a tumor suppressor factor in the human breast *(102,103)*. Primary breast cancers have low or no expression of ID4 protein *(104,105)* and also has been considered a putative tumor-suppressor gene that is methylated in most mouse and human leukemias but in only a minority of other human cancers *(105–108)*.

Other transcription factors also upregulated in the parous breast are *GTB2B* that encodes the general transcription factor IIB, one of the ubiquitous factors required for transcription initiation by RNA polymerase II and the *HOXD1. The HOXD1 or Homeo box D1* is the first and initially most anterior Hox genes expressed in the embryo. In Xenopus, the three PG1 genes, *Hoxa1*, *Hoxb1*, and *Hoxd1*, are expressed in a widely overlapping domain, which includes the region of the future hindbrain and its associated neural crest *(109)*. Of great interest is that transcription factors, encoded by the homeobox (HOX) genes that play a crucial role in Drosophila, Xenopus, and mammalian embryonic differentiation and development, are upregulating HOXC6, HOXD1, and HOXD8 expression in human neuroblastoma cells, which are chemically induced to differentiate. This indicates that HOX is associated with maturation toward a differentiated neuronal phenotype *(110)*. The upregulation of the homeo box D1 in the parous breast epithelial cell could also be an indicator of higher degree of differentiation and maturation reached by these cells when compared with the breast epithelial cells of the nulliparous breast or those breast epithelial cells either from parous or nulliparous breast with cancer.

The *protein inhibitor of activated STAT 1* encodes a member of the mammalian PIAS [protein inhibitor of activated STAT-1 (signal transducer and activator of transcription-1)] family and in the testis functions as a nuclear receptor transcriptional coregulator and may have a role in androgen receptor initiation and maintenance of spermatogenesis *(111)*. Therefore, in the breast STAT 1 may have a differentiation controlling function after parity. Other genes also implicated in cell lineage determination and differentiation that are also upregulated in the parous breast epithelia are the *Zinc finger protein 16* and the *twist homolog-Basic helix-loop-helix (bHLH)*.

A group of genes that are downregulated after the process of pregnancy are those controlling methylation such as the *histone deacetylase- and the methyl-CpG binding-protein*. It is well known that DNA methylation is the major modification of eukaryotic genomes and plays an essential role in mammalian development; however, the role of this process in the silencing of genes that are part of the signature induced by pregnancy requires further evaluation.

As part of the chromatin remodeling occurring after pregnancy we have reported that the *suppressor of hairy wing homolog 4* is significantly upregulated in the epithelial cells of the parous women *(29–31)*. This gene transcript, shown in Drosophila *(112)*, can bind chromatin insulators and is thought to regulate gene expression by establishing higher-order domains of chromatin organization. Chromatin insulators, or boundary elements, affect promoter-enhancer interactions and buffer transgenes from position effects *(113–115)*. Whereas we do not know how the suppressor of Hairy-wing can regulate the chromatin organization of the breast epithelial cells it is possible that mechanisms of this nature work in silencing or repressing certain genes that control proliferation. At the same time they may increase repair of damage and specific response to hormones. A similar function in chromatin remodeling could be played by the *suppressor of Ty homolog 3* that has been found to be significantly upregulated in the parous breast epithelial cells *(29–31)*. Suppressor of Ty (SPT) genes was originally identified through a genetic screen for mutations in the yeast *Saccharomyces cerevisiae* that restore gene expression disrupted by the insertion of the transposon Ty *(116)*. Suppressor of Ty homolog 3 could be considered part of the unique signature to the parous breast and be functionally involved in the protective effect of pregnancy.

Three genes that are also part of the signature of the parous breast are *Ephrin B3 carcinoembryonic antigen related cell adhesion molecule 1, and the BCR2 and CDKNIA interacting protein or BCCIP*. The *Ephrin B3* is upregulated in breast epithelial cells of parous women and is part of the family of proteins involved in signaling pathway networks with the WNT signaling pathway during embryogenesis and tissue regeneration *(117–121)*. The *carcinoembryonic antigen related cell adhesion molecule 1* is also upregulated in parous breast epithelial cells, and is part of a family of proteins implicated in various intercellular-adhesion and intracellular-signaling-mediated effects that govern the growth and differentiation of normal cells *(122,123)*. In vitro, CEACAM1 regulates proliferation, migration, and differentiation of murine endothelial cells *(124)* and it has been found to be downregulated in colorectal, prostate, and breast cancer, functioning as a tumor suppressor. The *BCR2 and CDKNIA interacting protein or BCCIP* is critical for BRCA2- and RAD51-dependent responses to DNA damage and homologous recombination repair *(125–127)*.

6. CONCLUDING REMARKS

Early first full-term pregnancy induces in the breast epithelia a specific genomic profile that can be identified in the postmenopausal breast and that is a signature that makes epithelial cells different from those of parous breast tissue from women with breast cancer as well as from those nulliparous women either with and without breast cancer. This genomic signature allows to evaluate the degree of mammary gland differentiation induced by pregnancy and it could be the signature postulated for the stem cell 2. Importantly enough this signature could help to predict in which woman parity has been protective, and furthermore, it can be used as a biomarker for evaluating preventive agents.

Acknowledgments: This study was supported by Grant RO1-CA093599 from the National Cancer Institute, USA.

REFERENCES

1. Russo J and Russo IH. Development of the human mammary gland. In: Neville MC, Daniel C, eds. The Mammary Gland. New York: Plenum, 1987:67–93.
2. Russo J, Rivera R and Russo J. Influence of age and parity on the development of the human breast. Breast Cancer Res Treat 1992;23:211–218.
3. Russo J and Russo IH. The cellular basis of breast cancer susceptibility. Oncol Res 1999;11:169–178.
4. Russo J and Russo IH. Development pattern of human breast and susceptibility to carcinogenesis. Eur J Cancer Prev 1993;2:85–100.
5. Russo J, Romero AL and Russo IH. Architectural pattern of the normal and cancerous breast under the influence of parity. J Cancer Epidemiol Biomarkers Prev 1994;3:219–224.
6. Russo J, Ao X, Grill C and Russo IH. Pattern of distribution of cells positive for estrogen receptor a and progesterone receptor in relation to proliferating cells in the mammary gland. Breast Cancer Res Treat 1999;53:217–227.
7. Russo J and Russo IH. Role of hormones in human breast development – The menopausal breast. In: Wren BG, ed. Progress in the Management of Menopause. London: Parthenon, 1997:184–193.
8. Russo J and Russo IH. Role of differentiation in the pathogenesis and prevention of breast cancer. Endocr Relat Cancer 1997;4:7–21.
9. Kumar V, Stack GS, Berry M, Jin JR and Chambon P. Functional domains of the human estrogen receptor. Cell 1978;51:941–951.
10. King RJB. Effects of steroid hormones and related compounds on gene transcription. Clin Endocrinol 1992;36:1–14.
11. Soto AM, and Sonnenschein C. Cell proliferation of estrogen-sensitive cells – The case for negative control. Endocr Rev 1987;48:52–58.
12. Huseby RA, Maloney TM, and McGrath CM. Evidence for a direct growth-stimulating effect of estradiol on human MCF-7 cells in vitro. Cancer Res 1987;144:2654–2659.
13. Huff KK, Knabbe C, Lindsey R, Kaufman D, Bronzert D, Lippman ME, Dickson RB. Multihormonal regulation of insulin-like growth factor-1-related protein in MCF-7 human breast cancer cells. Mol Endocrinol 1988;2:200–208.
14. Dickson RB, Huff KK, Spencer EM and Lippman ME. Introduction of epidermal growth factor related polypeptides by 17b-estradiol in MCF-7 human breast cancer cells. Endocrinology 1986;118:138–142.
15. Page MJ, Field JK, Everett P and Green CD. Serum regulation of the estrogen responsiveness of the human breast cancer cell line MCF-7. Cancer Res 1983;43:1244–1250.
16. Katzenellenbogen BS, Kendra KL, Norman MJ and Berthois Y. Proliferation, hormonal responsiveness and estrogen receptor content of MCF-7 human breast cancer cells growth in the short-term and long-term absence of estrogens. Cancer Res 1987;47:4355–4360.
17. Aakvaag A, Utaacker E, Thorsen T, Lea OA and Lahooti H. Growth control of human mammary cancer cells (MCF-7 cells) in culture: Effect of estradiol and growth factors in serum containing medium. Cancer Res 1990;50:7806–7810.
18. Dell'aquilla ML, Pigott DA, Bonaquist DL and Gaffney EV. A factor from plasma derived human serum that inhibits the growth of the mammary cell line MCF-7- characterization and purification. J Natl Cancer Inst 1984;72:291–298.
19. Russo IH and Russo J. Role of hormones in cancer initiation and progression. J Mammary Gland Biol Neoplasia 1997;3:49–61.
20. Russo J, Reina D, Frederick J and Russo IH. Expression of phenotypical changes by human breast epithelial cells treated with carcinogens in vitro. Cancer Res 1988;48:2837–2857.
21. Russo J, Calaf G and Russo IH. A critical approach to the malignant transformation of human breast epithelial cells. CRC Crit Rev Oncogenesis 1993;4:403–417.
22. Russo J, Tay LK and Russo IH. Differentiation of the mammary gland and susceptibility to carcinogenesis: A Review. Breast Cancer Res Treat 1982;2:5–73.

23. Russo J, Gusterson BA, Rogers AE, Russo IH, Welling SR and Van Zwieten MJ. Comparative study of human and rat mammary tumorigenesis. Lab Invest 1990;62:244–278.
24. Russo J and Russo I.H. Biological and molecular bases of mammary carcinogenesis. Lab Invest 1987;57:112–137.
25. Russo IH and Russo J. Mammary gland neoplasia in long-term rodent studies. Environ Health Perspect 1996;104:938–967.
26. MacMahon B, Cole P, Lin TM, et al. Age at first birth and breast cancer risk. Bull Natl Health Org 1970;43:209.
27. Vessey MD, McPherson K, Roberts MM, Neil A and Jones L. Fertility and the risk of breast cancer. Br J Cancer 1985;52:625–628.
28. Russo J, Mills MJ, Moussali MJ and Russo IH. Influence of human breast development on the growth properties of primary cultures. In Vitro Cell Dev Biol 1989;25:643–649.
29. Balogh GA, Heulings R, Mailo DA, et al. Genomic signature induced by pregnancy in the human breast. Int J Oncol 2006;28:399–410.
30. Russo J, Balogh GA, Heulings R, et al. Molecular basis of pregnancy induced breast cancer protection. Eur J Cancer Prev 2006;15:306–342.
31. Russo J, Balogh GA, Chen J, et al. The concept of stem cell in the mammary gland and its implication in morphogenesis, cancer and prevention. Front Biosci 2006;11:151–172.
32. Wellings SR, Jansen MM and Marcum RG. An atlas of sub-gross pathology of the human breast with special reference to possible pre-cancerous lesions. JNCI 1975;55:231–275.
33. Russo J and Russo IH. Differentiation and breast cancer development. In: Heppner G, ed. Advances in Oncobiology, Vol. 2. London: JAI Press, 1998:1–10.
34. Russo J, Lynch H, and Russo IH. Mammary gland architecture as a determining factor in the susceptibility of the human breast to cancer. Breast J 2001;7(5):278–291.
35. Milanese TR, Hartmann LC, Sellers TA, et al. Age-related lobular involution and risk of breast cancer. J Natl Cancer Inst 2006;98:1600.
36. Harvey JA, Santen RJ, Petroni GR, Smolkin, et al. Histology findings of mammographically dense breast tissue in postmenopausal women with and without hormone replacement therapy. Breast Cancer Res Treat 2004;88(Suppl 1):5008a.
37. Russo J, Mailo D, Hu YF, Balogh GA, Sheriff F and Russo IH. Breast differentiation and its implication in cancer prevention. Clin Cancer Res 2005;11:931s–936s.
38. Russo J and Russo IH. Biological and Molecular Basis of Breast Cancer. Heidelberg, Germany: Springer, 2004.
39. Cheng J, Cui R, Chen CH and Du J. Oxidized low-density lipoprotein stimulates p53-dependent activation of proapoptotic Bax leading to apoptosis of differentiated endothelial progenitor cells. Endocrinology 2007;148:2085–2094.
40. Shankar S and Srivastava RK. *Bax* and *Bak* genes are essential for maximum apoptotic response by curcumin, a polyphenolic compound and cancer chemopreventive agent derived from turmeric, *Curcuma longa*. Carcinogenesis 2007;28:1277–1286.
41. Lysiak JJ, Zheng S, Woodson R and Turner TT. Caspase-9-dependent pathway to murine germ cell apoptosis: Mediation by oxidative stress, BAX, and caspase 2. Cell Tissue Res 2007;328:411–419.
42. Eissing T, Waldherr S, Allgöwer F, Scheurich P and Bullinger E. Response to bistability in apoptosis: Roles of bax, bcl-2, and mitochondrial permeability transition pores. Biophys J 2007;92:3332–3334.
43. Geng Y, Akhtar RS, Shacka JJ, Klocke BJ, Zhang J, Chen X and Roth KA. p53 transcription-dependent and -independent regulation of cerebellar neural precursor cell apoptosis. Neuropathol Exp Neurol 2007;66:66–74.
44. Mori N, Murakami YI, Shimada S, et al. TIA-1 expression in hairy cell leukemia. Mod Pathol 2004;17(7):840–846.
45. Xie P, Hostager BS, Munroe ME, Moore CR and Bishop GA. Cooperation between TNF receptor-associated factors 1 and 2 in CD40 signaling. J Immunol 2006;176(9):5388–5400.
46. Bryce PJ, Oyoshi MK, Kawamoto S, Oettgen HC and Tsitsikov EN. TRAF1 regulates Th2 differentiation, allergic inflammation and nuclear localization of the Th2 transcription factor, NIP45. Int Immunol 2006;18(1):101–111.

Chapter 1 / The Genomic Basis of Breast Development and Differentiation

15

47. Zheng L, Bidere N, Staudt D, Cubre A, Orenstein J, Chan FK and Lenardo M. Competitive control of independent programs of tumor necrosis factor receptor-induced cell death by TRADD and RIP1. Mol Cell Biol 2006;26(9):3505–3513.

48. Thakar J, Schleinkofer K, Borner C and Dandekar T. RIP death domain structural interactions implicated in TNF-mediated proliferation and survival. Proteins 2006;63(3):413–423.

49. Guo Y, Srinivasula SM, Druilhe A, Fernandes-Alnemri T and Alnemri ES. Caspase-2 induces apoptosis by releasing proapoptotic proteins from mitochondria. J Biol Chem 2002; 277(16):13430–13437.

50. Mi J, Guo C, Brautigan DL and Larner JM. Protein phosphatase-1{alpha} regulates centrosome splitting through Nek2. Cancer Res 2007;67(3):1082–1089.

51. Boesten LS, Zadelaar SM, De Clercq S, et al. Mdm2, but not Mdm4, protects terminally differentiated smooth muscle cells from p53-mediated caspase-3-independent cell death. Cell Death Differ 2006;13:2089–2098.

52. Toledo F, Krummel KA, Lee CJ, et al. A mouse p53 mutant lacking the proline-rich domain rescues Mdm4 deficiency and provides insight into the Mdm2-Mdm4-p53 regulatory network. Cancer Cell 2006;9(4):273–285.

53. Francoz S, Froment P, Bogaerts S, et al. Mdm4 and Mdm2 cooperate to inhibit p53 activity in proliferating and quiescent cells in vivo. Proc Natl Acad Sci USA 2006;103(9):3232–3237.

54. Xiong S, Van Pelt CS, Elizondo-Fraire AC, Liu G and Lozano G. Synergistic roles of Mdm2 and Mdm4 for p53 inhibition in central nervous system development. Proc Natl Acad Sci USA 2006;103(9):3226–3231.

55. Steinman HA, Hoover KM, Keeler ML, Sands AT and Jones SN. Rescue of Mdm4-deficient mice by Mdm2 reveals functional overlap of Mdm2 and Mdm4 in development. Oncogene 2005; 24(53):7935–7940.

56. Colnaghi R, Connell CM, Barrett RM and Wheatley SP. Separating the anti-apoptotic and mitotic roles of survivin. J Biol Chem 2006;281(44):33450–33456.

57. Eichholtz-Wirth H, Fritz E and Wolz L. Overexpression of the 'silencer of death domain', SODD/ BAG-4, modulates both TNFR1- and CD95-dependent cell death pathways. Cancer Lett 2003;194(1):81–89.

58. Srivastava P, Russo J and Russo IH. Chorionic gonadotropin inhibits rat mammary carcinogenesis through activation of programmed cell death. Carcinogenesis 1997;18:1799–1808.

59. Srivastava P, Russo J and Russo IH. Inhibition of rat mammary tumorigenesis by human chorionic gonadotropin is associated with increased expression of inhibin. Mol Carcinogenesis 1999;26:1–10.

60. Russo J and Russo IH. Human chorionic gonadotropin in breast cancer prevention. In: Ethier SP, ed. Endocrine Oncology. Totowa, NJ: Humana, 2000:121–136.

61. Tay LK and Russo J. 7,12-Dimethylbenz (a) anthracene (DMBA) induced DNA binding and repair synthesis in susceptible and non-susceptible mammary epithelial cells in culture. J Natl Cancer Inst 1981;67:155–161.

62. Tay LK and Russo J. Formation and removal of 7,12-dimethylbenz(a)- anthracene-nucleic acid adducts in rat mammary epithelial cells with different susceptibility to carcinogenesis. Carcinogenesis 1981;2:1327–1333.

63. Materna V, Surowiak P, Markwitz E, Spaczynski M, Drag-Zalesinska M, Zabel M and Lage H. Expression of factors involved in regulation of DNA mismatch repair- and apoptosis pathways in ovarian cancer patients. Oncol Rep 2007;17(3):505–516.

64. Tudek B, Swoboda M, Kowalczyk P and Olinski R. Modulation of oxidative DNA damage repair by the diet, inflammation and neoplastic transformation. J Physiol Pharmacol 2006;57 Suppl 7:33–49.

65. Shi Q, Wang LE, Bondy ML, Brewster A, Singletary SE and Wei Q. Reduced DNA repair of benzo[a]pyrene diol epoxide-induced adducts and common XPD polymorphisms in breast cancer patients. Carcinogenesis 2004;25(9):1695–1700.

66. Wiese C, Hinz JM, Tebbs RS, et al. Disparate requirements for the Walker A and B ATPase motifs of human RAD51D in homologous recombination. Nucleic Acid Res 2006;34(9):2833–2843.

67. Gruver AM, Miller KA, Rajesh C, et al. The ATPase motif in RAD51D is required for resistance to DNA interstrand crosslinking agents and interaction with RAD51C. Mutagenesis 2005; 20(6):433–440.

68. Kawabata M, Kawabata T, Nishibori M. Role of recA/RAD51 family proteins in mammals. Acta Med Okayama 2005;59(1):1–9.
69. Gao Y, Ferguson DO, Xie W, et al. Interplay of p53 and DNA-repair protein XRCC4 in tumorigenesis, genomic stability and development. Nature 2000;404(6780):897–900.
70. Yan CT, Kaushal D, Murphy M, et al. XRCC4 suppresses medulloblastomas with recurrent translocations in p53-deficient mice. Proc Natl Acad Sci USA 2006;103(19):7378–7383.
71. Allen-Brady K, Cannon-Albright LA, Neuhausen SL and Camp NJ. A role for XRCC4 in age at diagnosis and breast cancer risk. Cancer Epidemiol Biomarkers 2006;15(7):1306–1310.
72. Balogh GA, Russo J, Mailo DA, Heulings R, Russo PA, Morrison P, Sheriff F and Russo IH. The breast of parous women without cancer has a different genomic profile compared to those with Cancer. Int J Oncol 2007;31:1165–1175.
73. Bomgarden RD, Yean D, Yee MC and Cimprich KA. A novel protein activity mediates DNA binding of an ATR-ATRIP complex. J Biol Chem 2004;279(14):13346–13353.
74. Zou L and Elledge SJ. Sensing DNA damage through ATRIP recognition of RPA-ssDNA complexes. Science 2003;300(5625):1542–1548.
75. Sinha DK, Pazik JE and Dao TL. Prevention of mammary carcinogenesis in rats by pregnancy: Effect of full-term and interrupted pregnancy. Br J Cancer 1988;57:390–394.
76. D'Cruz CM, Moody SE, Master SR, et al. Persistent parity-induced changes in growth factors, TGF-beta3, and differentiation in the rodent mammary gland. Mol Endocrinol 2002;16:2034–2051.
77. Sanghavi SK, Shankarappa R and Reinhart TA. Genetic analysis of toll/interleukin-1 receptor (TIR) domain sequences from rhesus macaque toll-like receptors (TLRs) 1-10 reveals high homology to human TLR/TIR sequences. Immunogenetics 2004;56(9):667–674.
78. Nukaya I, Yasumoto M, Iwasaki T, et al. Identification of HLA-A24 epitope peptides of carcinoembryonic antigen which induce tumor-reactive cytotoxic T lymphocyte. Int J Cancer 1999;80(1):92–97.
79. Vitale M, Pelusi G, Taroni B, et al. HLA class I antigen down-regulation in primary ovary carcinoma lesions: Association with disease stage. Clin Cancer Res 2005;11(1):67–72.
80. Yoon BI, Kim DY, Jang JJ and Han JH. Altered expression of thioredoxin reductase-1 in dysplastic bile ducts and cholangiocarcinoma in a hamster model. J Vet Sci 2006;7(3):211–216.
81. Yegorova S, Yegorov O and Lou MF. Thioredoxin induced antioxidant gene expressions in human lens epithelial cells. Exp Eye Res 2006;83:783–792.
82. Yoo MH, Xu XM, Carlson BA, Gladyshev VN and Hatfield DL. Thioredoxin reductase 1 deficiency reverses tumor phenotype and tumorigenicity of lung carcinoma cells. J Biol Chem 2006;281(19):13005–13008.
83. Rigobello MP, Vianello F, Folda A, Roman C, Scutari G and Bindoli A. Differential effect of calcium ions on the cytosolic and mitochondrial thioredoxin reductase. Biochem Biophys Res Commun 2006;343(3):873–878.
84. Kurochkin IV, Yonemitsu N, Funahashi SI and Nomura H. ALEX1, a novel human armadillo repeat protein that is expressed differentially in normal tissues and carcinomas. Biochem Biophys Res Commun 2001;280(1):340–347.
85. Komitova M and Eriksson PS. Sox-2 is expressed by neural progenitors and astroglia in the adult rat brain. Neurosci Lett 2004;369(1):24–27.
86. Miyagi S, Saito T, Mizutani K, et al. The Sox-2 regulatory regions display their activities in two distinct types of multipotent stem cells. Mol Cell Biol 2004;24(10):4207–4220.
87. Stevanovic M. Modulation of *SOX2* and *SOX3* gene expression during differentiation of human neuronal precursor cell line NTERA2. Mol Biol Rep 2003;30(2):127–132.
88. Ginis I, Luo Y, Miura T, et al. Differences between human and mouse embryonic stem cells. Dev Biol 2004;269(2):360–380.
89. Cremazy F, Berta P and Girard F. Genome-wide analysis of Sox genes in *Drosophila melanogaster*. Mech Dev 2001;109(2):371–375.
90. Koopman P, Schepers G, Brenner S and Venkatesh B. Origin and diversity of the SOX transcription factor gene family: Genome-wide analysis in *Fugu rubripes*. Gene 2004;328:177–186.
91. Bullejos M, Diaz de la Guardia R, Barragan MJ and Sanchez A. HMG-box sequences from microbats homologous to the human SOX30 HMG-box. Genetica 2000;110(2):157–162.

Chapter 1 / The Genomic Basis of Breast Development and Differentiation 17

92. De Martino SP, Errington F, Ashworth A, Jowett T and Austin CA. sox30: A novel zebrafish sox gene expressed in a restricted manner at the midbrain-hindbrain boundary during neurogenesis. Dev Genes Evol 1999;209(6):357–362.

93. Kelsh RN. Sorting out Sox10 functions in neural crest development. Bioessays 2006;28(8):788–798.

94. Schlierf B, Werner T, Glaser G and Wegner M. Expression of Connexin47 in oligodendrocytes is regulated by the Sox10 transcription factor. J Mol Biol 2006;361(1):11–21.

95. Ito Y, Wiese S, Funk N, et al. Sox10 regulates ciliary neurotrophic factor gene expression in Schwann cells. Proc Natl Acad Sci USA 2006;103(20):7871–7876.

96. Wissmuller S, Kosian T, Wolf M, Finzsch M and Wegner M. The high-mobility-group domain of Sox proteins interacts with DNA-binding domains of many transcription factors. Nucleic Acids Res 2006;34(6):1735–1744.

97. Girard M and Goossens M. Sumoylation of the SOX10 transcription factor regulates its transcriptional activity. FEBS Lett 2006;580(6):1635–1641.

98. Weiss J, Meeks JJ, Hurley L, Raverot G, Frassetto A and Jameson JL. Sox3 is required for gonadal function, but not sex determination, in males and females. Mol Cell Biol 2003; 23(22):8084–8091.

99. Watts GS, Oshiro MM, Junk DJ, et al. The acetyltransferase p300/CBP-associated factor is a p53 target gene in breast tumor cells. Neoplasia 2004;6(3):187–194.

100. Iwase H. Molecular action of the estrogen receptor and hormone dependency in breast cancer. Breast Cancer 2003;10(2):89–96.

101. Hayashi K, Goodison S, Urquidi V, Tarin D, Lotan R and Tahara E. Differential effects of retinoic acid on the growth of isogenic metastatic and non-metastatic breast cancer cell lines and their association with distinct expression of retinoic acid receptor beta isoforms 2 and 4. Int J Oncol 2003;22(3):623–629.

102. de Candia P, Akram M, Benezra R and Brogi E. Id4 messenger RNA and estrogen receptor expression: Inverse correlation in human normal breast epithelium and carcinoma. Hum Pathol 2006;37(8):1032–1041.

103. Roldan G, Delgado L and Muse IM. Tumoral expression of BRCA1, estrogen receptor alpha and ID4 protein in patients with sporadic breast cancer. Cancer Biol Ther 2006;5(5):505–510.

104. Umetani N, Mori T, Koyanagi K, et al. Aberrant hypermethylation of ID4 gene promoter region increases risk of lymph node metastasis in T1 breast cancer. Oncogene 2005;24(29):4721–4727.

105. Yu L, Liu C, Vandeusen J, et al. Global assessment of promoter methylation in a mouse model of cancer identifies ID4 as a putative tumor-suppressor gene in human leukemia. Nat Genet 2005;37(3):265–274.

106. Umetani N, Takeuchi H, Fujimoto A, Shinozaki M, Bilchik AJ and Hoon DS. Epigenetic inactivation of ID4 in colorectal carcinomas correlates with poor differentiation and unfavorable prognosis. Clin Cancer Res 2004;10(22):7475–7483.

107. de Candia P, Benera R and Solit DB. A role for Id proteins in mammary gland physiology and tumorigenesis. Adv Cancer Res 2004;92:81–94.

108. Chan AS, Tsui WY, Chen X, Chu KM, et al. Downregulation of ID4 by promoter hypermethylation in gastric adenocarcinoma. Oncogene 2003;22(44):6946–6953.

109. McNulty CL, Peres JN, Bardine N, van den Akker WM and Durston AJ. Knockdown of the complete Hox paralogous group 1 leads to dramatic hindbrain and neural crest defects. Development 2005;132(12):2861–2871.

110. Manohar CF, Salwen HR, Furtado MR and Cohn SL. Up-regulation of *HOXC6, HOXD1,* and *HOXD8* homeobox gene expression in human neuroblastoma cells following chemical induction of differentiation. Tumour Biol 1996;17(1):34–47.

111. Du JX, Yun CC, Bialkowska A and Yang VW. Protein inhibitor of activated STAT 1 interacts with and up-regulates activities of the pro-proliferative transcription factor Kruppel-like factor 5. J Biol Chem 2006;282:4782–4793.

112. Parnell TJ, Viering MM, Skjesol A, Helou C, Kuhn EJ and Geyer PK. An endogenous suppressor of hairy-wing insulator separates regulatory domains in Drosophila. Proc Natl Acad Sci USA 2003;100(23):13436–13441.

113. Byrd K and Corces VG. Visualization of chromatin domains created by the gypsy insulator of Drosophila. J Cell Biol 2003;162(4):565–574.
114. Pai CY, Lei EP, Ghosh D and Corces VG. The centrosomal protein CP190 is a component of the gypsy chromatin insulator. Cell 2004;16(5):737–748.
115. Yamaguchi Y, Narita T, Inukai N, Wada T and Handa H. SPT genes: Key players in the regulation of transcription, chromatin structure and other cellular processes. J Biochem 2001;129(2):185–191.
116. Burkett TJ and Garfinkel DJ. Molecular characterization of the *SPT23* gene: a dosage-dependent suppressor of Ty-induced promoter mutations from *Saccharomyces cerevisiae*. Yeast 1994;10(1):81–92.
117. Katoh Y and Katoh M. Comparative integromics on Ephrin family. Oncol Rep 2006;15(5):1391–1395.
118. Liu X, Hawkes E, Ishimaru T, Tran T and Sretavan DW. EphB3: An endogenous mediator of adult axonal plasticity and regrowth after CNS injury. J Neurosci 2006;26(12):3087–3101.
119. Benson MD, Romero MI, Lush ME, Lu QR, Henkemeyer M and Parada LF. Ephrin-B3 is a myelin-based inhibitor of neurite outgrowth. Proc Natl Acad Sci USA 2005; 102(30):10694–10699.
120. Yu G, Luo H, Wu Y and Wu J. Mouse ephrinB3 augments T-cell signaling and responses to T-cell receptor ligation. J Biol Chem 2003;278(47):47209–47216.
121. de Saint-Vis B, Bouchet C, Gautier G, Valladeau J, Caux C and Garrone P. Human dendritic cells express neuronal Eph receptor tyrosine kinases: Role of EphA2 in regulating adhesion to fibronectin. Blood 2003;102(13):4431–4440.
122. Gray-Owen SD and Blumberg RS. CEACAM1: Contact-dependent control of immunity. Nat Rev Immunol 2006;6(6):433–446.
123. Horst AK, Ito WD, Dabelstein J, et al. Carcinoembryonic antigen-related cell adhesion molecule 1 modulates vascular remodeling in vitro and in vivo. Clin Invest 2006;116(6):1596–1605.
124. Briese J, Schulte HM, Bamberger CM, Loning T and Bamberger AM. Expression pattern of osteopontin in endometrial carcinoma: Correlation with expression of the adhesion molecule CEACAM1. Int J Gynecol Pathol 2006;25(2):161–169.
125. Lu H, Guo X, Meng X, et al. The BRCA2-interacting protein BCCIP functions in RAD51 and BRCA2 focus formation and homologous recombinational repair. Mol Cell Biol 2005;25(5):1949–1957.
126. Meng X, Lu H and Shen Z. BCCIP functions through p53 to regulate the expression of p21Waf1/Cip1. Cell Cycle 2004;3(11):1457–1462.
127. Meng X, Liu J and Shen Z. Inhibition of G1 to S cell cycle progression by BCCIP beta. Cell Cycle 2004;3(3):343–348.

2 Mammary Glands, Stem Cells, and Breast Cancer

David L. Mack, Gilbert H. Smith, and Brian W. Booth

SUMMARY

The mammary gland is unique in that most of its development occurs after birth with dramatic changes in proliferation and differentiation taking place during puberty and pregnancy. Different subsets of mammary-specific stem/progenitor cells have been shown to drive the individual stages of mammary gland development, and their regulation requires coordination between localized signals and systemic hormones. That sophisticated integration and control is achieved through the function of the stem cell niche. The goal of this chapter is to review why somatic stem cells are thought to exist in the mouse mammary gland, how they are being isolated and assayed, how their fate is influenced by the surrounding microenvironment, and how aberrant regulation of this process might contribute to breast cancer. If the components of the niche could be defined, each might then be targeted as a method to modify the fate of stem or progenitor cells during normal organ regeneration or repaired after tumorigenesis has been initiated.

Key Words: Breast cancer; Mammary gland; Stem cells; Progenitors; Tumorigenesis

1. BREAST DEVELOPMENTAL BIOLOGY AND TUMORIGENESIS

The current view on breast cancer as a stem cell disease is founded on compelling evidence that many breast cancers may arise as clonal expansions from epithelial progenitors with an infinite lifespan *(1)*. It has been hypothesized that unique properties of mammary stem cells, such as self-renewal, make this population a prime target for transformation and tumorigenesis. Several experimental breast cancer models support this hypothesis. The most venerable is the mammary tumor virus model in mice *(2)*, where MMTV proviral insertions produce mutated mammary cells, which attain immortality (escape from growth senescence) and produce clones

From: *Current Clinical Oncology: Breast Cancer in the Post-Genomic Era,*
Edited by: A. Giordano and N. Normanno, DOI: 10.1007/978-1-60327-945-1_2,
© Humana Press, a part of Springer Science + Business Media, LLC 2009

of mammary cells with increased propensity to develop into mammary cancer. Serial transplantations of these preneoplastic lesions result in the formation of hyperplastic/dysplastic ductal trees, suggesting that multipotent cells are affected by MMTV transformation and that they pass on their neoplastic properties to their descendants *(3)*. Morphologically undifferentiated cells, reminiscent of stem/progenitor cells, are present in both premalignant and malignant mammary populations (Fig. 1). Reproductive history has a profound impact on breast

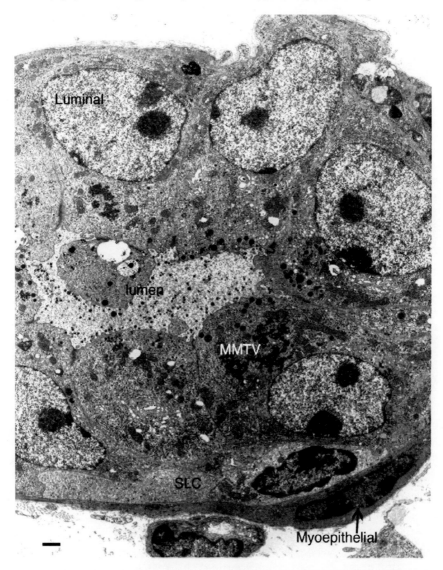

Fig. 1. This electron micrograph depicts an ultrathin section through one of the acini in an MMTV-induced alveolar hyperplasia. There is evidence of virus replication (MMTV) of secretory activity leading to secretory granule formation in the apical cytoplasm of the luminal cells and release into the lumen. An undifferentiated suprabasal cell (SLC) is present and proximal to it, a differentiated myoepithelial cell (*arrow*). Bar equals 1.0 mM.

Chapter 2 / Mammary Glands, Stem Cells, and Breast Cancer

tumorigenesis; thus, it is reasonable to assume that pregnancy and lactation have enduring effects on the cancer susceptibility of multipotent stem/progenitor cells.

Evidence that cancer stem cells sustain solid neoplasms has recently emerged *(1,4)*. Whether these "cancer stem cells" arise de novo or result from mutations within normal tissue stem/progenitor cells is presently unknown. A shift in the microenvironment of mammary epithelial cells as the result of pregnancy is a plausible mechanism by which to explain the greater refractivity of mammary tissue after early parity to cancer induction or progression. In a rat chemical carcinogenesis model, Nandi and his colleagues have argued that there is no difference in the susceptibility of the mammary epithelium between nulliparous and parous females to initiation (malignant transformation) by NMU; rather, it is a reduction in the incidence of progression of the "initiated" cells to frank malignancy. This difference in "progression" is completely reversible when the parous rodents are subjected to various hormonal regimens or given growth factors such as IGF-1 *(5)*. If this is correct, then epithelial (stem/progenitor) cell targets for carcinogenesis are the same but behave differently in their respective microenvironments (niches) during homeostatic tissue maintenance in the parous female.

1.1. Pregnancy Mediates Permanent Changes in Mammary Epithelial Cells

The basic principle for the dual phenomenon of pregnancy and breast cancer is that a gestation cycle induces massive proliferation and an endpoint differentiation of epithelial subtypes. Either permanent systemic changes following a full-term pregnancy (such as a decrease in circulating levels of hormones) or the alteration of the mammary tissue itself could explain the difference in breast cancer risk between nulliparous and parous women. Sivaraman and coworkers suggested that the hormonal milieu of pregnancy affects the developmental state of a subset of mammary epithelial cells and their progeny *(6)*.

Microarray evidence suggests that pregnancy mediates persistent changes in the gene expression profile in parous females *(7,8)*. These pregnancy-induced changes can be imitated through a transient administration of hormones, in particular estrogen and progesterone or human chorionic gonadotropin. Ginger et al. used subtractive hybridization as a method to identify differentially expressed genes between hormone-treated Wistar–Furth rats and their untreated controls. Twenty-eight days after the last treatment, they identified approximately 100 differentially expressed loci. In a more comprehensive study, D'Cruz and colleagues utilized oligonucleotide arrays to examine differences in the expression profile of approximately 5,500 genes between parous mice and their nulliparous controls. These initial results were verified by more laborious methods (northern blot analysis and in situ hybridization) and across several mouse strains as well as in two rat models.

1.2. The Origination of Parity-Induced Mammary Epithelial Cells During Late Pregnancy and Lactation

Using the Cre-lox technology, a mammary epithelial subtype, which is abundant in nonlactating and nonpregnant parous mice, was recently described *(9)*. These parity-induced mammary epithelial cells (PI-MECs) then permanently reside at the terminal ends of ducts (i.e., lobuloalveolar units) after postlactational remodeling. Two lines of evidence exist showing that the presence of PI-MECs in the involuted mammary gland is not an artifact caused by a deregulated activation of the promoter of our randomly integrated WAP-Cre construct. First, the WAP-Cre transgenic expression closely follows the activation of the endogenous WAP locus, and Ludwig and coworkers *(10)* have reported similar observations in genetically engineered mice that express Cre recombinase under the endogenous *Wap* gene promoter (i.e., WAP-Cre knock-in mutants). Second, limiting dilution transplantation assays with dispersed epithelial cells from nulliparous female mice demonstrate the existence of lobule-limited and duct-limited progenitors *(11)*. These studies were carried out with epithelial cells from WAP-LacZ transgenic mice, where LacZ is expressed from the whey acidic protein promoter in late pregnant mice. Lobule-limited outgrowths positive for LacZ expression were observed in the implanted fat pads at parturition. Similar lobule-limited outgrowths were developed when PI-MECs were inoculated in limiting dilution into the cleared mammary fat pads of subsequently impregnated hosts (Fig. 2). These structures like

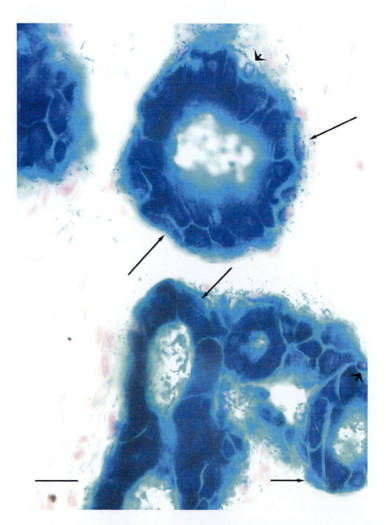

Fig. 2. The image shows a section through a lobule-limited LacZ-positive outgrowth in full-term pregnant host composed entirely of progeny from PI-MEC. The growth comprises both luminal and myoepithelial (*long arrows*) cells and small-undifferentiated light cells (*short arrows*). Bar equals 20 mM.

those described earlier *(11)* comprised both secretory luminal cells and myoepithelial cells and were 100% positive for LacZ activity indicating that they were developed entirely from PI-MECs. Therefore, it is likely that PI-MECs arise from the lobule-limited progenitor population discovered by Smith among the mammary epithelial cells present in nulliparous unbred females. In addition to luminal and myoepithelial progeny, PI-MECs produced both small (SLC) and large undifferentiated light cells (ULLC) in the lobules. SLCs and ULLCs have essential roles in mammary stem/progenitor cell function *(3)*. The existence of committed mammary alveolar precursors in mice and rats has been proposed earlier *(12,13)*.

1.3. PI-MECs Are Self-Renewing and Pluripotent

When fragments from glands containing PI-MECs were transplanted into epithelium-free fat pads in nulliparous hosts, PI-MECs contributed to ductal elongation in a very significant manner. The vast majority of resulting outgrowths contained LacZ-positive cells, and in >75% of the transplants, PI-MEC-derived cells were present throughout the *entire* ductal tree. These results clearly demonstrated that PI-MECs exhibit two important features of multipotent stem cells: self-renewal and contribution to diverse epithelial populations in ducts and alveoli. We demonstrated, for the first time, that the progeny from cells previously expressing an *alveolar* differentiation marker (i.e., WAP) could contribute to the formation of primary and secondary *ducts*. When the transplanted hosts were impregnated, the self-renewed PI-MECs at the tips of duct side branches proliferated during early pregnancy to form the new secretory acini. The transplantation procedure itself had no effect on the activation of the WAP-Cre and Rosa-LacZ transgenes because mammary fragments from nulliparous double transgenic donors never produced outgrowths with uniformly distributed LacZ-positive cells *(9)*. To establish an estimate of the self-renewing ability of PI-MECs, mammary fragments containing LacZ-positive cells were transferred through four transplant generations. Each successful transplant resulted in a 400-fold increase of the implanted epithelial population, which represents roughly an 8–9 (8.65)-fold doubling of the implanted cells *(9)*.

To determine to what extent the presence of neighboring LacZ-negative epithelial cells contributed to the self-renewing capacity of labeled PI-MECs, dispersed mammary epithelial cells from multiparous WAP-Cre/Rosa-LacZ females were inoculated at limiting dilutions into cleared fat pads, and the hosts were subsequently impregnated. All outgrowths contained LacZ-expressing cells, even though PI-MECs represented only 20% of the inoculated epithelial cells. Notably, no epithelial outgrowths were comprised entirely from unlabeled (LacZ-negative) cells. Both lobule-limited and duct-limited outgrowths were, however, entirely comprised from PI-MECs (and their LacZ-expressing descendents), as determined by serial sections through these structures. These results indicate that all luminal, myoepithelial and cap cells of terminal buds may be derived from PI-MECs and their progeny. This conclusion was confirmed by demonstrating that the LacZ-positive cells in these structures could be doubly stained for mammary cell lineage markers for myoepithelium (smooth muscle actin, Fig. 3), estrogen receptor alpha (ER-α), or progesterone receptor (PR). Thus, PI-MECs are not only self-renewing, but they are pluripotent as well, giving rise to progeny that differentiate along all the epithelial cell lineages of the mammary gland.

1.4. WAP-TGF-$\beta1$ Expression Aborts Self-Renewal of PI-MECs in Transplants

The reproductive capacity of the mammary epithelial stem cell is reduced coincident with the number of symmetric divisions it must perform. In a study using WAP-TGF-$\beta1$ transgenic

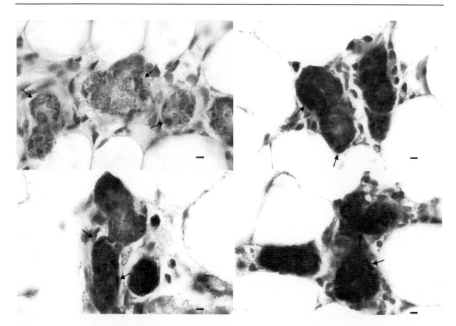

Fig. 3. This composite shows LacZ-negative acini stained for SMA in the upper left panel and LacZ-positive acini in the remaining three panels. The *arrows* indicate the myoepithelial cells demonstrated by positive SMA-staining. The LacZ-positive cells appear as dark gray in this grayscale figure. Bars equal 5 mM.

mice, it was observed that mammary epithelial stem cells were prematurely aged due to ectopic expression of TGF-β1 under the regulation of the *WAP* gene promoter *(14)*. To assess whether TGF-β1 expression in PI-MECs abolishes their capacity to self-renew, mammary epithelia from WAP-TGF-β1/WAP-Cre/Rosa-LacZ triple transgenic mice were transplanted into wild-type recipients. It is important to note that the percentage of labeled cells in the triple transgenic glands after a single parity was indistinguishable from that observed in WAP-Cre/Rosa-LacZ double transgenic controls. As expected, mammary tissue implants and dispersed cells from the triple transgenic females, after either a single pregnancy or multiple gestation cycles, failed to produce full lobular development in full-term pregnant hosts. Perhaps more importantly, LacZ-positive cells were not observed in the ducts in these transplant outgrowths either in nulliparous or early pregnant hosts. LacZ-expressing cells did appear in the transplant population and were present in the lobular structures during late pregnancy in these transplants (after 15 days to parturition). In summary, the results of these studies demonstrate that the PI-MECs that develop during pregnancy and survive subsequent tissue remodeling in the absence of lactation in WAP-TGF-β1 females were incapable or severely limited in their ability to self-renew in transplants and could not contribute to ductal development in subsequent transplant outgrowths. Therefore, self-renewal (expansion outside of a stem cell niche) and proliferation competence (asymmetric divisions within a niche) appear to be properties independently affected by autocrine TGF-β1 expression in the PI-MECs.

By definition, the self-renewal of stem cells occurs by two different processes. In asymmetric divisions, the most common activity of stem cells residing in a niche, the stem cell is preserved and one daughter becomes committed to a particular cell fate. Alternatively, a stem

Chapter 2 / Mammary Glands, Stem Cells, and Breast Cancer   25

cell may divide symmetrically and expand to produce two or more stem cell daughters that retain stem cell properties. This latter form of self-renewal is essential for expansion of the stem cell population during allometric growth of the tissue (i.e., during ductal growth and expansion in the postpubertal female or when the mammary epithelial implant is growing in the transplanted mammary fat pad). The negative effect of TGF-β1 on the expansive self-renewal of PI-MECs supports our earlier observation regarding protection from mouse mammary tumor virus (MMTV)-induced mammary tumorigenesis in WAP-TGF-β1 transgenic females *(14)*. This might suggest that the cellular targets for MMTV-mediated neoplastic transformation are PI-MECs because multiple pregnancies accelerate MMTV-induced oncogenesis *(3)*.

1.5. PI-MECs and Mammary Tumorigenesis

Pregnancy has a dual effect on human breast cancer (protection or promotion), depending on the age of an individual, the period after a pregnancy and the genetic predisposition. In genetically engineered strains that are highly susceptible to mammary tumorigenesis and exhibit accelerated tumor development in postpartum or parous females, one might expect that PI-MECs serve as targets for neoplastic transformation. The unique growth properties of PI-MECs (i.e., responsiveness to pregnancy hormones, survival during involution, and ability to self renew) make this epithelial subtype a potential target for pregnancy-associated tumorigenesis. Transgenic mice expressing the wild-type Her2/neu (ErbB2) oncogene under transcriptional regulation of the MMTV-LTR seem to be suitable for studying the involvement of PI-MECs in pregnancy-associated mammary tumorigenesis since this animal model exhibits a relatively long latency of tumorigenesis (T50 of 205 days). Using this animal model, we demonstrated that (a) multiparous females consistently exhibited accelerated tumorigenesis compared with their nulliparous littermate controls in a mixed genetic background and (b) PI-MECs were, indeed, primary targets of neoplastic transformation in this model *(15)*. The de novo generation and amplification of a large number of hormone-responsive and apoptosis-resistant epithelial cells (i.e., PI-MECs) during the first and subsequent reproductive cycles might, therefore, account for the significantly increased cancer susceptibility of parous MMTV-neu transgenic females.

To further substantiate that PI-MECs are primary targets for neoplastic transformation in MMTV-neu transgenic mice, we eliminated or greatly impaired the growth of PI-MECs by deleting the *Tsg101* gene in cells that transiently activated WAP-Cre (i.e., females that carry two transgenes, MMTV-neu and WAP-Cre, in a homozygous *Tsg101* conditional knockout background). The complete deletion of *Tsg101* can serve as an excellent negative "selection marker" for WAP-Cre expressing cells since this gene is indispensable for the survival of normal, immortalized, and fully transformed cells *(16)*. In multiparous MMTV-neu females, impaired genesis or elimination of PI-MECs resulted in a significantly reduced tumor onset, suggesting that restraining the growth and survival of differentiating alveolar cells during pregnancy (and therefore PI-MECs in parous mice) eliminates the cellular basis for transformation in this model.

1.6. Some PI-MECs Are Asymmetrically Dividing Long-Label Retaining Cells

It was proposed over 30 years ago that somatic stem cells avoid accumulation of genetic errors resulting from DNA synthesis prior to dividing by selectively retaining their template

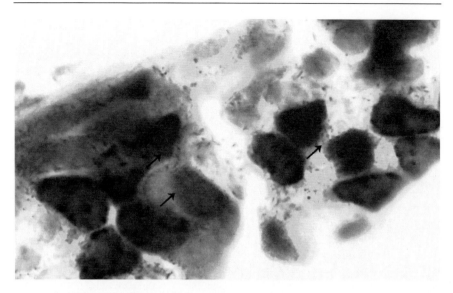

Fig. 4. PI-MEC long-label-retaining (3H-thymidine) with autoradiographic grains were doubly labeled with 5BrdU (darker nuclei) in transplant labeled with thymidine 7 weeks earlier following a 2-day pulse with 5BrdU and produced 5BrdU-labeled-only (*arrows*) daughters after a 6-day chase.

DNA strands and passing the newly synthesized strands to their committed daughters *(17)*. Therefore, somatic epithelial stem/progenitor cells labeled by DNA analogs during their inception will become long-label retaining epithelial cells (LREC). Label retention has long been considered to be a characteristic of somatic stem cells and this propensity to retain DNA label has been explained by postulating that somatic stem cells seldom divide and are mainly proliferatively quiescent. Recent studies have, however, shown that in multiple tissues long-label-retaining cells are actively dividing and asymmetrically retain their labeled template DNA strands while passing the newly synthesized DNA to their differentiating progeny *(18,19)*. Interestingly, PI-MECs that have proliferated extensively in transplants give rise to LacZ-positive progeny, which retain the original DNA label for long periods and when pulsed with a second alternative DNA label prove to be actively traversing the cell cycle and thus become doubly labeled incorporating the second label into new DNA strands. Subsequent to a short chase period the second label is transferred along with the new DNA strands to LacZ-positive progeny (Fig. 4). This evidence demonstrates that during self-renewal PI-MECs produce progeny (in addition to luminal and myoepithelial offspring) that behave as asymmetrically dividing stem/progenitor cells responsible for the steady-state maintenance of the diverse LacZ-positive mammary epithelial population in the resulting outgrowth.

2. STEM CELL BIOLOGY IN THE MAMMARY GLAND

Stem cells have the ability to produce progeny that are different from themselves and to self-renew. The presence of mammary stem cells in mice was proven in the 1950s when it was demonstrated that any portion of the mouse mammary gland, regardless of age or parity

Chapter 2 / Mammary Glands, Stem Cells, and Breast Cancer

status, could regenerate a functional gland when transplanted into a fat pad cleared of endogenous epithelium in prepubescent female recipients *(20–22)*. This model has become a powerful tool in the study of mammary stem cells as both tissue fragments and dispersed cells can regenerate an entire mammary gland. This is especially important because before any cell can be considered a stem cell, it must fulfill the following functional criteria, regardless of its biochemistry. It must self-renew, differentiate into at least one other cell type and participate significantly in the generation and maintenance of its tissue.

The study of human mammary stem cells has been hampered until recently by the lack of in vivo models. The generation of immunocompromised animals that minimizes tissue rejection has advanced study immensely. More recently Kuperwaser and colleagues have developed a new in vivo model in which they "humanize" a mouse mammary fat pad by transplanting human fibroblasts into the cleared murine fat pad *(23)*. The human fibroblasts are allowed to establish prior to the addition of human mammary epithelial cells allowing for the epithelium to engraft in a more natural environment.

In the mouse mammary gland three distinct classes of mammary progenitor cells have been identified: multilineage progenitors, ductal-limited progenitor cells, and lobule-limited progenitor cells *(12,24)*. These classes are distinguished by their functional properties evident during pregnancy. Multilineage progenitor cells have the capacity to generate any epithelial subtype; ductal-only progenitor cells do not develop secretory lobules during subsequent pregnancies following transplantation while lobule-limited progenitor cells develop functional secretory alveoli during pregnancy but do not generate a complex ductal network.

Stem cell isolation in the hematopoietic system has been at the forefront for years. Efficient flow cytometric techniques for stem cell isolation have allowed characterization of these cells. Using techniques based on the hematopoietic system, four types of mammary progenitor cells have been identified in humans based on cell surface marker expression phenotypes: multilineage, myoepithelial-restricted, and two classes of luminal-restricted [reviewed in *(25)]*. A number of different candidate markers have been investigated including CD10/CALLA, ESA (epithelial specific antigen), MUC-1 and the cytokeratins 8, 9, 18, and 19. Myoepithelial-restricted cells are isolated based on an EpCAM^{low}MUC1$^-$CD49f$^+$phenotype. Luminal-restricted progenitors are isolated based on expression of MUC1 and either K19$^+$K14$^-$ or K19$^-$K14$^-$ phenotypes.

A valuable in vitro tool for studying mammary stem cells is the newly developed "mammosphere" culture system where anchorage-independent cells generate clonal floating sphere structures *(26)*. Mammospheres formed under these conditions possess multilineage progenitors that self-renew and begin to differentiate to form luminal and myoepithelial cells. We have used this system to demonstrate that lobule-limited PI-MECs self-renew in culture *(27)*. Mammospheres can be transplanted and recapitulate an entire gland. A small number of cells within mammospheres also segregate BrdU-labeled DNA suggesting asymmetric cell divisions (Fig. 5). Mammosphere cultures that were exposed to differentiating conditions, such as activation of the Notch or Hedgehog pathways, showed an increase in secondary mammospheres formed after dissociation as well as an increase in branching morphogenesis and cellular proliferation *(26,28)*. This indicates that both Notch and Hedgehog are involved in the self-renewal and differentiation pathways in mammary stem cells. These molecular pathways, along with the Wnt pathway, are involved in the maintenance of the hematopoietic stem cell hierarchy *(29)*.

Two different methods have been used to demonstrate that a single cell can regenerate a mouse mammary gland by acting as a multilineage mammary stem cell. Kordon and Smith *(12)* showed first in 1998 through serial transplantation studies that a single retrovirally tagged mammary cell formed a mammary gland comprised of ductal and luminal components of

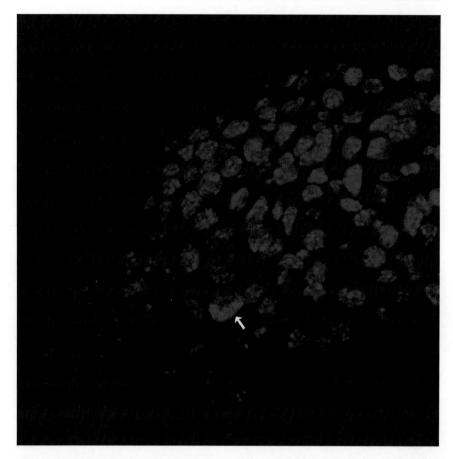

Fig. 5. A mammosphere after 10 days in anchorage-independent culture conditions. The arrow shows a BrdU labeled nucleus.

both luminal and myoepithleial lineages. Later in 2006, two groups published their findings where they demonstrated that by transplanting a single, visually confirmed cell that was fluorescently sorted on the basis of being CD24$^+$ Sca-1^{low}CD49f^{high}CD29^{high} and not expressing CD45, Ter119, or CD31 they were able to generate a mammary gland *(30,31)*. CD24 acts as a P-selectin ligand and may modulate integrin function while CD29 is β1-integrin and CD49f is α6-integrin. CD29 and CD49f are markers for basal epithelia suggesting that the basal epithelial compartment contains the mammary stem cells. Furthermore, only luminal epithelial cells are ERα$^+$, which have almost no fat pad outgrowth potential.

2.1. Cancer Stem Cells

Stem cells are believed to be the targets of tumorigenesis in the mammary gland. Most DNA mutations rely on replication and cellular division. It is hypothesized that stem cells protect themselves against such mutations through asymmetric division *(17)*. Since the

Chapter 2 / Mammary Glands, Stem Cells, and Breast Cancer

majority of breast cancers are heterogeneous this argues that malignant transformation originates in cells that can generate progeny of different lineages.

Cancer stem cells do not have to arise from normal somatic stem cells. Another theory of mammary tumor heterogeneity is that the different types of mammary cells (luminal, basal, myoepithelial) vary in degrees of susceptibility to genetic mutations and transformation. Transit amplifying cells or differentiated cells may generate cancer stem cells if a genetic mutation reactivates a self-renewal pathway, although there is as of yet no direct evidence of this occurring [reviewed in *(29)*].

Approximately 15–21% of human breast cancers present a basal phenotype characterized by the lack of expression of ER, PR, and erbB2 *(32–34)*. These "triple negative" breast cancers have a poor prognosis. Compared with patients having other forms of breast cancer, these patients are more likely to have a recurrence within 5 years and the mortality rates are correspondingly higher. Triple negative tumors are associated with BRCA1 and usually occur in younger women. BRCA1 (breast cancer 1) mutations are synonymous with basal breast cancer. It has been hypothesized that BRCA1 acts as a stem cell regulator and loss of BRCA1 in a conditional knockout model demonstrates a proliferation defect during pregnancy. BRCA1 tumors often have mutated p53 and Trp53, key cell cycle regulators *(35)*.

In 2003, Al-Hajj and colleagues isolated tumor-initiating cells as determined by xenotransplatation into immunocompromised NOD/SCID mice. The tumor-initiating cells isolated from eight pleural effusions and one primary tumor had an EpCam$^+$ CD44$^+$ CD24$^{-/low}$ phenotype. They found that the frequency of tumor-initiating cells within that subpopulation of the tumor cells was <1% *(1)*. This observation agrees with other human tumor types including colon, brain, and pancreatic cancers. However, clinical studies have confirmed through both breast cancer cell lines and breast tumors that the CD44$^+$/CD24$^-$ phenotype is not associated with patient outcome or metastasis. In light of these and other studies the question that has arisen is as follows: are CD44$^+$/CD24$^-$ cells better at adapting to the mouse mammary environment or are they really more tumorigenic in humans *(36)*?

The human breast stem cell niche in both normal and tumor tissues has been characterized as CD44$^+$CD24$^-$ and PROCR$^+$ (a basal marker) but CD10$^-$ (a myoepithelial marker) *(37)*. Gene expression profile analysis showed that CD44$^+$CD24$^-$ PROCR$^+$ CD10$^-$ cells from normal tissue are more similar to CD44$^+$CD24$^-$ PROCR$^+$ CD10$^-$ tumor cells than to normal CD24$^+$ cells *(38)*.

Mammosphere initiating cells from the MCF-7 and MDA-MB-231 cell lines that are CD44+CD24low/– have an increased radio resistance. CD133+ glioma stem cells display similar resistance due to improved DNA damage repair as compared to nonstem cells *(39)*. "Differentiation therapy" of BMP4 can eliminate glioma stem cells, and other molecular therapies have shown promise in eliminating leukemia stem cells *(40)*. Better understanding of mammary stem cells, both normal and tumor-initiating, will help to devise new therapies that will allow elimination of tumor-initiating cells through molecular targeting.

Pregnancy has a dual effect on human breast cancer (protection or promotion), depending on the age of an individual, the period after a pregnancy, and the genetic predisposition *(41)*. In genetically engineered strains of mice that are highly susceptible to mammary tumorigenesis and exhibit accelerated tumor development in postpartum or multiparous females, one might expect that PI-MECs serve as targets for neoplastic transformation. PI-MECs represent reporter gene marked lobule-limited mammary epithelial stem/progenitor cells that persist following pregnancy, lactation, and involution. These pluripotent cells exist in nulliparous glands *(11,27)* but do not express the reporter gene, which is activated by Cre-lox recombination upon expression of Cre from the whey acidic protein (WAP) promoter *(42,43)*, hence parity-identified. The unique growth properties of PI-MECs (i.e., responsiveness to pregnancy hormones, survival during involution, and ability to self-renew) make this epithelial subtype a potential target for pregnancy-associated tumorigenesis *(14)*. Transgenic mice expressing the wild-type neu oncogene under the transcriptional regulation of the MMTV-LTR are suitable for studying the involvement of PI-MECs in pregnancy-associated mammary tumorigenesis since this animal model exhibits a relatively long latency of tumorigenesis (T50 of 205 days) *(15)*. MMTV-neu mice generate ERα-negative lesions that exhibit pathological features similar to a subset of human breast cancers. More importantly, the overexpression of neu/erbB2/HER2 has been observed in a significant subset of pregnancy-associated breast cancers in humans *(44,45)*. Using this animal model, Henry et al., *(15)* demonstrated that (a) multiparous females consistently exhibited accelerated tumorigenesis compared with their nulliparous littermate controls in a mixed genetic background and (b) PI-MECs were, indeed, primary targets of neoplastic transformation in this model. Interestingly, the significantly fewer lesions that arose in nulliparous controls originated from hormone-responsive cells that transiently activated WAP-Cre (i.e., an epithelial subpopulation that represents only 1–4% of all epithelial cells in the virgin gland) during estrus. The de novo generation and amplification of a large number of hormone-responsive and apoptosis-resistant epithelial cells (i.e., PI-MECs) during the first and subsequent reproductive cycles might, therefore, account for the significantly increased cancer susceptibility of parous MMTV-neu transgenic females.

We have hypothesized that if PI-MECs are the targets for MMTV-neu induced tumors then neu-transformed PI-MECs might represent a subpopulation of tumor-initiating stem cells responsible for maintenance and expansion of the MMTV-neu-induced tumorigenic population. We mixed increasing dilutions of MMTV-neu tumor cells collected from WAP-Cre/Rosa26R/MMTV-neu females with normal wild-type mammary epithelial cells from FVB/N mice. These mixtures were inoculated into the epithelium-divested mammary fat pads of immunocompromised female hosts. Our results demonstrate that some MMTV-neu-initiated tumor cells are capable of interacting with the normal epithelium contributing to normal mammary gland growth and regeneration, and in the process produce both luminal and myoepithelial epithelial progeny.

3. INFLUENCE OF THE MICROENVIRONMENT ON STEM CELL BIOLOGY AND CANCER

Stem and progenitor cells in most adult tissues reside in specialized, highly regulated microenvironments called stem cell niches *(46–48)*. In general terms, niches are made up of signaling cells, characteristic of extracellular matrix (ECM), soluble mediators, and the stem cell *(49,50)* (Fig. 6). The niche interprets a myriad of signals and controls whether stem cells remain quiescent, expand via symmetric division, or self-renew while contributing to the pool of progenitor cells by dividing asymmetrically. A constant dialogue made up of physical and molecular interactions between stem cells and the "support" cells of the niche shelters stem cells from differentiation or apoptotic stimuli that might deplete their stores. Homeostasis is maintained by the niche by balancing the need for additional differentiated progeny with the long-term protection against overproduction, which if not properly controlled may lead to cancer. One might even argue that adult or somatic stem cells have limited function outside their niche and that the justification for studying the niche emerges from its ability to impose function on its resident stem cells.

The idea of a niche as a specialized microenvironment sheltering stem cells was first proposed by Schofield almost 30 years ago in the context of mammalian hematology *(51)*. However, most of the early evidence supporting the niche as a physical entity came from

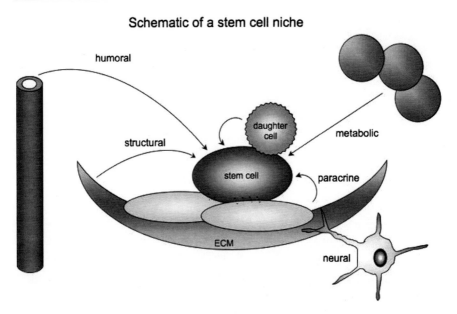

Fig. 6. Schematic of a generic somatic stem cell niche showing the various elements that participate in regulating the fate of the resident stem cell. The distance from the ultimate stem cell position may determine the relative strength of each of these signals and thus contribute to the differentiation of the daughter cell. *ECM* extracellular matrix.

invertebrate models, like the gonads of *Drosophila* and *C. elegans*. In both cases the germ cells reside at the distal tip of a tapered organ and depend on the interaction with surrounding somatic cells to maintain their undifferentiated state *(52–54)*. The idea that heterologous cell types compose the niche has now been well documented and drives much of our search for similar cell-based niche components in mammalian tissues. Whether normal stem cell function requires multiple cell types has recently been brought into question. Two reports showed that a posterior midgut population of cells in *Drosophila* could renew and differentiate into enterocytes and enteroendocrine cells in a clonal fashion *(55,56)*. These cells do not appear to be in contact with a heterologous cell type but do sit on the basement membrane. In addition, two papers showed the successful transplantation of single mammary stem/progenitor cells that generated full ductal outgrowths *(30,31)*. These data suggest that the extracellular matrix and other noncellular constituents might be sufficient to regulate stem cell function in some tissues.

In the murine mammary gland a pool of stem cells produces a branching bilayered epithelial tissue with an inner luminal epithelial layer and an outer myoepithelial layer bounded by a basement membrane surrounded by a fatty stroma of adipocytes with vasculature, nerves, and lymph vessels. What is special about the mammary niche is its ability to generate these structures by coordinating local stimuli with systemic hormonal stimuli to generate new mammary structures. Three groups have shown that putative mammary stem cells are ERα-negative *(57–59)* so it would follow that a subset of the support cells within or nearby the niche would be estrogen and/or progesterone responsive. However, because the location of niches in situ has not yet been identified, formal proof remains to be provided. In a recent review on how hormones influence the mammary niche, Brisken and Duss proposed that the pubertal niche and the adult niche are overlapping entities in terms of what cells compose them. A hormone receptor positive sensor cell and the stem cell are identical in both but any additional niche cells that are recruited in response to estrogens versus progesterones are different *(60)*. They further speculated about whether there is a "special" subpopulation of receptor positive sensor cells that directly control the niche or whether their inductive effect is indirect and mediated through a sensed depletion of mammary progenitors. These hints should allow for a better stage-specific characterization of the mammary niche.

Despite knowing the combination of stem/progenitor cell surface markers outlined in the previous section, the physical location of the mammary niche remains elusive. Several reports have suggested that the cap region of the terminal end buds (TEBs) in mice is one possible location of the stem cell niche during estrogen-dependent ductal outgrowth [reviewed in *(60)*]. During ductal elongation the cap cells are able to directly interact with the stroma because the basal lamina is degraded locally suggesting that some stromal cells participate in this process. Bolstering this idea is the observation that wild-type epithelium does not grow out in an EGFR-deficient fat pad but EGFR-deficient epithelium does reconstitute a wild-type fat pad *(61)*. This result coupled with the fact that EGFR mRNA is enriched in the stem cell compartment *(59)* and is an important downstream effector of ERα signaling via paracrine amphiregulin *(62)* argues that the pubertal niche has a stromal component. However, since the TEBs and cap cells no longer exist after the completion of the ductal tree, the cap region is an unlikely location for the adult stem cell niche.

Proliferation and differentiation (secondary side branching) resulting from the stimulation of the adult mammary niche are driven primarily by the cyclic release of progesterone during the estrous cycle. Unlike estrogen and its receptor, progesterone can stimulate proliferation of both PR-positive and PR-negative luminal epithelial cells *(63)*. At least part of progesterone's paracrine effects are thought to be mediated through the *r*eceptor *a*ctivator of NF-κB *l*igand (RANKL) *(64,65)* and Wnt-4 *(58)*. The Wnt signal is believed to act directly on the stem cell within the niche and trigger an asymmetric division *(40–43)* followed by the differentiating daughter's expansion induced by RANKL *(60)*.

In general terms of the location of the adult niche, some older data suggested that the mammary ducts of mice and rats may contain stem cells. In virgin mice, putative stem cells were found in ducts rather than alveoli, and these were shown to regenerate ductal epithelium as well as to form new alveolar buds *(66)*. Sca-1 was proposed as a marker of mammary stem cells in mice when its expression was observed in ducts as well as in invading TEBs *(67)*. Earlier work from our laboratory corroborated this idea by showing that rudimentary ducts from postgestational mice, when transplanted into cleared fat pads of TGF-β1 transgenic mice, grew out and retained the capacity to reactivate lobular structures at late pregnancy *(9)*. In addition, ductal niches appear to respond specifically to the MMTV-c-myc transgene by amplifying the stem cell compartment *(50)*, which supported the previous findings in humans *(68)* that an entire TDLU represents the progeny from a single early ductal progenitor. Recent evidence employing microdissection to collect organoids from reduction mammoplasties demonstrated that the terminal ducts are one of the major sites of stem cells in adults *(69)*. Cells from these isolated structures produced self-renewing mammospheres, multilineage colonies in 2D culture and TDLU-like structures in 3D ECM cultures, while cells from the lobules did not display any of these capacities. A further subdivision of these human ductal cells revealed a subpopulation that double stain positive for both K14 and K19. K14 typically marks myoepithelial cells and K19 is expressed mostly on luminal cells. The expression of both lineage markers in the same cell suggests that it might identify a subpopulation of stem or progenitor cells in the human breast. It has even been proposed that

Chapter 2 / Mammary Glands, Stem Cells, and Breast Cancer

K19 functions as a "switch keratin," enabling a cell to transition from one type of cytoskeleton to the other *(70)*. The same K14⁺/K19⁺ cells also express chondroitin sulfate, K6a, K15, and SSEA-4 *(69)*, which overlap nicely with stem cell markers from other tissues, including brain, hair follicle, and prostate *(71–74)*. This set of putative stem cell markers coincides with the EpCam⁺/CD49f⁺ population discussed earlier. Taken together, these data suggest the likely location of the mammary stem cell niche to be most closely associated with the ducts. However, the data published to date do not rule out the possibility of other niches and it is unknown whether the niche in the postpubertal virgin gland remains the same throughout adulthood or after pregnancy. The fact that the parity-induced mammary epithelial cells (PI-MECs) produced luminal and myoepithelial lineages in ductal-limited and lobule-limited outgrowths when employed in limiting dilution transplantation experiments using parous mammary tissue from WapCreRosa26stopβGal mice *(9)* and the fact that PI-MECs survive involution suggest that new niches might be established during the extensive proliferation of pregnancy. This same population of cells was later shown to be enriched for CD24+/CD49f+ cells corroborating their stem/progenitor status *(43)*.

Unlike other tissues, where the niche has been associated with a particular anatomical structure, the fact that any portion of the mammary gland can be transplanted and generate a complete outgrowth capable of full lactation indicates that the mammary niche resides at regular intervals throughout the gland. Studies from other animal model systems have shown that adult stem cells are generally focal in their distribution and not necessarily colocalized with the majority of the transiently amplifying cells [for review see *(75)*]. For example, stem cells have been shown to reside in the hair follicle bulge and the proximal ducts of the prostate, both separate from the main site of proliferation in each tissue. In an attempt to ascertain how many niches (or stem cells) are responsible for generating a mouse mammary gland, several groups have tried to estimate stem cell frequency by serial dilution transplantation experiments. The estimates range from 1 mammary repopulating unit (MRU) in 200 dissociated cells *(76)* to 1 in 5,000 cells *(31)*.

Many human stem cell studies are forced to use ex vivo culture of putatively enriched stem cell or progenitor populations before transplantation into animal hosts. Several of these studies, upon first glance, appear to contain contradictory results about the repopulating ability of certain marked stem or progenitor populations *(30,31,67)*. Confusion in these reports revolves around the Sca-1 status, inclusion in the side population, and whether endothelial cells were excluded from study. Most of the discrepancies in these papers can be explained if one considers the different culture conditions used. It has been suggested that any manipulation of mammary epithelial cells in culture selects for immature progenitors or transit amplifying cells with repopulating activity, but not stem cells. This might suggest that bona fide stem cells will not exist outside their niche; that stem cells are defined by their place in the niche. This idea originated in tissues where downstream progenitors (immediate daughters of the ultimate stem cell) can occupy vacated niches and reacquire stem cell traits. For example, the melanocyte stem cell niche in mice is located in the base of the hair bulb in the transient portion of the hair follicle. Stem cells occupy the very bottom of the follicle and as they divide their progeny ascend and line the sides of the follicle, becoming increasingly differentiated with increasing distance from the niche. When the stem cell is selectively ablated experimentally, committed progenitors traversed the interstitial space, took up residence in the vacated niche, and began to function like stem cells *(77)*. Similarly, when endogenous skeletal muscle satellite cells were killed by irradiation, transplanted myoblasts derived from explanted, quiescent satellite cells could fuse with the existing muscle fiber and regenerate it after successive damage with snake venom *(78)*. This same mechanism was also suggested when glands resulting from transplantation of epithelial cell into cleared fat pads underwent multiple rounds of pregnancy (9).

The dominance of the niche over the stem cell's autonomous phenotype has also been demonstrated in several reports involving cells crossing lineage "boundaries" to regenerate "foreign" tissues. Mice that received bone marrow transplants from syngeneic donors, using transgenes as markers for self and nonself, revealed that bone marrow-derived cells could participate in repair of muscle damage (79–83). In three of the five studies, bone marrow-derived cells resided in the satellite cell position on muscle fibers after irradiation and were able to respond appropriately to damage cues brought on by the physiological response to exercise, but the conversion from bone marrow stem (progenitor) cell to muscle cell was not complete. Interestingly, myoblasts derived from satellite cells can easily and completely undergo myogenesis in culture after serum withdrawl but marrow-derived cells could only be pushed toward the myoblast fate by culturing them in myoblast-conditioned media or by coculturing them with a myoblast cell line (83). These experiments might suggest that the muscle microenvironment is important in maintaining the ability of nonmuscle-derived cells to exhibit myogenic characteristics. In addition, recent work from our lab has shown that the mammary microenvironment is dominant over testicular stem cells. Germinal stem cells from WapCreRosaLacZ mouse testis enriched for CD49f (α6-integrin) expression, when mixed with mammary epithelial cells, were able to self-renew and give rise to cells that expressed either myoepithelial or luminal cell markers and more importantly, showed evidence of milk production (84). Taken together, these experiments demonstrate that the lineage of adult tissue-specific stem cells can be redirected if given the right microenvironment. Therefore, consideration of the stem cell niche requires a reversal of the reductionist approach often adopted by molecular biologists. Indeed, it demands the reassembly and integration of the reductionist data at the level of the tissue or organ since at this level, structure is function.

4. CLOSING REMARKS

Stem cells are defined by how they act physiologically in the context of heterologous cells, i.e., the microenvironment or stem cell niche that balances protecting stem cells from exhaustion and protecting the host from unregulated stem cell growth. In addition to this complex model, it has been demonstrated recently that not only normal tissues, but also neoplastic lesions contain heterogeneous (hierarchical) types of stem cells (85). The discovery and genetic labeling of a parity-induced mammary epithelial cell population that is specific for parous females makes it possible to further examine the concept of stem cell hierarchy in the mammary gland and the homeostasis of mammary stem cells within the niche. In addition, our study of this progenitor population provides direct evidence for the proof of principle that a stem/progenitor cell may be the target of carcinogenic events and also that progression to frank malignancy is dependent upon the continued ability of the affected cell to expansively proliferate.

REFERENCES

1. Al-Hajj M, Wicha MS, Benito-Hernandez A, Morrison SJ, Clarke MF. Prospective identification of tumorigenic breast cancer cells. Proc Natl Acad Sci USA 2003;100:3983–8.
2. Callahan R, Smith GH. MMTV-induced mammary tumorigenesis: gene discovery, progression to malignancy and cellular pathways. Oncogene 2000;19:992–1001.
3. Smith GH. Stem cells and mammary cancer in mice. Stem Cell Rev 2005;1:215–23.

Chapter 2 / Mammary Glands, Stem Cells, and Breast Cancer

4. Singh SK, Clarke ID, Terasaki M, et al. Identification of a cancer stem cell in human brain tumors. Cancer Res 2003;63:5821–8.
5. Thordarson G, Slusher N, Leong H, et al. Insulin-like growth factor (IGF)-I obliterates the pregnancy-associated protection against mammary carcinogenesis in rats: evidence that IGF-I enhances cancer progression through estrogen receptor-alpha activation via the mitogen-activated protein kinase pathway. Breast Cancer Res 2004;6:R423–R436.
6. Sivaraman L, Medina D. Hormone-induced protection against breast cancer. J Mammary Gland Biol Neoplasia 2002;7:77–92.
7. D'Cruz CM, Moody SE, Master SR, et al. Persistent parity-induced changes in growth factors, TGF-beta3, and differentiation in the rodent mammary gland. Mol Endocrinol 2002;16:2034–51.
8. Ginger MR, Gonzalez-Rimbau MF, Gay JP, Rosen JM. Persistent changes in gene expression induced by estrogen and progesterone in the rat mammary gland. Mol Endocrinol 2001;15:1993–2009.
9. Boulanger CA, Wagner KU, Smith GH. Parity-induced mouse mammary epithelial cells are pluripotent, self-renewing and sensitive to TGF-beta1 expression. Oncogene 2005;24:552–60.
10. Ludwig T, Fisher P, Murty V, Efstratiadis A. Development of mammary adenocarcinomas by tissue-specific knockout of Brca2 in mice. Oncogene 2001;20:3937–48.
11. Smith GH. Experimental mammary epithelial morphogenesis in an in vivo model: evidence for distinct cellular progenitors of the ductal and lobular phenotype. Breast Cancer Res Treat 1996;39:21–31.
12. Kordon EC, Smith GH. An entire functional mammary gland may comprise the progeny from a single cell. Development 1998;125:1921–30.
13. Kamiya K, Gould MN, Clifton KH. Quantitative studies of ductal versus alveolar differentiation from rat mammary clonogens. Proc Soc Exp Biol Med 1998;219:217–25.
14. Boulanger CA, Smith GH. Reducing mammary cancer risk through premature stem cell senescence. Oncogene 2001;20:2264–72.
15. Henry MD, Triplett AA, Oh KB, Smith GH, Wagner KU. Parity-induced mammary epithelial cells facilitate tumorigenesis in MMTV-neu transgenic mice. Oncogene 2004;23:6980–5.
16. Krempler A, Henry MD, Triplett AA, Wagner KU. Targeted deletion of the Tsg101 gene results in cell cycle arrest at G1/S and p53-independent cell death. J Biol Chem 2002;277:43216–23.
17. Cairns J. Mutation selection and the natural history of cancer. Nature 1975;255:197–200.
18. Potten CS, Owen G, Booth D. Intestinal stem cells protect their genome by selective segregation of template DNA strands. J Cell Sci 2002;115:2381–8.
19. Smith GH. Label-retaining epithelial cells in mouse mammary gland divide asymmetrically and retain their template DNA strands. Development 2005;132:681–7.
20. DeOme KB, Faulkin LJ Jr, Bern HA, Blair PB. Development of mammary tumors from hyperplastic alveolar nodules transplanted into gland-free mammary fat pads of female C3H mice. Cancer Res 1959;19:515–20.
21. Daniel CW, Deome KB. Growth of mouse mammary glands in vivo after monolayer culture. Science 1965;149:634–6.
22. Daniel CW, Young LJ. Influence of cell division on an aging process. Life span of mouse mammary epithelium during serial propagation in vivo. Exp Cell Res 1971;65:27–32.
23. Proia DA, Kuperwasser C. Reconstruction of human mammary tissues in a mouse model. Nat Protoc 2006;1:206–14.
24. Smith GH, Boulanger CA. Mammary stem cell repertoire: new insights in aging epithelial populations. Mech Ageing Dev 2002;123:1505–19.
25. Stingl J, Caldas C. Molecular heterogeneity of breast carcinomas and the cancer stem cell hypothesis. Nat Rev Cancer 2007;7:791–9.
26. Dontu G, Jackson KW, McNicholas E, Kawamura MJ, Abdallah WM, Wicha MS. Role of Notch signaling in cell-fate determination of human mammary stem/progenitor cells. Breast Cancer Res 2004;6:R605–R615.
27. Booth BW, Boulanger CA, Smith GH. Alveolar progenitor cells develop in mouse mammary glands independent of pregnancy and lactation. J Cell Physiol 2007;212:729–36.
28. Liu S, Dontu G, Mantle ID, et al. Hedgehog signaling and Bmi-1 regulate self-renewal of normal and malignant human mammary stem cells. Cancer Res 2006;66:6063–71.

29. Molyneux G, Regan J, Smalley MJ. Mammary stem cells and breast cancer. Cell Mol Life Sci 2007;64:3248–3260.
30. Stingl J, Eirew P, Ricketson I, et al. Purification and unique properties of mammary epithelial stem cells. Nature 2006;439:993–7.
31. Shackleton M, Vaillant F, Simpson KJ, et al. Generation of a functional mammary gland from a single stem cell. Nature 2006;439:84–8.
32. Perou CM, Sorlie T, Eisen MB, et al. Molecular portraits of human breast tumours. Nature 2000;406:747–52.
33. Sorlie T, Perou CM, Tibshirani R, et al. Gene expression patterns of breast carcinomas distinguish tumor subclasses with clinical implications. Proc Natl Acad Sci USA 2001;98:10869–74.
34. Sorlie T, Tibshirani R, Parker J, et al. Repeated observation of breast tumor subtypes in independent gene expression data sets. Proc Natl Acad Sci USA 2003;100:8418–23.
35. Foulkes WD, Stefansson IM, Chappuis PO, et al. Germline BRCA1 mutations and a basal epithelial phenotype in breast cancer. J Natl Cancer Inst 2003;95:1482–5.
36. Fillmore C, Kuperwasser C. Human breast cancer stem cell markers CD44 and CD24: enriching for cells with functional properties in mice or in man? Breast Cancer Res 2007;9:303.
37. Mahendran R, McIlhinney R, O'Hare M, Monaghan P, Gusterson B. Expression of the common acute lymphoblastic leukaemia antigen (CALLA) in the human breast. Mol Cell Probes 1989;3:39–44.
38. Shipitsin M, Campbell LL, Argani P, et al. Molecular definition of breast tumor heterogeneity. Cancer Cell 2007;11:259–73.
39. Bao S, Wu Q, McLendon RE, et al. Glioma stem cells promote radioresistance by preferential activation of the DNA damage response. Nature 2006;444:756–60.
40. Piccirillo SG, Reynolds BA, Zanetti N, et al. Bone morphogenetic proteins inhibit the tumorigenic potential of human brain tumour-initiating cells. Nature 2006;444:761–5.
41. Medina D. Mammary developmental fate and breast cancer risk. Endocr Relat Cancer 2005;12:483–95.
42. Wagner KU, Boulanger CA, Henry MD, Sgagias M, Hennighausen L, Smith GH. An adjunct mammary epithelial cell population in parous females: its role in functional adaptation and tissue renewal. Development 2002;129:1377–86.
43. Matulka LA, Triplett AA, Wagner KU. Parity-induced mammary epithelial cells are multipotent and express cell surface markers associated with stem cells. Dev Biol 2007;303:29–44.
44. Pal S, Pegram M. HER2 targeted therapy in breast cancer…beyond Herceptin. Rev Endocr Metab Disord 2007;8:269–77.
45. Dhesy-Thind B, Pritchard K, Messersmith H, O'Malley F, Elavathil L, Trudeau M. HER2/neu in systemic therapy for women with breast cancer: a systematic review. Breast Cancer Res Treat 2007;109:209–29.
46. Lin H. The stem-cell niche theory: lessons from flies. Nat Rev Genet 2002;3:931–40.
47. Rizvi AZ, Wong MH. Epithelial stem cells and their niche: there's no place like home. Stem Cells 2005;23:150–65.
48. Wilson A, Trumpp A. Bone-marrow haematopoietic-stem-cell niches. Nat Rev Immunol 2006;6:93–106.
49. Chepko G, Dickson RB. Ultrastructure of the putative stem cell niche in rat mammary epithelium. Tissue Cell 2003;35:83–93.
50. Chepko G, Slack R, Carbott D, Khan S, Steadman L, Dickson RB. Differential alteration of stem and other cell populations in ducts and lobules of TGFalpha and c-Myc transgenic mouse mammary epithelium. Tissue Cell 2005;37:393–412.
51. Schofield R. The relationship between the spleen colony-forming cell and the haemopoietic stem cell. Blood Cells 1978;4:7–25.
52. Xie T, Spradling AC. A niche maintaining germ line stem cells in the Drosophila ovary. Science 2000;290:328–30.
53. Kiger AA, White-Cooper H, Fuller MT. Somatic support cells restrict germline stem cell self-renewal and promote differentiation. Nature 2000;407:750–4.

Chapter 2 / Mammary Glands, Stem Cells, and Breast Cancer

54. Crittenden SL, Bernstein DS, Bachorik JL, et al. A conserved RNA-binding protein controls germline stem cells in Caenorhabditis elegans. Nature 2002;417:660–3.
55. Ohlstein B, Spradling A. The adult Drosophila posterior midgut is maintained by pluripotent stem cells. Nature 2006;439:470–4.
56. Micchelli CA, Perrimon N. Evidence that stem cells reside in the adult Drosophila midgut epithelium. Nature 2006;439:475–9.
57. Stumpf WE, Narbaitz R, Sar M. Estrogen receptors in the fetal mouse. J Steroid Biochem 1980;12:55–64.
58. Brisken C, Heineman A, Chavarria T, et al. Essential function of Wnt-4 in mammary gland development downstream of progesterone signaling. Genes Dev 2000;14:650–4.
59. Asselin-Labat ML, Shackleton M, Stingl J, et al. Steroid hormone receptor status of mouse mammary stem cells. J Natl Cancer Inst 2006;98:1011–14.
60. Brisken C, Duss S. Stem cells and the stem cell niche in the breast: an integrated hormonal and developmental perspective. Stem Cell Rev 2007;3:147–56.
61. Wiesen JF, Young P, Werb Z, Cunha GR. Signaling through the stromal epidermal growth factor receptor is necessary for mammary ductal development. Development 1999;126:335–44.
62. Ciarloni L, Mallepell S, Brisken C. Amphiregulin is an essential mediator of estrogen receptor alpha function in mammary gland development. Proc Natl Acad Sci USA 2007;104:5455–60.
63. Brisken C, Park S, Vass T, Lydon JP, O'Malley BW, Weinberg RA. A paracrine role for the epithelial progesterone receptor in mammary gland development. Proc Natl Acad Sci USA 1998;95:5076–81.
64. Mulac-Jericevic B, Lydon JP, DeMayo FJ, Conneely OM. Defective mammary gland morphogenesis in mice lacking the progesterone receptor B isoform. Proc Natl Acad Sci USA 2003;100:9744–9.
65. Brisken C, Ayyannan A, Nguyen C, et al. IGF-2 is a mediator of prolactin-induced morphogenesis in the breast. Dev Cell 2002;3:877–87.
66. Sonnenberg A, Daams H, Van der Valk MA, Hilkens J, Hilgers J. Development of mouse mammary gland: identification of stages in differentiation of luminal and myoepithelial cells using monoclonal antibodies and polyvalent antiserum against keratin. J Histochem Cytochem 1986;34:1037–46.
67. Welm BE, Tepera SB, Venezia T, Graubert TA, Rosen JM, Goodell MA. Sca-1(pos) cells in the mouse mammary gland represent an enriched progenitor cell population. Dev Biol 2002;245:42–56.
68. Tsai YC, Lu Y, Nichols PW, Zlotnikov G, Jones PA, Smith HS. Contiguous patches of normal human mammary epithelium derived from a single stem cell: implications for breast carcinogenesis. Cancer Res 1996;56:402–4.
69. Villadsen R, Fridriksdottir AJ, Ronnov-Jessen L, et al. Evidence for a stem cell hierarchy in the adult human breast. J Cell Biol 2007;177:87–101.
70. Stasiak PC, Purkis PE, Leigh IM, Lane EB. Keratin 19: predicted amino acid sequence and broad tissue distribution suggest it evolved from keratinocyte keratins. J Invest Dermatol 1989;92:707–16.
71. Dravida S, Pal R, Khanna A, Tipnis SP, Ravindran G, Khan F. The transdifferentiation potential of limbal fibroblast-like cells. Brain Res Dev Brain Res 2005;160:239–51.
72. Ohyama M, Terunuma A, Tock CL, et al. Characterization and isolation of stem cell-enriched human hair follicle bulge cells. J Clin Invest 2006;116:249–60.
73. Schmelz M, Moll R, Hesse U, et al. Identification of a stem cell candidate in the normal human prostate gland. Eur J Cell Biol 2005;84:341–54.
74. Hudson DL, Guy AT, Fry P, O'Hare MJ, Watt FM, Masters JR. Epithelial cell differentiation pathways in the human prostate: identification of intermediate phenotypes by keratin expression. J Histochem Cytochem 2001;49:271–8.
75. Fuchs E, Tumbar T, Guasch G. Socializing with the neighbors: stem cells and their niche. Cell 2004;116:769–78.
76. Moraes RC, Zhang X, Harrington N, et al. Constitutive activation of smoothened (SMO) in mammary glands of transgenic mice leads to increased proliferation, altered differentiation and ductal dysplasia. Development 2007;134:1231–42.
77. Nishimura EK, Jordan SA, Oshima H, et al. Dominant role of the niche in melanocyte stem-cell fate determination. Nature 2002;416:854–60.

78. Collins CA, Olsen I, Zammit PS, et al. Stem cell function, self-renewal, and behavioral heterogeneity of cells from the adult muscle satellite cell niche. Cell 2005;122:289–301.
79. Dreyfus PA, Chretien F, Chazaud B, et al. Adult bone marrow-derived stem cells in muscle connective tissue and satellite cell niches. Am J Pathol 2004;164:773–9.
80. Ferrari G, Cusella-De Angelis G, Coletta M, et al. Muscle regeneration by bone marrow-derived myogenic progenitors. Science 1998;279:1528–30.
81. Fukada S, Miyagoe-Suzuki Y, Tsukihara H, et al. Muscle regeneration by reconstitution with bone marrow or fetal liver cells from green fluorescent protein-gene transgenic mice. J Cell Sci 2002;115:1285–93.
82. LaBarge MA, Blau HM. Biological progression from adult bone marrow to mononucleate muscle stem cell to multinucleate muscle fiber in response to injury. Cell 2002;111:589–601.
83. Sherwood RI, Christensen JL, Conboy IM, et al. Isolation of adult mouse myogenic progenitors: functional heterogeneity of cells within and engrafting skeletal muscle. Cell 2004;119:543–54.
84. Boulanger CA, Mack DL, Booth BW, Smith GH. Interaction with the mammary microenvironment redirects spermatogenic cell fate in vivo. Proc Natl Acad Sci USA 2007;104:3871–6.
85. Hope KJ, Jin L, Dick JE. Acute myeloid leukemia originates from a hierarchy of leukemic stem cell classes that differ in self-renewal capacity. Nat Immunol 2004;5:738–43.

3

The Genetics of Breast Cancer: Application in Clinical Practice

*Antonio Russo, Valentina Agnese,
Sergio Rizzo, Laura La Paglia,
and Viviana Bazan*

SUMMARY

Breast cancer (BC) is a complex and heterogeneous disease caused by interaction of both genetic and nongenetic risk factors. The biological diversity of sporadic BCs consists in the development of several BC subtypes, which are systematically different from one another and which present specific genetic and phenotypic features. Recently, with the advent of cDNA microarrays it has been possible to associate a distinctive "molecular portrait" to a single BC subtype and, consequently, improve BC taxonomy. From a clinical point of view, the gene expression profiles could supply the classic pathological experiment with the aim to select patients with a better prognosis and that could have a benefit from a specific chemotherapy treatment. Recently a new role in BC progression has been identified in a group of small, noncoding RNAs, the MicroRNA (miRNA), which regulate gene expression. Of particular interest is the identification of different miRNA expression levels according to the five molecular BC subtypes identified by experiments on microarray gene expression. About 3–8% of all breast cancers are hereditary, and it is estimated that the main contributors to this type of cancer are mutations in autosomal dominant genes segregating with the disease. Nowadays, *BRCA1* and *BRCA2* are considered as the two main BC susceptibility genes, although the involvement of additional low penetrance genes implicated in particular syndromes should not be overlooked. Epidemiologic studies reported that women who are *BRCA1* mutation carriers have a 45–60% cumulative risk to develop BC before age 35–40, and the average cumulative risk in *BRCA1*-mutation carriers by age 70 years is 65% whereas the corresponding risk to develop this neoplasm for *BRCA2* mutation carriers is estimated to be 25–40% and 45%, respectively. Oncogenetic counseling requires a "multidisciplinary approach," involving geneticists, oncologists, and psychologists and is offered by many diagnostic clinical

From: *Current Clinical Oncology: Breast Cancer in the Post-Genomic Era,*
Edited by: A. Giordano and N. Normanno, DOI: 10.1007/978-1-60327-945-1_3,
© Humana Press, a part of Springer Science + Business Media, LLC 2009

genetic services. Nowadays, risk evaluation regarding BC patients is performed with the use of specific mathematical models, such as BRCAPro, the Couch and the Myriad models.

Key Words: Sporadic and hereditary breast cancer; Molecular profile; MicroRNA; Founder mutation; Oncogenetic counseling

1. INTRODUCTION

Breast cancer (BC) is the most frequently diagnosed malignancy and one of the leading causes of death in Western women. It is a complex and heterogeneous disease caused by interaction of both genetic and nongenetic risk factors. Whereas the vast majority of BC cases are sporadic and not attributable to inherited traits, family history suggesting an inherited component in the development of some BC is one of the best known risk factors. Sporadic BCs result from a serial stepwise accumulation of acquired and uncorrected mutations in somatic genes, without any germline mutation playing a role. Recent studies have identified particular expression patterns that can classify tumors into new groups and aid in the prediction of the natural history of the disease and the therapeutic response. This wealth of information may also form the basis for the development of new therapeutic strategies.

2. SPORADIC BREAST CANCER

2.1. The Advent of Breast Cancer Molecular Portrait

The biological diversity of sporadic BCs consists in the development of several BC subtypes, which are systematically different from one another and which present specific genetic and phenotypic features. For this reason the clinical prognosis and outcome of BC patients is often incompletely explained by known pathological factors such as histological grade, ER/PgR status, and *HER2/neu* expression (*HER2*). In actual clinical practice, this leads to doubts regarding the treatment of lymph-node negative BC patients by surgery and radiotherapy alone or by toxic and expensive chemotherapy.

Recently, with the advent of cDNA microarrays it has been possible to associate a distinctive "molecular portrait" to a single BC subtype and, consequently, improve BC taxonomy (*1–3*). In 2000, Perou and collaborators were the first authors to identify four principal BC subtypes by means of the comparison between the different gene expression patterns of 65 BCs, 1 fibroadenoma, and 3 normal BC samples (*1*). In particular, the study focused on the analysis of 496 genes termed the "intrinsic" gene set because they showed the greatest variation between tumors from different patients compared with samples from the same patient; it identified the basal-like subtype characterized by the overexpression of keratin 5/6 and 17, the Erb-B2 subtype with the *ErbB2* gene overexpression, the normal breast-like subtypes with overexpression of basal epithelial and adipose cell genes and the underexpression of luminal epithelial cell genes, and the luminal subtype characterized by the overexpression of ER and luminal epithelial cell markers. In a following study Sorlie et al., analyzing the gene expression pattern of 456 intrinsic genes in a larger group of 85 patients, reclassified the luminal subtype in luminal A, B, and C subtypes, which showed an overexpression of the ER gene, an underexpression of luminal specific genes, and an overexpression of an unknown novel set of genes shared with the basal and ERBB2 subtypes (*2*), respectively. Finally, in 2003, the same authors analyzed the gene expression patterns of 534 intrinsic genes in 115 BC samples and 7 nonmalignant breast tissues and identified 2 major luminal epithelial/ER+ subtypes: the ER+ luminal A subtype and the luminal B subtype, which overexpress not only ER, but also the HER2 gene *(3)*. These latest results have been confirmed by other experiments involving gene expression and immunohistochemistry *(4–6)*, confirming the classification of BC into five principal subtypes with specific immunophenotypic markers and therapeutic features (Table 1). These consist in the basal-like subtype, which is positive for the keratin of basal cells (keratins 5/6 and 17) and responsive to chemotherapy; the HER2+/ER− subtype, which has no expression of *ER* and *PgR* but which overexpresses the *erbB2* gene and is responsive to chemotherapy and target therapy with the anti-HER2 antibody, the anti-EGFR antibody and EGFR inhibitors; the so-far insufficiently studied normal breast-like subtype, which is apparently brought about by tissue contamination; the luminal B subtype, which shows overexpression of ER, PgR, and sometimes of HER2 and which is responsive to endocrine therapy and to target therapy against HER2; and, finally, the luminal A subtype, which is ER+ and PgR+ and responsive to endocrine therapy only. These five molecular subtypes have also been identified among different ethnic groups of patients *(7)*, in inflammatory BC *(8)* and in metastatic lesions *(9)*.

Although at present there is considerable interest in this BC classification, up till now, no acceptable international definition of such neoplasias exists. This is mainly due to the fact that the identification of the different BC sub-types is based on microarray gene expression and the resulting gene signature is hard to reproduce. Furthermore, it is improbable that diagnostic practice might be disposed to consider experiments involving the extraction of RNA from formalin-fixed tissues. Therefore, several attempts to define an immunohistochemical surrogate for basal-like cancers have been described. For example, Nielsen and coworkers

Table 1

Schematic representation of the characteristic genes, IHC markers, and therapeutic features of each BC subtype

BC subtypes	*Characteristic genes*	*IHC markers*	*Therapeutic features*
Basal like	*CK 5/6/17; BRCA1mut* (80–90%)	ER−; PgR−; HER2−; CK5/6+; often EGFR+; ↑Ki-67	Responsive to chemotherapy
HER2+/ER−	*HER2/c-erb B2*	ER−; PgR−; HER2+; ↑Ki-67	Responsive to chemoterapy, anti-HER2 antibody, anti-EGFR antibody, EGFR inhibitors
Normal breast-like	Adipose tissue enriched pattern potentially due to normal tissue contamination		
Luminal A	*ER*	ER+ and/or PgR+; HER2−; ↓Ki-67	Responsive to endocrine therapy
Luminal B	*ER cluster*	ER+ and/or PgR+; sometimes HER2+; ↓Ki-67	Variable response to chemotherapy. Responsive to endocrine therapy

BC breast cancer, *IHC* immunohistochemestry, *CK* cytokeratin, *ER* estrogen receptor, *PgR* progesterone receptor, *EGFR* epidermal growth factor receptor have proposed an immunohistochemical panel of BC subtypes where the basal-like phenotype is defined as the one lacking both ER and HER2 expression and expressing CK 5/6 and EGFR *(6)*. Unfortunately not all immunohistochemical experiments offer the same quality in terms of specificity and sensibility and thus they are not suitable for use in diagnostic practice.

2.2. Triple-Negative and Basal-Like Tumors: Clinical Implications

Many risk factors have been identified as contributing to the development of the different BC subtypes. In particular, the basal-like type has a higher frequency in *BRCA1* genetic mutation carriers *(10)* and in premenopausal Afro-American women *(11,12)*. Furthermore, from the histopathological point of view, basal-like tumors have different characteristics, such as a high histological grade, a high mitotic index, the presence of central necrotic areas, pushing borders and conspicuous lymphocytic infiltrate *(13–17)*. Moreover, more than 90% of metaplastic breast carcinomas and the majority of medullary carcinomas show a basal-like phenotype *(18–20)*. From the clinical point of view, BC cells with a basal-like phenotype appear to have a predilection for hematogenous dissemination, for brain and lung metastases *(16,21)* and present *TP53* mutations *(2)*. This is according to the evidence that BCs with basal-like phenotypes are more aggressive than other types and seem to be associated with a poorer outcome and prognosis *(2,6,22,23)*.

With regard to the molecular markers of each subtype, it seems that the basal-like phenotype overlaps the class of BC triple negative. In actual fact, about 56–84% of triple negative BCs are not basal-like and, more specifically, do not overexpress CKs and EGFR, and about 15–54% of basal-like BCs are not triple negative; in fact, they overexpress at least one of ER, PR or HER2. The evidence that triple negative BCs expressing a basal phenotype present a shorter disease-free survival period than those without the expression of basal markers *(24,25)* suggests that triple negative cancer should not be considered as a synonym for basal-like cancer. Apart from this, there is a link between the BRCA1 pathway and triple-negative and basal-like BCs *(26,27)*. In fact, most BCs with sporadic mutations in *BRCA1*, and especially those diagnosed under the age of 50, present immunohistochemical and gene expression features, which are typical of triple-negative phenotypes *(14,28)* and basal-like *(3)*. Furthermore, it has been demonstrated that tumors with basal-like phenotypes present an alteration of the BRCA1 pathway, which is not limited to the single mutation only *(27,29,30)*. In fact, in these tumors the levels of the BRCA1 protein are significantly lower in those of high histological grade, lacking ER and PR; this downregulation might be due both to epigenetic phenomena such as promoter methylation *(31,32)* and to transcriptional silencing phenomena brought about by the expression of BRCA1 negative regulators, for example, the ID4 factor *(30)*.

From a clinical point of view, the selection of patients with basal-like BCs based on the BRCA1 status could suggest the use of cross-linking agents or targeted therapy to the polyADP-ribose polymerase enzyme (PARP) instead of taxanes *(27,29,33–36)*. In fact, trials of both approaches are currently underway in women with BC. The Triple Negative Trial (TNT) compares carbiplatin with docetaxel in women with advanced sporadic triple-negative BCs, while the BRCA trial tests the same hypothesis in a more genetically defined advanced BC population with germline *BRCA1* or *BRCA2* mutations. Finally, since PARP inhibitor clinical trials have shown encouraging results, phase II clinical trials in *BRCA1/BRCA2*-associated BCs have recently been started.

Chapter 3 / The Genetics of Breast Cancer: Application in Clinical Practice

In summary of what has been said so far, the gene expression profiles could supply the classic pathological experiment with the aim to select patients with a better prognosis and that could have a benefit from a specific chemotherapy treatment. Different gene expression markers have been identified to predict the likelihood to chemotherapy response *(37)* and the studies on different BC molecular subtypes have shown that basal-like and HER2 subtypes are more sensitive to paclitaxel and doxorubicin-containing neoadjuvant chemotherapy compared with luminal and normal-like tumors *(38)*. Finally, a recent study used the microarray experiment to identify the cell signaling pathways rather than discrete genes with the aim to characterize the biological behavior of the tumor and to choose the most effective combination of therapies *(39)*.

2.3. Genomic Profiling in Clinical Practice

Several attempts to define a panel of gene expression with a prognostic role and an immunohistochemical surrogate for basal-like cancers have been described. For example, van't Veer and coworkers, analyzing the different expression level of 25,000 genes in 98 lymphnode negative BC, identified a panel of 70 genes with an expression pattern that allowed highly accurate classification of patients with a poor prognosis form those with a good one *(40)*. The custom-made microarray assay that arose from the 70-genes panel has been approved by the Food and Drug Administration (FDA) on February 2007 and it is called Mammaprint *(41)*. With this assay it is possible to establish, by the use of a score, whether a patient has a "low risk" or a "high risk" of BC recurrence. The Mammaprint assay is currently being validated in the MINDACT Trial (Microarray in Node negative Disease may Avoid ChemoTherapy). In addition, Genomic Health Incorporated and investigators of the NSABP (National Surgical Adjuvant Breast and Bowel Project) have developed a 21-gene expression-based recurrence score assay for ER-positive, lymph-node negative tamoxifen treated BC, known as Oncotype DxTM *(42)*. This assay is currently incorporated in the TAILORx [Trial Assigning IndividuaLized Options for Treatment (Rx)] trial by which patients with ER-positive or ER-negative, HER2 negative and lymph-node negative BC are randomized to hormone therapy and/or chemotherapy according to the recurrence score. The TAILORx and MINDACT trials, two prospective multicenter phase III trials evaluating tumor profile in BC are currently accruing patients (Table 2). Besides, Gianni and coworkers showed that the Oncotype DXTM assay is strongly correlated with pathologic complete response in patients treated with neoadjuvant paclitaxel and doxorubicin *(37)*.

Table 2
Schematic representation of the two multicenter phase III
trials evaluating the principal custom-made assays

	MINDACT	*TAILORx*
Cohort	600	11.000
Treatment arms	Low-risk: E; high-risk: CT/E; discordant clinical and genomic risk: randomized to CT	Low-risk: E; high-risk: CT/E; indeterminate risk: randomized to CT/E or E
Assay	Mammaprint	Oncotype DXTM
Specimen	Paraffin-embedded tumor samples	Frozen or fresh tumor samples

CT chemotherapy, *E* endocrine

2.4. MicroRNA Expression Identifies BC Molecular Subtypes

Recently a new role in BC progression has been identified in a group of small, noncoding RNAs, the MicroRNA (miRNA), which regulate gene expression *(43)*. miRNAs are transcribed as long RNA precursors (pre-miRNAs) by the RNase III enzyme complex Drosha-Pasha/DGCR8 *(44–50)*. Pre-miRNAs are exported from the nucleus by exportin-5 *(51)*, processed by the RNase III enzyme Dicer, and incorporated into an Argonaut containing the RNA-induced silencing complex (RISC) *(52)*. Within this silencing complex, miRNA pair to the mRNA through an imperfect match at the 3′-untranslated region (3′UTR) causing mRNA destabilization and translational repression *(53,54)*. Two different studies have shown a correlation between BC and the deregulation of several miRNA *(55,56)* while, for the first time, another study has found that the different miRNA expression in BC is correlated with HER2 and estrogen receptor (ER) status *(57)*. Of particular interest is the identification of different miRNA expression levels according to the five molecular BC subtypes identified by experiments on microarray gene expression *(58)*. This most recent study thus represents the first integrated analysis of miRNA expression and of mRNA expression and genomic changes and may serve as a basis for functional studies of the role of miRNAs in the etiology of BCs and for future clinical applications. In addition, the study of miRNA expression signature in BC may have a major advantage with respect to the study of gene expression profiling. In fact, one of the difficulties of the latter tecnique is that the number of genes that can be analysed can be challenging. In contrast, the number of miRNAs is relatively limited compared with mRNAs, and thus miRNA profiles present opportunities for a more simple tumor "bar-coding" approach. In miRNA profiling studies the association of certain miRNAs with traditional molecular markers, such as ER and HER2, and their role in BC proliferation, invasion and metastasis have been observed. These observations suggest that miRNAs may have the potential to provide novel therapeutic strategies for BC treatment. It is yet to be seen how emerging miRNA data will translate into a clinical setting for the BC diagnosis and treatment. However, a better understanding of their pathways will help to a better BC classification, prognostication and direct treatments and also help identify targets for developing further treatment.

3. HEREDITARY BREAST CANCER

3.1. The Genetics of Susceptibility to Breast Cancer

About 3–8% of all breast cancers are hereditary breast cancers (HBCs), and it is estimated that the main contributors to this type of cancer are mutations in autosomal dominant genes segregating with the disease *(59)*. Nowadays *BRCA1* and *BRCA2* are considered as the two main BC susceptibility genes, although the involvement of additional low penetrance genes implicated in particular syndromes should not be overlooked *(60)*. Breast cancer due to inherited susceptibility shows several clinical and pathological features and differs significantly from sporadic cases. These characteristics might help the oncologist to choose a more suitable therapeutic management of the patient and could be useful in identifying individuals more likely to carry germline mutations.

3.2. HBC Susceptibility Genes

The first BC gene to be discovered was *BRCA1*. It was first detected in 1990 and completely sequenced in 1994 *(61,62)*. *BRCA1* maps on chromosome 17q21; it is a large gene of 24 exons, of which 22 are coding, and encodes a 220-kDa tumor suppressor protein *(63)*.

Chapter 3 / The Genetics of Breast Cancer: Application in Clinical Practice   45

Because of its interactions with other proteins, BRCA1 has been involved in several cellular functions, such as DNA repair, cell cycle control, transcription regulation, tumor suppressor activity, and also centrosome dynamics, stress response, apoptosis, and ubiquitination *(64,65)*.

BRCA1 has a role in double-strand breaks (DSB) repair, indirectly, through the interaction with RAD51, the human ortholog of the bacterial RecA, and BRCA2 *(66,67)*. Additional repair proteins interact with BRCA1 and colocalize within the same foci as the MRN (Mre11/Rad51/NBS1) complex in the mechanism of homologous recombination (HR) *(68)*. Recent data indicate that BRCA1 contributes to DNA damage repair through its interaction with certain enzymes, which alter the chromatin structure, such as the SWI/SNF proteins *(69)*. Different phosphorylation sites have been discovered, each of which permits the protein to participate and to regulate different steps of cell cycle control *(70)*. Several reports suggest the involvement of the protein in transcription regulation, since it is associated with p53 and CtIP *(71,72)*.

If all this consistent pattern of interactions is taken into consideration, it would appear that loss-of-function mutations of *BRCA1* give rise to pleiotropic phenotypes, including problems regarding correct cellular growth, increased apoptosis, alterating and defecting response to damage to DNA structure, abnormal centrosome duplication, and defective cell cycle checkpoints *(73,74)*. Since the tumor suppressor function of BRCA1 alone is not sufficient to justify all these phenotypes, it might therefore be hypothesized that such mutations in *BRCA1* are associated with the formation of genomic instability, subjecting cells to a high risk of tumor transformation.

The *BRCA2* locus is on chromosome 13q12-q13 and was cloned in 1995 *(75)*. Human BRCA2 is a large protein of 3,418 amino acids (aa). It is an ubiquitous cell cycle-regulated protein localizing to the nucleus in normal cells *(76)*. It has 27 exons, of which 26 are coding. Like *BRCA1*, exon 11 takes more than 50% of the coding region. The protein product is characterized by the presence of several distinct functional regions, such as the NLS domains and the BRC repeats. This latter region is the major site for the direct interaction of the protein with the RAD51 recombination and DNA repair protein. This interaction is direct, as in vitro demonstrated with recombinant protein fragments. Moreover, one of the other targets of the protein is BRCA1: BRCA1 and BRCA2 colocalize in another distinct region from the one reported to bind RAD51, in mitotic and meiotic cells *(77)*. The discovery of the interaction and colocalization between BRCA2, BRCA1, and RAD51 leads to the clear deduction of a synergic aspect of their collaboration in the DNA repairing process.

BRCA2 has also been implicated in transcription regulation *(78)*. In a study regarding a yeast two-hybrid system, Futamura et al. reported that the BRCA2 protein is involved in a mitotic checkpoint in vivo after it has been phosphorylated by hBUBR1 *(79)*.

In the last 10 years, several studies have focused attention on other possible low penetrance BC susceptibility genes, which might predispose to BC in women with a family history *(80,81)*.

3.3. Lifetime Risk for HBC

Epidemiologic studies reported that women who are *BRCA1* mutation carriers have a 45–60% cumulative risk to develop BC before age 35–40, and the average cumulative risk in *BRCA1*-mutation carriers by age 70 years is 65% (95% confidence interval 44–78%) whereas the corresponding risk to develop this neoplasm for *BRCA2* mutation carriers is estimated to be 25–40% and 45% (31–56%), respectively *(82,83)*. Moreover, the risk of developing a second contralateral BC is similar to that previously reported for *BRCA1/2* mutation carriers *(84,85)*.

3.4. BRCA Founder Mutations

High-risk BC families usually present a large spectrum of different types of mutations, whereas some ethnic groups are characterized by the presence of a "founder mutation." The comparison of haplotypes among families with the same mutation can establish whether alleles derive from an older or more recent single mutational event or they have arisen independently *(86)*.

Among Ashkenazy Jewish population, three founder mutations have been found: these are *BRCA1-185delAG*, with a frequency of 1%, the *5382insC BRCA1* mutation, with a frequency of 0.13%, and *6174delT* in the *BRCA2* gene, with a frequency of 1.52% *(87,88)*. The overall rate of these three founder mutations is 2.6% (1/40) compared with the rate of 0.2% (1/500) of *BRCA1/2* mutation carriers in the general population *(87,89)*.

Founder mutations have also been found in several European countries, the majority of which are high penetrance. Eleven recurrent mutations with a founder effect have been reported in the Finnish population, and represent 84% of all the mutations found in the *BRCA1/2* genes *(90)*. Two other founder mutations were reported in Iceland: *BRCA1 G5193A*, and *BRCA2 999del5*; the latter is the most common mutation with a founder effect in this population *(91,92)*. In a French study conducted in 2004, two founder mutations were identified in high-risk families: *3600del11* and *G1710X*, in the *BRCA1* gene, representing 37% and 15%, respectively, of all identified mutations *(93)*.

The first mutation with a founder effect in the Italian population was identified by Baudi et al. in 2001 *(94)*. Four of 24 analyzed patients had the *5083del19* mutation.

Many other recurrent mutations have been identified in other countries such as the USA, Japan, the Philippines, and Pakistan *(95–98)*.

3.5. Oncogenetic Counseling

Oncogenetic counseling requires a "multidisciplinary approach," involving geneticists, oncologists, and psychologists and is offered by many diagnostic clinical genetic services. This is a multistep process that involves genetic counseling, automated DNA analysis techniques, and different statistical and software models, aimed at evaluating the BC risk and the likelihood of *BRCA* mutations (Fig. 1). Nowadays, risk evaluation regarding BC patients is performed with the use of specific mathematical models, such as *BRCAPro*, the *Couch* and the *Myriad* models *(99–102)*. All these models require the reconstruction of the familial pedigree going back for at least three generations from the "proband." Furthermore, both paternal and maternal family history should be included, since most of the genes involved in the risk of developing BC could derive equally from the mother and the father. This "risk assessment" step is followed by a genetic test, when required.

The American Society of Clinical Oncology (ASCO) has proposed several features indicating HBC: these include the pathologic history of the individual, early onset age, presence of bilateral breast cancer, personal or family history of male breast cancer, multiple cases of early-onset BC, individuals belonging to the Ashkenazy Jewish population, or other information regarding the ethnic family background; nevertheless, the autosomal pattern of inheritance and the presence of other malignancies associated with *BRCA* mutations (ASCO 2003) should be considered.

The genetic test is definitely recommended when there is a family history supporting the pathological condition of the index case, and moreover when the result might be of help in the diagnosis or the medical or surgical management of the patient or of the family members at increased risk of BC *(103, 104)*.

Chapter 3 / The Genetics of Breast Cancer: Application in Clinical Practice

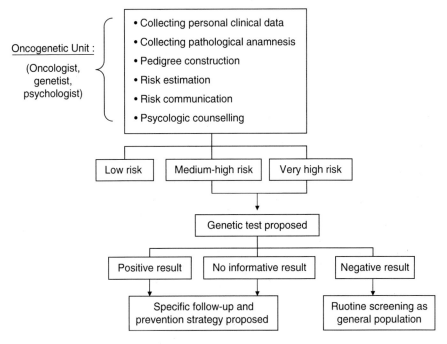

Fig. 1. Scheme of the genetic counseling and clinical management proposed to affected or healthy individuals with a BC family history.

The genetic testing for *BRCA1/2* genes provides automatic sequencing of all codifying exons and of the exon-intron boundaries. There are no hot spots, so that the mutations are distributed throughout the whole gene.

The result of the genetic testing for the identification of germinal mutations is only able to indicate the probability, but not the certainty, that a cancer will develop; not in all individuals with a positive test for *BRCA1/2* gene mutations, malignancies will occur.

It is possible to classify a sequence variant based on its relationship with the disease as following:

- Deleterious mutations, characterized by high-penetrance *(105)* (usually point mutations). These are clearly associated with the disease. Generally they bring about the formation of a truncated protein *(106,107)*, although several missense mutations and "splicing variants," which have already been reported as having a clear correlation with the disease, should be added to these.
- Missense mutations, defined as *splicing variants*, found in the flanking region of the exon, that cause the formation of alternative splice sites. These are considered as "suspected deleterious," because of their unknown but potentially pathologic biological significance.
- Unknown Variants (UV), point mutations in which no pathological association has been reported. In this case the result of the genetic test is uninformative and more investigative analyses are required in order to clarify the roles played in the risk of developing BC.
- Polymorphisms, point mutations presenting a frequency more of 1%, with no clinico-pathological significance.

Recent techniques such as Multiple Ligation-dependent Probe Amplification techniques (MLPA) allow to detect also wide insertions and deletions involving one or more whole exons.

3.6. HBC: Clinical and Histopathological Features

With regard to the morphology of BC, it has been shown that the ductal invasive histotype is the most common of all hereditary BC forms, both in *BRCA* mutation carriers and noncarriers. A study conducted by Armes et al., comparing two early onset tumor populations (before the age of 40), respectively, with and without *BRCA1* or *BRCA2* mutations, confirmed the histological differences occurring between them. The histology of phenotypes in *BRCA1* carriers is characterized by high grade, high mitotic counts, syncytial growth pattern, and confluent necrosis.

Other studies report that atypical medullary carcinoma is overrepresented in *BRCA1* mutation carriers, and pleomorphic lobular carcinomas and extensive intraduct carcinomas are more common in *BRCA2* mutation carriers *(108)*. Besides the higher proportion of medullary histology, a higher frequency of ductal carcinoma has also been reported *(109–111)*. A slightly increased incidence of lobular or tubulolobular carcinomas has been shown among *BRCA2*-associated tumors *(108,112)*. Nevertheless, the data are still inconsistent, and in most cases the differences between *BRCA2*-associated tumors and sporadic cancers are not particularly significant *(113,114)*.

Breast cancers in patients with *BRCA1* germline mutations are more often negative for estrogen receptor, progesterone receptor, and HER-2, and are more likely to be positive for p53 protein compared with controls. In contrast, *BRCA2* tumors do not show a significant difference in the expression of any of these proteins compared with controls *(115)*.

To date, different studies have reported HER2/neu status in *BRCA1*-associated tumors, the majority of which report that they are generally HER-2/neu expression-negatives *(111)*. Moreover, tumors with low levels of amplification displayed a reduction of chromosome 17 to one copy *(116)*. Different theories have been proposed to explain the low amplification rate, such as simple physical codeletion of one allele of *HER-2/neu* and nearby sequences during loss of heterozygosity (LOH) at the *BRCA1* locus *(66,117)*. Low amplification rates were also reported for *BRCA-2* associated tumors.

Characteristic patterns of gene expression measured by DNA microarrays have been used to classify tumors into clinically relevant subgroups. Recently, Sorlie et al. evidenced a basal differentiation of the epithelium for *BRCA1* tumors defined as "basal-like" types *(3)*. This type of tumor is notably characterized by the expression of different markers of mioepithelial and basal cells, such as basal keratins and P-cadherin, by the overexpression of other markers such as the Epidermal Growth Factor Receptor (EGFR), in addition to the specific morphological, proliferative, and prognostic features that characterize it. Other studies support this relation between the expression of a basal subgroup of BC tumors and mutations in *BRCA1* gene *(40)*.

3.7. Practice Points (Adapted from NCCN Guidelines for HBC Clinical Management)

Women
- Monthly breast self exam >18 years
- Clinical breast exam >25 yearrs every 6 months
- Annual mammogram and breast MRI >25 years or individualized if early age of onset
- Optional reducing mastectomy depending on case and counseling

Chapter 3 / The Genetics of Breast Cancer: Application in Clinical Practice 49

- Optional risk reducing salpingo oophorectomy 35–40 years based on reproductive desire or after completing child bearing
- TransVaginal UltraSound + CA-125 every 6 months, >35 years or earlier for OC early age of onset
- Consider chemoprevention options
- Consider Imaging and screening studies
- Advise about risk relatives, and consider about counseling option

Men
- Monthly breast self-exam
- Clinical breast exam every 6 months
- Consider baseline or annual mammogram if gynecomastia or parenchymal/glandular breast density
- Advise about risk relatives, and consider about counseling option
- Adhere to screening guidelines for prostate cancer

REFERENCES

1. Perou CM, Sorlie T, Eisen MB, et al. Molecular portraits of human breast tumours. Nature 2000;406(6797):747–52.
2. Sorlie T, Perou CM, Tibshirani R, et al. Gene expression patterns of breast carcinomas distinguish tumor subclasses with clinical implications. Proc Natl Acad Sci USA 2001;98(19):10869–74.
3. Sorlie T, Tibshirani R, Parker J, et al. Repeated observation of breast tumor subtypes in independent gene expression data sets. Proc Natl Acad Sci USA 2003;100(14):8418–23.
4. Abd El-Rehim DM, Ball G, Pinder SE, et al. High-throughput protein expression analysis using tissue microarray technology of a large well-characterised series identifies biologically distinct classes of breast cancer confirming recent cDNA expression analyses. Int J Cancer 2005;116(3):340–50.
5. Hu Z, Fan C, Oh DS, et al. The molecular portraits of breast tumors are conserved across microarray platforms. BMC Genomics 2006;7:96.
6. Nielsen TO, Hsu FD, Jensen K, et al. Immunohistochemical and clinical characterization of the basal-like subtype of invasive breast carcinoma. Clin Cancer Res 2004;10(16):5367–74.
7. Yu K, Lee CH, Tan PH, Tan P. Conservation of breast cancer molecular subtypes and transcriptional patterns of tumor progression across distinct ethnic populations. Clin Cancer Res 2004;10(16):5508–17.
8. Van Laere SJ, Van den Eynden GG, Van der Auwera I, et al. Identification of cell-of-origin breast tumor subtypes in inflammatory breast cancer by gene expression profiling. Breast Cancer Res Treat 2006;95(3):243–55.
9. Weigelt B, Hu Z, He X, et al. Molecular portraits and 70-gene prognosis signature are preserved throughout the metastatic process of breast cancer. Cancer Res 2005;65(20):9155–8.
10. King MC, Marks JH, Mandell JB. Breast and ovarian cancer risks due to inherited mutations in BRCA1 and BRCA2. Science 2003;302(5645):643–6.
11. Carey LA, Perou CM, Livasy CA, et al. Race, breast cancer subtypes, and survival in the Carolina Breast Cancer Study. JAMA 2006;295(21):2492–502.
12. Chlebowski RT, Chen Z, Anderson GL, et al. Ethnicity and breast cancer: factors influencing differences in incidence and outcome. J Natl Cancer Inst 2005;97(6):439–48.
13. Fulford LG, Easton DF, Reis-Filho JS, et al. Specific morphological features predictive for the basal phenotype in grade 3 invasive ductal carcinoma of breast. Histopathology 2006;49(1):22–34.
14. Lakhani SR, Reis-Filho JS, Fulford L, et al. Prediction of BRCA1 status in patients with breast cancer using estrogen receptor and basal phenotype. Clin Cancer Res 2005;11(14):5175–80.
15. Livasy CA, Karaca G, Nanda R, et al. Phenotypic evaluation of the basal-like subtype of invasive breast carcinoma. Mod Pathol 2006;19(2):264–71.

16. Tsuda H, Takarabe T, Hasegawa F, Fukutomi T, Hirohashi S. Large, central acellular zones indicating myoepithelial tumor differentiation in high-grade invasive ductal carcinomas as markers of predisposition to lung and brain metastases. Am J Surg Pathol 2000;24(2):197–202.
17. Tsuda H, Takarabe T, Hasegawa T, Murata T, Hirohashi S. Myoepithelial differentiation in high-grade invasive ductal carcinomas with large central acellular zones. Hum Pathol 1999;30(10):1134–9.
18. Jacquemier J, Padovani L, Rabayrol L, et al. Typical medullary breast carcinomas have a basal/myoepithelial phenotype. J Pathol 2005;207(3):260–8.
19. Reis-Filho JS, Milanezi F, Steele D, et al. Metaplastic breast carcinomas are basal-like tumours. Histopathology 2006;49(1):10–21.
20. Vincent-Salomon A, Gruel N, Lucchesi C, et al. Identification of typical medullary breast carcinoma as a genomic sub-group of basal-like carcinomas, a heterogeneous new molecular entity. Breast Cancer Res 2007;9(2):R24.
21. Rodriguez-Pinilla SM, Sarrio D, Honrado E, et al. Prognostic significance of basal-like phenotype and fascin expression in node-negative invasive breast carcinomas. Clin Cancer Res 2006;12(5):1533–9.
22. Abd El-Rehim DM, Pinder SE, Paish CE, et al. Expression of luminal and basal cytokeratins in human breast carcinoma. J Pathol 2004;203(2):661–71.
23. Fan C, Oh DS, Wessels L, et al. Concordance among gene-expression-based predictors for breast cancer. N Engl J Med 2006;355(6):560–9.
24. Rakha EA, El-Sayed ME, Green AR, Lee AH, Robertson JF, Ellis IO. Prognostic markers in triple-negative breast cancer. Cancer 2007;109(1):25–32.
25. Tischkowitz M, Brunet JS, Begin LR, et al. Use of immunohistochemical markers can refine prognosis in triple negative breast cancer. BMC Cancer 2007;7:134.
26. Hoadley KA, Weigman VJ, Fan C, et al. EGFR associated expression profiles vary with breast tumor subtype. BMC Genomics 2007;8:258.
27. Turner N, Tutt A, Ashworth A. Hallmarks of 'BRCAness' in sporadic cancers. Nat Rev Cancer 2004;4(10):814–19.
28. Foulkes WD, Stefansson IM, Chappuis PO, et al. Germline BRCA1 mutations and a basal epithelial phenotype in breast cancer. J Natl Cancer Inst 2003;95(19):1482–5.
29. Turner NC, Reis-Filho JS. Basal-like breast cancer and the BRCA1 phenotype. Oncogene 2006;25(43):5846–53.
30. Turner NC, Reis-Filho JS, Russell AM, et al. BRCA1 dysfunction in sporadic basal-like breast cancer. Oncogene 2007;26(14):2126–32.
31. Esteller M, Silva JM, Dominguez G, et al. Promoter hypermethylation and BRCA1 inactivation in sporadic breast and ovarian tumors. J Natl Cancer Inst 2000;92(7):564–9.
32. Osin P, Lu YJ, Stone J, et al. Distinct genetic and epigenetic changes in medullary breast cancer. Int J Surg Pathol 2003;11(3):153–8.
33. Bartz SR, Zhang Z, Burchard J, et al. Small interfering RNA screens reveal enhanced cisplatin cytotoxicity in tumor cells having both BRCA network and TP53 disruptions. Mol Cell Biol 2006;26(24):9377–86.
34. Rottenberg S, Nygren AO, Pajic M, et al. Selective induction of chemotherapy resistance of mammary tumors in a conditional mouse model for hereditary breast cancer. Proc Natl Acad Sci USA 2007;104(29):12117–22.
35. Turner N, Tutt A, Ashworth A. Targeting the DNA repair defect of BRCA tumours. Curr Opin Pharmacol 2005;5(4):388–93.
36. Xing D, Orsulic S. A mouse model for the molecular characterization of brca1-associated ovarian carcinoma. Cancer Res 2006;66(18):8949–53.
37. Gianni L, Zambetti M, Clark K, et al. Gene expression profiles in paraffin-embedded core biopsy tissue predict response to chemotherapy in women with locally advanced breast cancer. J Clin Oncol 2005;23(29):7265–77.
38. Rouzier R, Perou CM, Symmans WF, et al. Breast cancer molecular subtypes respond differently to preoperative chemotherapy. Clin Cancer Res 2005;11(16):5678–85.
39. Yu K, Ganesan K, Miller LD, Tan P. A modular analysis of breast cancer reveals a novel low-grade molecular signature in estrogen receptor-positive tumors. Clin Cancer Res 2006;12(11, Part 1):3288–96.

Chapter 3 / The Genetics of Breast Cancer: Application in Clinical Practice 51

40. van 't Veer LJ, Dai H, van de Vijver MJ, et al. Gene expression profiling predicts clinical outcome of breast cancer. Nature 2002;415(6871):530–6.

41. Glas AM, Floore A, Delahaye LJ, et al. Converting a breast cancer microarray signature into a high-throughput diagnostic test. BMC Genomics 2006;7:278.

42. Paik S, Shak S, Tang G, et al. A multigene assay to predict recurrence of tamoxifen-treated, node-negative breast cancer. N Engl J Med 2004;351(27):2817–26.

43. Bartel DP. MicroRNAs: genomics, biogenesis, mechanism, and function. Cell 2004;116(2):281–97.

44. Denli AM, Tops BB, Plasterk RH, Ketting RF, Hannon GJ. Processing of primary microRNAs by the microprocessor complex. Nature 2004;432(7014):231–5.

45. Gregory RI, Yan KP, Amuthan G, et al. The Microprocessor complex mediates the genesis of microRNAs. Nature 2004;432(7014):235–40.

46. Griffiths-Jones S. The microRNA Registry. Nucleic Acids Res 2004;32(Database issue): D109–D111.

47. Griffiths-Jones S. miRBase: the microRNA sequence database. Methods Mol Biol 2006; 342:129–38.

48. Han J, Lee Y, Yeom KH, Kim YK, Jin H, Kim VN. The Drosha-DGCR8 complex in primary microRNA processing. Genes Dev 2004;18(24):3016–27.

49. Landthaler M, Yalcin A, Tuschl T. The human DiGeorge syndrome critical region gene 8 and its D. melanogaster homolog are required for miRNA biogenesis. Curr Biol 2004;14(23):2162–7.

50. Lee Y, Ahn C, Han J, et al. The nuclear RNase III Drosha initiates microRNA processing. Nature 2003;425(6956):415–19.

51. Lund E, Guttinger S, Calado A, Dahlberg JE, Kutay U. Nuclear export of microRNA precursors. Science 2004;303(5654):95–8.

52. Du T, Zamore PD. microPrimer: the biogenesis and function of microRNA. Development 2005;132(21):4645–52.

53. Olsen PH, Ambros V. The lin-4 regulatory RNA controls developmental timing in *Caenorhabditis elegans* by blocking LIN-14 protein synthesis after the initiation of translation. Dev Biol 1999;216(2):671–80.

54. Petersen CP, Bordeleau ME, Pelletier J, Sharp PA. Short RNAs repress translation after initiation in mammalian cells. Mol Cell 2006;21(4):533–42.

55. Iorio MV, Ferracin M, Liu CG, et al. MicroRNA gene expression deregulation in human breast cancer. Cancer Res 2005;65(16):7065–70.

56. Volinia S, Calin GA, Liu CG, et al. A microRNA expression signature of human solid tumors defines cancer gene targets. Proc Natl Acad Sci USA 2006;103(7):2257–61.

57. Mattie MD, Benz CC, Bowers J, et al. Optimized high-throughput microRNA expression profiling provides novel biomarker assessment of clinical prostate and breast cancer biopsies. Mol Cancer 2006;5:24.

58. Blenkiron C, Goldstein LD, Thorne NP, et al. MicroRNA expression profiling of human breast cancer identifies new markers of tumor subtype. Genome Biol 2007;8(10):R214.

59. Arver B, Du Q, Chen J, Luo L, Lindblom A. Hereditary breast cancer: a review. Semin Cancer Biol 2000;10(4):271–88.

60. Pathology of familial breast cancer: differences between breast cancers in carriers of BRCA1 or BRCA2 mutations and sporadic cases. Breast Cancer Linkage Consortium. Lancet 1997; 349(9064):1505–10.

61. Hall JM, Lee MK, Newman B, et al. Linkage of early-onset familial breast cancer to chromosome 17q21. Science 1990;250(4988):1684–9.

62. Miki Y, Swensen J, Shattuck-Eidens D, et al. A strong candidate for the breast and ovarian cancer susceptibility gene BRCA1. Science 1994;266(5182):66–71.

63. Cornelis RS, Neuhausen SL, Johansson O, et al. High allele loss rates at 17q12-q21 in breast and ovarian tumors from BRCA1-linked families. The Breast Cancer Linkage Consortium. Genes Chromosomes Cancer 1995;13(3):203–10.

64. Mani A, Gelmann EP. The ubiquitin-proteasome pathway and its role in cancer. J Clin Oncol 2005;23(21):4776–89.

65. Shinagawa H, Miki Y, Yoshida K. BRCA1-mediated ubiquitination inhibits topoisomerase II alpha activity in response to oxidative stress. Antioxid Redox Signal 2008;10(5):939–49.

66. Scully R, Chen J, Plug A, et al. Association of BRCA1 with Rad51 in mitotic and meiotic cells. Cell 1997;88(2):265–75.
67. Zhang J, Willers H, Feng Z, et al. Chk2 phosphorylation of BRCA1 regulates DNA double-strand break repair. Mol Cell Biol 2004;24(2):708–18.
68. Paull TT, Rogakou EP, Yamazaki V, Kirchgessner CU, Gellert M, Bonner WM. A critical role for histone H2AX in recruitment of repair factors to nuclear foci after DNA damage. Curr Biol 2000;10(15):886–95.
69. Bochar DA, Wang L, Beniya H, et al. BRCA1 is associated with a human SWI/SNF-related complex: linking chromatin remodeling to breast cancer. Cell 2000;102(2):257–65.
70. Xu B, O'Donnell AH, Kim ST, Kastan MB. Phosphorylation of serine 1387 in Brca1 is specifically required for the Atm-mediated S-phase checkpoint after ionizing irradiation. Cancer Res 2002;62(16):4588–91.
71. Ouchi T, Monteiro AN, August A, Aaronson SA, Hanafusa H. BRCA1 regulates p53-dependent gene expression. Proc Natl Acad Sci USA 1998;95(5):2302–6.
72. Wong AK, Ormonde PA, Pero R, et al. Characterization of a carboxy-terminal BRCA1 interacting protein. Oncogene 1998;17(18):2279–85.
73. Venkitaraman AR. Functions of BRCA1 and BRCA2 in the biological response to DNA damage. J Cell Sci 2001;114 (Part 20):3591–8.
74. Brodie SG, Deng CX. BRCA1-associated tumorigenesis: what have we learned from knockout mice? Trends Genet 2001;17(10):S18–S22.
75. Wooster R, Neuhausen SL, Mangion J, et al. Localization of a breast cancer susceptibility gene, BRCA2, to chromosome 13q12–13. Science 1994;265(5181):2088–90.
76. Bertwistle D, Swift S, Marston NJ, et al. Nuclear location and cell cycle regulation of the BRCA2 protein. Cancer Res 1997;57(24):5485–8.
77. Wong AK, Pero R, Ormonde PA, Tavtigian SV, Bartel PL. RAD51 interacts with the evolutionarily conserved BRC motifs in the human breast cancer susceptibility gene *brca2*. J Biol Chem 1997;272(51):31941–4.
78. Fuks F, Milner J, Kouzarides T. BRCA2 associates with acetyltransferase activity when bound to P/CAF. Oncogene 1998;17(19):2531–4.
79. Futamura M, Arakawa H, Matsuda K, et al. Potential role of BRCA2 in a mitotic checkpoint after phosphorylation by hBUBR1. Cancer Res 2000;60(6):1531–5.
80. Antoniou AC, Pharoah PD, McMullan G, et al. A comprehensive model for familial breast cancer incorporating *BRCA1, BRCA2* and other genes. Br J Cancer 2002;86(1):76–83.
81. Hopper JL. More breast cancer genes? Breast Cancer Res 2001;3(3):154–7.
82. Antoniou A, Pharoah PD, Narod S, et al. Average risks of breast and ovarian cancer associated with BRCA1 or BRCA2 mutations detected in case series unselected for family history: a combined analysis of 22 studies. Am J Hum Genet 2003;72(5):1117–30.
83. Ferla R, Calo V, Cascio S, et al. Founder mutations in *BRCA1* and *BRCA2* genes. Ann Oncol 2007;18 Suppl 6:vi93–vi98.
84. Cancer risks in BRCA2 mutation carriers. The Breast Cancer Linkage Consortium. J Natl Cancer Inst 1999;91(15):1310–16.
85. Easton DF, Ford D, Bishop DT. Breast and ovarian cancer incidence in BRCA1-mutation carriers. Breast Cancer Linkage Consortium. Am J Hum Genet 1995;56(1):265–71.
86. Friedman LS, Szabo CI, Ostermeyer EA, et al. Novel inherited mutations and variable expressivity of BRCA1 alleles, including the founder mutation 185delAG in Ashkenazi Jewish families. Am J Hum Genet 1995;57(6):1284–97.
87. Neuhausen S, Gilewski T, Norton L, et al. Recurrent BRCA2 6174delT mutations in Ashkenazi Jewish women affected by breast cancer. Nat Genet 1996;13(1):126–8.
88. Struewing JP, Abeliovich D, Peretz T, et al. The carrier frequency of the BRCA1 185delAG mutation is approximately 1 percent in Ashkenazi Jewish individuals. Nat Genet 1995;11(2):198–200.
89. Roa BB, Boyd AA, Volcik K, Richards CS. Ashkenazi Jewish population frequencies for common mutations in BRCA1 and BRCA2. Nat Genet 1996;14(2):185–7.
90. Sarantaus L, Huusko P, Eerola H, et al. Multiple founder effects and geographical clustering of BRCA1 and BRCA2 families in Finland. Eur J Hum Genet 2000;8(10):757–63.

Chapter 3 / The Genetics of Breast Cancer: Application in Clinical Practice 53

91. Bergthorsson JT, Jonasdottir A, Johannesdottir G, et al. Identification of a novel splice-site mutation of the BRCA1 gene in two breast cancer families: screening reveals low frequency in Icelandic breast cancer patients. Hum Mutat 1998;Suppl 1:S195–S197.

92. Thorlacius S, Olafsdottir G, Tryggvadottir L, et al. A single BRCA2 mutation in male and female breast cancer families from Iceland with varied cancer phenotypes. Nat Genet 1996; 13(1):117–19.

93. Muller D, Bonaiti-Pellie C, Abecassis J, Stoppa-Lyonnet D, Fricker JP. BRCA1 testing in breast and/or ovarian cancer families from northeastern France identifies two common mutations with a founder effect. Fam Cancer 2004;3(1):15–20.

94. Baudi F, Quaresima B, Grandinetti C, et al. Evidence of a founder mutation of BRCA1 in a highly homogeneous population from southern Italy with breast/ovarian cancer. Hum Mutat 2001; 18(2):163–4.

95. De Leon Matsuda ML, Liede A, Kwan E, et al. BRCA1 and BRCA2 mutations among breast cancer patients from the Philippines. Int J Cancer 2002;98(4):596–603.

96. Ikeda N, Miyoshi Y, Yoneda K, et al. Frequency of BRCA1 and BRCA2 germline mutations in Japanese breast cancer families. Int J Cancer 2001;91(1):83–8.

97. Khoo US, Chan KY, Cheung AN, et al. Recurrent BRCA1 and BRCA2 germline mutations in ovarian cancer: a founder mutation of BRCA1 identified in the Chinese population. Hum Mutat 2002;19(3):307–8.

98. Rashid MU, Zaidi A, Torres D, et al. Prevalence of BRCA1 and BRCA2 mutations in Pakistani breast and ovarian cancer patients. Int J Cancer 2006;119(12):2832–9.

99. Claus EB, Risch N, Thompson WD. Autosomal dominant inheritance of early-onset breast cancer. Implications for risk prediction. Cancer 1994;73(3):643–51.

100. Berry DA, Iversen ES Jr, Gudbjartsson DF, et al. BRCAPRO validation, sensitivity of genetic testing of BRCA1/BRCA2, and prevalence of other breast cancer susceptibility genes. J Clin Oncol 2002;20(11):2701–12.

101. Berry DA, Parmigiani G, Sanchez J, Schildkraut J, Winer E. Probability of carrying a mutation of breast-ovarian cancer gene BRCA1 based on family history. J Natl Cancer Inst 1997; 89(3):227–38.

102. Parmigiani G, Berry D, Aguilar O. Determining carrier probabilities for breast cancer-susceptibility genes BRCA1 and BRCA2. Am J Hum Genet 1998;62(1):145–58.

103. Hallowell N, Murton F, Statham H, Green JM, Richards MP. Women's need for information before attending genetic counselling for familial breast or ovarian cancer: a questionnaire, interview, and observational study. BMJ 1997;314(7076):281–3.

104. Lynch HT, Lemon SJ, Durham C, et al. A descriptive study of BRCA1 testing and reactions to disclosure of test results. Cancer 1997;79(11):2219–28.

105. Tommasi S, Crapolicchio A, Lacalamita R, et al. BRCA1 mutations and polymorphisms in a hospital-based consecutive series of breast cancer patients from Apulia, Italy. Mutat Res 2005; 578(1–2):395–405.

106. Fedier A, Steiner RA, Schwarz VA, Lenherr L, Haller U, Fink D. The effect of loss of Brca1 on the sensitivity to anticancer agents in p53-deficient cells. Int J Oncol 2003;22(5):1169–73.

107. Judkins T, Hendrickson BC, Deffenbaugh AM, Scholl T. Single nucleotide polymorphisms in clinical genetic testing: the characterization of the clinical significance of genetic variants and their application in clinical research for BRCA1. Mutat Res 2005;573(1–2):168–79.

108. Armes JE, Egan AJ, Southey MC, et al. The histologic phenotypes of breast carcinoma occurring before age 40 years in women with and without BRCA1 or BRCA2 germline mutations: a population-based study. Cancer 1998;83(11):2335–45.

109. Eerola H, Heikkila P, Tamminen A, Aittomaki K, Blomqvist C, Nevanlinna H. Histopathological features of breast tumours in BRCA1, BRCA2 and mutation-negative breast cancer families. Breast Cancer Res 2005;7(1):R93–R100.

110. Jacquemler J, Eisinger F, Guinebretiere JM, Stoppa-Lyonnet D, Sobol H. Intraductal component and BRCA1-associated breast cancer. Lancet 1996;348(9034):1098.

111. Johannsson OT, Idvall I, Anderson C, et al. Tumour biological features of BRCA1-induced breast and ovarian cancer. Eur J Cancer 1997;33(3):362–71.

112. Marcus JN, Watson P, Page DL, et al. Hereditary breast cancer: pathobiology, prognosis, and BRCA1 and BRCA2 gene linkage. Cancer 1996;77(4):697–709.
113. Barkardottir RB, Sarantaus L, Arason A, et al. Haplotype analysis in Icelandic and Finnish BRCA2 999del5 breast cancer families. Eur J Hum Genet 2001;9(10):773–9.
114. Hedenfalk I, Duggan D, Chen Y, et al. Gene-expression profiles in hereditary breast cancer. N Engl J Med 2001;344(8):539–48.
115. Lakhani SR, Van De Vijver MJ, Jacquemier J, et al. The pathology of familial breast cancer: predictive value of immunohistochemical markers estrogen receptor, progesterone receptor, HER-2, and p53 in patients with mutations in BRCA1 and BRCA2. J Clin Oncol 2002;20(9):2310–18.
116. Grushko TA, Blackwood MA, Schumm PL, et al. Molecular-cytogenetic analysis of *HER-2/neu* gene in BRCA1-associated breast cancers. Cancer Res 2002;62(5):1481–8.
117. Marroni F, Aretini P, D'Andrea E, et al. Penetrances of breast and ovarian cancer in a large series of families tested for BRCA1/2 mutations. Eur J Hum Genet 2004;12(11):899–906.

4 Alterations in Cell Cycle Regulatory Genes in Breast Cancer

Annalisa Roberti, Marcella Macaluso, and Antonio Giordano, MD

SUMMARY

Breast cancer is one of the most commonly diagnosed cancers worldwide. The underlying mechanisms accountable for aberrant cell proliferation and tumor growth involve multiple pathways, which include components of the cell cycle machinery. Proto-oncogene activation, loss of tumor suppressor genes, and growth sustained by growth factors and steroids may affect breast cancer initiation and progression. The regulation of cell cycle checkpoints is critical for the proper and orchestrated transition from one phase of the cell cycle to the next. The deregulation of these checkpoints plays a key role in the transformation process, allowing the cells to continuously cycle under conditions inadequate for normal cell proliferation. A key regulatory pathway determining cell cycle proliferation rate is the cyclin/cyclin-dependent kinase (CDK)/p16Ink4A/ retinoblastoma protein (pRb) axis. Alterations affecting components of this pathway through overexpression, mutation, and epigenetic gene silencing are almost universal in human cancer. In breast cancer, these include the overexpression of *cyclins D1* and *cyclin E*, decreased expression of the *p27Kip1* CDK inhibitor, and silencing of the *p16Ink4A* gene through promoter methylation. Understanding the biology of breast cancer may improve the possibility to overcome this pathology. The chance to have strong prognostic and/or predictive markers will be an immensely useful tool to identify patients at higher risk of relapse and to select the most appropriate systemic treatment for individual breast cancer patients.

Key Words: Breast cancer; Cell cycle control; G1/S transition; Cyclins, Cyclin-dependent kinases (CDKs); CDK inhibitors; RB pathway

From: *Current Clinical Oncology: Breast Cancer in the Post-Genomic Era,*
Edited by: A. Giordano and N. Normanno, DOI: 10.1007/978-1-60327-945-1_4,
© Humana Press, a part of Springer Science + Business Media, LLC 2009

1. CELL CYCLE: AN OVERVIEW

1.1. Cell Cycle Phases and Checkpoints

During an organism's development, the destiny of its individual cells is dictated by signals that each cell receives from its own environment. The cells may encounter five different fates: they can differentiate, become quiescent or senescent, proliferate, or undergo apoptosis. A finely regulated molecular network operates in the cells in order to manage and integrates the multiplicity of internal and external signals to settle on a cell's fate. Once a cell has been formed by the process of cell division it must "decide" whether it will once again start a new proliferating cycle or withdraw from the cell cycle in a nonproliferative state, named quiescent state G0. This choice is strongly influenced by the presence and amount of mitogenic or antimitogenic stimulation, respectively, in the surrounding environment. The majority of cells in the human body reside in nonproliferating, "out-of-cycle" states and only a minority population is actively cycling. These cycling cells are mainly located in stem-transit amplifying compartments of self-renewing tissues such as cervix, colon, or skin. On the other hand, most functional cells (e.g., hepatocytes) reside in a quiescent (G0), reversibly arrested state, or have irreversibly withdrawn from the mitotic cell division cycle into terminally differentiated states (e.g., neurons, myocytes, or surface colonic epithelial cells) *(1)*. Cell fate is mainly determined in a discrete window of time, during which the cell is responsive to extracellular signals; this critical point is called the *restriction point* or *R point*. If the cell should decide at the R point to undertake a proliferating path it commits itself to proceed in a highly structured cycle of growth and division, the *cell cycle*. An eukaryotic cell cannot divide into two daughter cells unless it replicates its genome (DNA) and then separates the duplicated genome. To achieve these tasks, cells must perform DNA synthesis and mitosis. The cell cycle is an ordered set of events that may be recapped into four central phases, namely G1 phase (or Gap1), S phase, G2 phase (Gap2), and mitosis (M phase). During G1 phase, the cells grow and prepare all the macromolecules required for the subsequent synthesis of DNA. In S phase the chromosome will be duplicate with fidelity. After this process the cells will enter in a second Gap phase (G2) in which they continue to grow and prepare for mitosis, the phase in which the cells will be actually divided. The decision to undertake a proliferation cycle begins at the onset of G1 and ends just before the last part of G1; this window of time represents the R point. At this point the cell takes an irreversible choice, since a cell that enters S phase will invariably proceed through the rest of the phases, even if mitogenic stimulation is not longer present in the surrounding setting. Metabolic, genetic, and physiological emergencies, however, may cause a delay in the cell cycle or may even cause the cell to withdraw from the cell cycle. The faithful replication of a cell's genome during S phase and the accurate allocation of the resulting DNA to daughter cells during mitosis are critical steps that guarantee the cell correct proliferation. Defects in these pathways have grievous consequences not only for the single cell but also for the entire organism. To avoid these dangerous consequences the cell has acquired rigorous quality control mechanisms, which tightly regulate progression through the cell cycle. These monitoring mechanisms, commonly named *checkpoints* (Fig. 1) work to ensure the proper sequence of cell cycle events and allow the cell to interrupt or delay the cell cycle if something goes wrong. A cell can advance into the next phase of the cycle if and only if it has properly completed all the required events in the previous phase and any potential problem has been fixed successfully. Moreover, the checkpoints ensure that once a given step of the cell cycle has been concluded, it is not repeated until the next cell cycle. Any pathways working in the cell cycle are strongly related to each other and the aim of this dependence is to guarantee a complete and accurate distribution of the genome to daughter cells. When cells have

Chapter 4 / Alterations in Cell Cycle Regulatory Genes in Breast Cancer

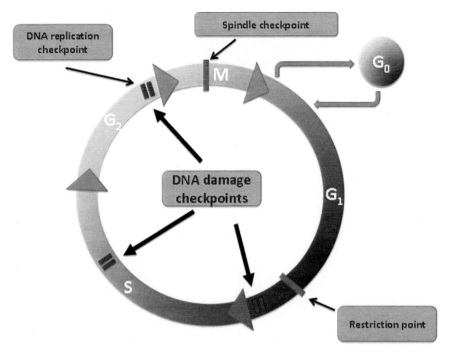

Fig. 1. Cell cycle phases and checkpoints. The cell cycle is the cyclical process by which a cell that has just divided grows, replicates its DNA, and then divides again. Four distinct, ordered stages constitute a cell cycle. DNA synthesis (S) and mitosis (M) separated by two "gap" phases (G_2 and G_1) of preparation and growth. The time period in which a cell is responsive to extracellular signal is called Restriction point. It represents an important G1 checkpoint, and cells that progress through this point are committed to proceed in the cell cycle. If a cell is not ready or external conditions are not appropriate for the S phase, the cell may enter G_0 phase, a quiescent stage. When cells acquire genomic damage they activate DNA damage checkpoints that according to the cell cycle stage are classified into G1/S (G1) checkpoint, intra-S phase checkpoint, and G2/M checkpoint. They slow or pause the cell cycle in order to repair any damage before cells proceed in the next step of the cell cycle. The DNA replication checkpoint arrests cells in G2/M transition until DNA replication is successfully completed. The spindle checkpoint arrests cell cycle at M phase until all chromosomes are aligned on spindle. This checkpoint is important for equal chromosomes distribution.

acquired DNA damages, cells activate *DNA damage checkpoints* that slow or pause the cell cycle in order to remedy the DNA mistakes when possible and promote cell death (apoptosis) in unrepaired cells. According to the cell cycle stages, there are at least three DNA damage checkpoints: G1/S checkpoint, intra-S phase checkpoint, and G2/M checkpoint. The *G1 checkpoint* is the first defense against genomic stress and DNA damage. Inhibiting the onset of DNA replication, this checkpoint ensures that a cell cannot advance from G1 into S phase if the genome needs to be repaired. Replication errors and DNA damage incurred during S phase have to be checked before the cell advances into M phase. Both S-phase and G2 checkpoints are designed to guarantee fidelity in DNA transmission. To ensure integrity of the genome and the fidelity of chromosome segregation, the cells have acquired multiple levels of control. Following any kind of events that may interfere with DNA synthesis, the cell responds by activating the *DNA replication checkpoint*, which arrests the cell cycle at G2/M transition until DNA replication is successfully complete. Highly efficient checkpoints are the *spindle checkpoint* and the *morphogenesis checkpoint*. The spindle checkpoint arrests the cell cycle at M phase until all chromosomes are aligned on the spindle. This checkpoint is very important for equal distribution of chromosomes. The morphogenesis checkpoint detects abnormality in the cytoskeleton and arrests the cell cycle at the G2/M transition. Any uncorrected errors that escape these restriction points will be inherited by the daughter cells, thus bringing about the so-called *mitotic catastrophe*. All the checkpoints examined require an orchestrated protein interaction pathway. Mutations in genes encoding for proteins involved at every step in cell cycle checkpoints may be related to cancer development and progression, since checkpoint failures allow the cell to continue dividing despite damages to its integrity.

1.2. Cyclins and Cyclin–CDK Complexes: Cell Cycle Progression

At the restriction point the cell makes the most important decision concerning its fate: to grow or not. A wrong choice may be responsible for the uncontrolled cell proliferation that leads to cancer development. Therefore, it is extremely important to understand the cell cycle machinery, its thorough regulation in normal physiology and its deregulation during oncogenesis. In eukaryotes, cell cycle progression is mediated by sequential activation and inactivation of particular serine/threonine kinases, altogether called *cyclin-dependent kinases (CDKs)*. The wording indicates that these enzymes never act alone, but their catalytic activity is dependent on their association with the *cyclin* proteins. By phosphorylating multiple distinct targets, cyclin–CDK complexes may create covalent modifications that operate by turning specific regulatory proteins on or off, generating a chain of events that culminate in the execution of specific cell cycle steps. The CDK catalytic subunit remains relatively uniform throughout the cell cycle, while the abundance of regulatory subunits the cyclins undergo periodic fluctuations in order to drive the cell through the different stages of the cell cycle *(2)*. Cyclins are so named because their concentration varies in a cyclical fashion during the cell cycle; their gradual accumulation is followed by their rapid degradation and moreover has a critical role in the ensuring that the cell cycle continues in the appropriate direction (Fig. 2). There are several different families of cyclins, which are active at different points of the cell cycle and exclusively pair with specific CDK or sets of CDKs in a phase-dependent manner. Moreover, there are several "orphan" cyclins for which no CDK partner has been identified. During the most part of G1 phase, *D-type cyclins* (D1, D2, and D3) form enzymatically active complexes with CDK4 and CDK6. After the R point in late G1, the *E-type cyclins* (E1 and E2) pair and activate CDK2. The Cyclin E/CDK2 complex phosphorylates p27^{Kip1} (an Cyclin D inhibitor), tagging it for degradation, and promotes the expression of Cyclin A, allowing progression to S phase. The *A-type cyclins* (A1and A2) are required for cell progression through the S phase. They start to accumulate during S phase and are destroyed during mitosis. Cyclin A has two CDK partners; at the beginning of S phase it replaces cyclin E as the partner of CDK2, while later in S it leaves CDK2 to associate with CDK1. The amount of the mitotic cyclin, named *Cyclin B*, increases through the cell cycle until mitosis: in late G2, cyclin B takes the place of cyclin A, switching cyclin A–CDK1complex into the so called mitosis promoting factor (MPF). This is a good example of how the binding with different cyclins may regulate the substrate specificity of the CDKs. The same catalytic domain may

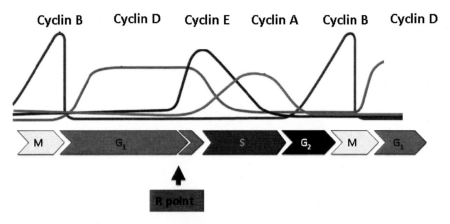

Fig. 2. Cyclin fluctuation through cell cycle phases: Cyclins have time-changed level during cell cycle and they are gradually accumulated and rapidly degraded in a cell cycle phase-dependent fashion. The scheduled availability of different cyclins in specific cell cycle phase imposes to the cell to move through cell cycle in a preestablished direction. Cyclin B is a mitotic cyclin. The amount of cyclin B rises through the cell cycle until mitosis, where it falls all at once following its degradation. Cyclin E expression increases promptly after a cell moves forward the restriction point and collapses when the cell passes S phase, while cyclin A increases concurrently with the cell entry in S phase. The cyclin D level represents an exception to this programmed fluctuation plans. Its levels are closely regulated by external conditions. Cyclin D is available in other cell cycle phases beside G1, after G1/S transition cyclin D is exported in the cytoplasm where it can no longer influence cell cycle.

have different targets depending on the binding with different regulatory subunits. This allows the cell cycle machinery to move through the different phases by a well-regulated and synchronized time schedule (Fig. 3). The cyclic fluctuation in the cyclin levels is tightly coordinated with cell cycle execution program; the sole exception is presented by D-type cyclins. The levels of these cyclins do not show the typical fluctuation pattern displayed by the other cyclins; instead, its regulation seems to be dictated by external signals. Mitogenic stimulation induces a signal-transduction cascade that ultimately leads to the induction of D-type cyclins. These molecules have the primary function of linking extracellular signals to the cell cycle machinery (3). Given that their expression is considerably influenced by the extracellular presence of mitogens, it is plausible to conclude that the presence of D-type cyclins represents the input signal to trigger the cell cycle machinery. The mitogen-dependent expression of D-type cyclins and their activity during early G1 exactly match with the period during which the cells are responsive to extracellular signals (restriction point). Thus, after cells pass through the R point, the activation of the remaining cyclin–CDK complexes takes place in a self-governing manner, no longer influenced by extracellular signals.

1.3. Cell Cycle Entry: Regulation of G1/S Transition

D-type cyclins are critical modulators of the G1/S transition. Given the central role played by these proteins, the cells have acquired multiple regulation levels designed in order to ensure that the cell cycle is launched only if actually needed. D-type cyclins have the

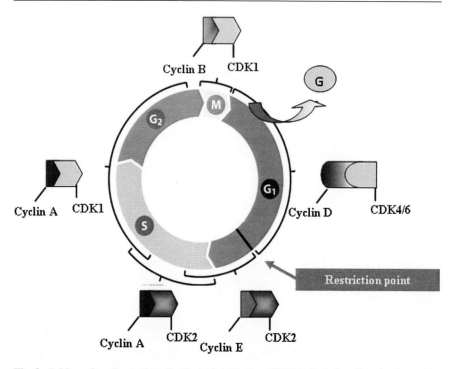

Fig. 3. Pairing of cyclins and cyclin-dependent kinases (CDKs) through cell cycle phases: the cell cycle is driven by the activity of cyclin-CDK complexes. Cyclins pair with and activate specific CDK or set of CDKs in a phase-dependent manner. During much of G1 D1-type cyclins form active complexes with CDK4 and CDK6. At the R point cyclin E pairs and activates CDK2, promoting the expression of cyclin A. Cyclin A has two CDK partners: at the beginning of S phase replace cyclin E in the CDK2 binding, while later in S cyclin A dissociates to CDK2 and binds CDK1. CDK1 pairs with cyclin B, forming the mitosis-promoting factor that remains activate until mitosis is completed. The binding with different regulatory subunits (cyclins) regulates the CDKs specificity for the different catalytic targets, allowing the cell cycle to proceed in a well-regulated time schedule.

unique role of acting as a link between extracellular proliferation and growth signals and the cell cycle machinery. The distribution of the various D-type cyclins in different tissues is not uniform, with cyclin D2 and D3 being more prominent in hematopoietic lineage cells, whereas cyclin D1 appears to be especially important in mammary epithelial cells and the nervous system (4). During G1, D-type cyclin expression is regulated by several mitogenic factors and is controlled by multiple signaling pathways, in turn activated by different sets of cellular surface receptors. This may in part explain the typical tissue-specific distribution of each of them. Transcription factors that induce cyclin D expression include signal transducers and activators of transcription (STATs), nuclear factor (NF)-κB, and some varieties of activator proteins (AP)-1. E2F and PARPγ transcription factors, conversely, inhibit cyclin D expression (5). Moreover, D-type cyclins have to be fleeting proteins to guarantee that the

Chapter 4 / Alterations in Cell Cycle Regulatory Genes in Breast Cancer 61

subunit pool shrinks rapidly when cells are deprived of mitogens. D-type cyclins undergo posttranscriptional regulation by different mechanisms, which influence their translation as well as their stability, location and association with CDK complexes. Intracellular levels of cyclin D are controlled by proteasome-mediated proteolysis after ubiquitination. During S phase, cyclin D is excluded from the nucleus and rapidly degraded following its phosphorylation by glycogen synthase kinase 3β (GSK-3β) *(6)*. AKT, on the other hand, is a positive regulator of cyclin D; it stabilizes cyclin D by inhibiting GSK-3β *(7)*.

Another layer of control governing the activity of the cyclin–CDK complex and therefore regulating the advance through the cell cycle is imposed by a class of proteins termed CDK inhibitors (CDKIs). Two CDKI gene families have been defined based on their structure and CDK specificities: the *INK4 gene family* and the *Cip/Kip* family. Both of them have the ability to block the CDKs activity at various points in the cell cycle, although by different regulatory strategies. The *INK4* (*inhibitors* of CDK4) gene family encodes p16INK4a, p15INK4b, p18INK4c, and p19INK4d, all of which bind to CDK4 and CDK6 and inhibit their kinase activities, preventing their association with D-type cyclins. In contrast, the Cip/Kip family members, p21$^{WAF1/Cip1}$, p27^{Kip1}, and p57^{Kip2} are able to bind both cyclin and CDK subunits and can modulate the activities of cyclin D-, E-, A-, and B–CDK complexes (Fig. 4).

p16INK4a is encoded by the *p16* tumor suppressor gene, which inhibits the activity of the cyclin D-dependent kinase. Its inhibitory effect is based on p16INK4a ability to form complexes with CDK4/6 in order to prevent the formation of CDK4/6–cyclin D complex and S phase entry, respectively *(8)*. A recent model proposed by Russo and coworkers explains how p16INK4a exerts its inhibitory function generating conformational distortions both in cyclin-binding and kinase catalytic sites of CDK4/6. In this way p16, not only indirectly prevents the binding of D-type cyclins, but also inhibits the preassembled CDK4/6–cyclin D complexes, by inhibiting directly the catalytic activity *(9)*. The genetic locus encoding for p16Ink 4a also encodes in an Alternative Reading Frame, for p14ARF protein. The latter provides an essential link between the cell cycle and p53-mediated apoptosis. The p14/19ARF protein can increase p53 levels by neutralizing Mdm2, which in turn mediates p53 degradation through an ubiquitin-dependent pathway. Indeed, p14/19ARF directly binds to Mdm2 and block its ability to interact productively with p53, by inhibiting Mdm2's ubiquitin ligase activity and by repressing Mdm2 capacity to export p53 from the nucleus to the cytoplasm, where it is degraded *(10)*.

p15INK4b has a central role in mediating cell cycle arrest triggered by tumor growth factor-β (TGF-β). TGF-β induces *p15INK4b* expression and stabilizes the respective protein. This allows p15 to bind CDK4 and CDK6, resulting in their inactivation *(11)*. The other members of the INK4 class, *p18Ink4c* and *p19Ink4d*, are expressed during fetal development and seem to play a key role in terminal differentiation *(12)*. If, the INK4 proteins are specialized to inhibit cyclin D–CDK4/6 complexes, active in early G1, on the other hand, the three Cip/Kip CDKIs can interact whit cyclin D–CDK4/6 complexes as well as with the remaining cyclin–CDK complexes, active throughout the next phases of the cell cycle.

The way by which Cip/Kip proteins act seems to be contradictory. While they inhibit the action of cyclin E–CDK2, cyclin A–CDK2/1, and cyclin B–CDK1/CDK1, they actually stimulate the formation of cyclin D–CDK4/6 complexes *(13)*.

p21Cip1/Waf1 was identified simultaneously by two independent research groups, who on the basis of its established functions, named it CDK-interacting protein 1 (Cip1) and Waf1 (wild-type p53-activated fragment 1), respectively. p21 is a multifunctional protein able to inhibit cell cycle progression at different levels.

The principal role of p21Cip1/Waf1 in cell cycle regulation lies in its ability to inhibit cyclin A, E/CDK2 activity, required for G1/S transition, and therefore promote G1 arrest.

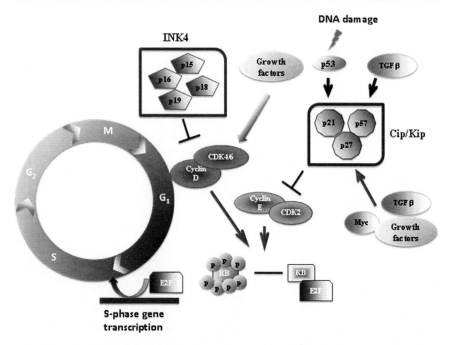

Fig. 4. Regulation of G1/S transition: The transition from G1 to S phase may be considered as a "point of no return" beyond which the cell is committed to dividing. Numerous regulatory mechanisms govern this critical point, integrating extracellular signals and transducing them in a transcriptional response. INK4 CKIs act on D-type cyclins/CDKs, while Cip/Kip proteins inhibit both cyclin D/CDKs and cyclin E/CDKs. TGF β, Myc, and growth factors may exert their cell cycle regulatory function by influencing CDKIs activity and thus the cell cycle progression. An important link between cell cycle and DNA damage checkpoint is guaranteed through the p53-dependent activation of p21. This allows cells to slow or arrest cell cycle progression until the damage has been repaired. Cyclin/CDK complexes phosphorylate and inhibit Rb proteins. Rb inhibits cell proliferation by inactivating the E2F-dependent transcription of genes involved in cell proliferation.

Furthermore, p21 can interact with PCNA, an elongation factor for the DNA polymerase δ, as well as a component of the DNA repair machinery *(14)*. The binding of p21 inhibits the ability of PCNA to act in DNA replication but not in DNA repair. p21 may inhibit cell cycle progression in two ways: (a) by inhibiting a variety of cyclin/CDK complexes and (b) by inhibiting DNA synthesis through PCNA binding. If the genome becomes damaged during the G1 phase, p21 will block the advance through the S phase, inhibiting E–CDK2 complexes, until the damage has been repaired. If the damage ensues during DNA replication, p21 by inhibiting PCNA halts DNA synthesis until DNA repair has been completed. In addition, as the name indicates, p21Cip1/Waf1 (wild-type p53-activated fragment 1) is under the control of p53 tumor suppressor gene. In DNA damaged cells, p21Cip1/Waf1 is responsible for p53-dependent G1 arrest. In response to DNA damage, the p53 is stabilized and activated

Chapter 4 /Alterations in Cell Cycle Regulatory Genes in Breast Cancer

as a transcription factor. The *p21* promoter region contains a p53-binding site that allows p53 to activate *p21* transcription and thus p21-mediated cell cycle arrest *(15)*. Like p21, p27 and p57 bind to a variety of cyclin/CDK complexes through a conserved amino-terminal domain, while divergence in the remaining sequences among them suggests that each protein could have distinct functions and regulatory abilities.

p27 has been implicated in mediating several growth inhibitory signals including transforming growth factor-β (TGF-β) and contact inhibition. In mitogen-starved cells and other quiescent states p27 expression is usually high and the protein is rapidly downregulated as cells enter the cell cycle. *p27* binds and inhibits cyclin E–CDK2 and cyclin A–CDK2 complexes in the early G1 phase of the cell cycle, but also assembles cyclin D1–CDKs in the cytoplasm and facilitates the import of cyclin D1-complexes into the nucleus. The cyclin–CDK complex to which p27 is bound determines its functional activity. During period of cell proliferation, p27 binds cyclin D1–CDK4/CDK6 complexes in a noninhibitory fashion. Antiproliferative signals, including TGF-β and cell to cell contact, mobilized the stored p27 so that it can bind and inhibit the cyclin E–CDK2 complex. The removal of p27 from the cyclin E–CDK2 complex is an essential step for S-phase entry. By binding cyclin D1–CDK4, p27 is sequestrated from cyclin E–CDK2, reducing its CDK2 inhibitory function and allowing the cell to proceed to the replication phase *(16)*. Since CDK2 is a nuclear protein, p27 exerts its inhibitory function on cyclin E–CDK2 complex in the nucleus; cytoplasmic localization of p27 would therefore keep it away from its target *(17)*, representing one of the principal ways by which p27 function may be compromised in uncontrolled growing cells. The abundance of p27 through the cell cycle is mainly regulated at the posttranscriptional level, although transcriptional control also contributes to protein regulation. p27 activity is regulated by a well-articulated phosphorylation network that modulates protein function by altering its subcellular localization, protein–protein interactions, and stability. As the cell exits quiescence and progresses through the S phase, p27 protein levels drop due to decreased translation of p27 mRNA and targeted proteolysis *(18)*. A site-specific phosphorylation labels p27 for degradation as well as for protein subcellular localization. Mitogenic signaling pathways promote the cytoplasmic localization and subsequent degradation of p27 via phosphorylation of the protein at specific sites. This will increase the activity of nuclear cyclin E–CDK2 complex, resulting in the additional p27 phosphorylation and consequent degradation, and then a positive feedback loop for enhancement of cyclin E–CDK2 activity and cell cycle progression *(19)*.

In contrast to the ubiquitous expression of p21 and p27, p57 displays a tissue-restricted expression pattern suggesting a specialized role in cell cycle control. Different lines of evidence emphasize the central role of p57 in cell cycle regulation during embryonic development *(20)*.

While antiproliferative signals, as well as DNA damage, may activate *Cip/Kip* expression, thereby blocking cell cycle advance, mitogens act by inhibiting CDKIs and promoting cell proliferation. Phosphorylation of various amino acids controls many aspect of Cip/Kip protein biology, not only by modifying Cip/Kip proteins' affinity for specific cyclin–CDK complexes, but by impacting their stability and subcellular localization. The Cip/Kip proteins' phosphorylation induced by mitogenic signaling pathways promotes cytoplasmatic retention of p21 and p27. Different kinds of mitogens stimulate tyrosine kinase receptor RTKs, which in turn activate the phosphatidylinositol 3-kinase (PI3K) pathway. Akt/PKB, the important kinase activated downstream of mitogen-activated PI3K, phosphorylates p21, as well as p27, thereby causing them to be exported in the cytoplasm where they can no longer engage and inhibit cyclin–CDK complexes. In addition to promot Cip/Kip cytoplasmatic localization, protein phosphorylation also regulates its degradation. Cip/Kip proteins have different phosphorylation sites each of them responding to different regulatory pathways and tagging the proteins for a specific destiny.

1.4. Rb Protein: the "Master Switch" of Cell Cycle Progression

Cyclins and CDKs coordinate the cell's progression through the different phases of the cell cycle. By a well-articulated network of interactions, these complexes catch extracellular signals and translate them into a proliferative or resting cell behavior. Once the cell goes beyond the restriction point it is marked for a proliferative destiny, and this "decision" is carried out by switching pRB proteins from an active to an inactive form. pRb protein is therefore considered the "guardian" of the restriction point, and represents the main break at the G1-S transition. The pRb tumor suppressor protein is an essential component of the cell cycle machinery, integrating both positive and negative signals for cellular growth and proliferation with the transcription machinery.

pRB, the tumor suppressor product of the retinoblastoma susceptibility gene, was so named because mutation in both alleles of the *RB1* gene are involved in the pathogenesis of retinoblastoma. Consistently, considering its central role in cell cycle regulation, alterations in the pRb pathway have been found to be present in most, if not all, human tumors. pRb is one of the members of three structurally related proteins, pRB, p107, and p130, which together are often called "pocket proteins." Although these three proteins share many structural features and the ability to work as negative regulators of cell proliferation, they are not functionally and temporally redundant.

To appreciate the functional impact of pRB family proteins in cell cycle control, it is important to identify some of the structural features of these proteins. pRB can be divided into a number of functional regions, each of them affect different protein-binding capacities. The three pocket proteins consist of an amino-terminal domain, a pocket region composed of two conserved domains (A and B) separated by a spacer region, and a carboxy-terminal domain. The pocket domain, the most highly conserved in the three proteins, is responsible for pRB protein interaction with the transcription factors, cyclin and CDKs. The surface residues of pRB that are conserved across species and in human p107 and pRb2 proteins cluster in two regions: the LXCXE binding site in the B domain and the interface between the A and B domains.

The B domain is necessary for the binding with proteins containing a conserved LXCXE amino acid motif, such as the viral oncoproteins SV40 large T, adenovirus E1A, and human papillomavirus E7. Other proteins that interact with pRB and may utilize this motif include the D-type cyclins and a type 1 serine/threonine protein phosphatase (PP1), crucial for guaranting the functional integrity of the protein. The pocket region is also able to bind proteins lacking the typical LXCXE amino acid motif, the most important of which is a class of transcription factors known as E2Fs, through which pRB exerts its growth suppressive function. A dozen distinct phosphorylation sites have been found in the spacer region, all of which can be phosphorylated during the G1 phase. pRB phosphorylation is an important mechanism of control since it can influence pRb relationships with the interacting proteins. The carboxy-terminal domain contains the NLS (nuclear localization signal) sequences and, hence it is responsible for the nuclear localization of the proteins *(21,22)*.

pRB undergoes phosphorylation in concert with cell cycle progression. In G0, the protein is basically unphosphorylated; as the cell advances through G1, pRb becomes hypophosphorylated and, while proceeding through the restriction point, pRB acquires new phosphate groups shifting in an extremely phosphorylated form (hyperphosphorylated). pRb remains in its hyperphosphorylated state in the remaining phases of the cell cycle until, in the late M, all the phosphate groups are stripped by the protein phosphatase PP1, and its unphosphorylated form overlaps with the beginning of a new cell cycle. In its unphosphorylated form pRb is active and carries out its role as a tumor suppressor by inhibiting cell cycle progression. Phosphorylation inactivates pRB; thus, after the cell passes

Chapter 4 /Alterations in Cell Cycle Regulatory Genes in Breast Cancer

though the restriction point, the hyperphosphorylated form of the protein is no longer able to stop cell progression, and this condition is preserved until the cell completes the entire cycle. pRb phosphorylation is governed by the cyclin–kinase complexes, which work in coordination with each other during the different phases of the cell cycle.

pRb is activated near the end of G1 phase. When it is time for a cell to enter S phase, complexes of CDK and cyclin phosphorylate pRb, inhibiting its activity. The initial phosphorylation, performed by cyclin D/CDK4/6, is a necessary but not sufficient condition for the functional inactivation of pRB. A hyperphosphorylated form is required to allow the cell to pass through the restriction point. The complete inactivation of pRB is driven by cyclin E–CDK2 complexes consistently with the increase in *cyclin E* expression at this point. Once a cell advances through the R point, pRB is maintained in a hyperhosphorylated form by the remaining cyclin–CDK complexes acting throughout S, G2, and M phases, until it becomes once again dephosphorylated.

The ability of pRB to function as a negative cell growth regulator is due to its capacity to bind and sequester a group of transcription factors termed E2Fs, preventing them from interacting with the cell's transcription machinery. In this way, pRB can function as a transcriptional modulator that limits the expression of many genes necessary for cell cycle progression. E2F factors regulate the expression of many genes (E2F-responsive genes) encoding for proteins involved in cell cycle progression and DNA synthesis, such as cyclins E and *A, cdc2* (CDK1), *B-myb, dihydrofolate reductase, thymidine kinase*, and *DNA polymerase α (23)*.

When pRb, and its two cousins, p107 and p130, are in their unphosphorylated or hypophosphorylated state, they bind E2Fs; however, in its inactive hyperphosphorylated state they dissociate from E2Fs, leading them to transcribe their responsive genes.

In G0 and early G1, the inactive forms of pRB protein associate with E2Fs, preventing them to promote gene transcription; as such, E2F-dependent genes remain repressed during the G1 phase.

Rb phosphorylation by CDK4 and/or 6 partially relieves its inhibitory effect on E2F transcription factors and causes a conformational change in pRB, which exposes Ser 567, a CDK2 substrate. E2F then induces the transcription of *cyclin E*, which forms complexes with CDK2. These complexes further phosphorylate pRB, thereby completely eliminating its inhibitory effect on E2F. Once free of pRB control, E2F factors induce transcription of E2F-regulated genes, the products of which are necessary for the cell to advance from G1 to S phase *(24,25)*. Hence, the inactivation of pRB leads to an increase in *cyclin E* expression, which in turn drives further pRB inactivation. This relationship generates a self-reinforcing positive feedback that is triggered as the cell passes through the R point. The creation of a regulatory positive-feedback mechanism ensures the cell to move rapidly and irreversibly to complete the cell cycle.

The E2F family of transcription factors is composed of eight different members (E2F1-8), which cooperate with one another to regulate the cell cycle. Based on their function, the genes that belong to this family have been divided into two subgroups: activating (E2F-3a) and repressive (E2F 3b-5; 6-8). E2F activity is dependent upon its dimerizzation with DP proteins. Once assembled, E2F–DP complexes recognize and bind a sequence at the promoter's region of different genes, which seems to be highly conserved. E2F transcription factors may exert two opposite effects on transcription control. When bound to the promoter region of the genes in the absence of any associated pocket proteins, they can engage proteins that promote a transcriptionally active chromatin structure, such as histoneacetylase, and recruit RNA polymerase to initiate transcription. In cycle-arrested cell, the hypophosphorylated form of RB binds and blocks the transactivation domain of E2Fs repressing transcription. Simultaneously, the pocket protein is able to inhibit E2F-dependent transcription by recruiting chromatin remodeling factors to E2F responsive elements, including histone deacetylase and methylase and Swi/Snf complexes *(26)*, generating a transcriptionally unfitting chromatin structure (Fig. 5).

A variety of mitogenic signaling pathways control the cell cycle progression by converging in the phosphorylation of pRB. Extracellular "hints" are collected and elaborated by the cell cycle machinery, which, by acting upon the pRB pathway, turns the cell cycle progression on or off. Mitogenic imputes promote cell growth through signaling network that propagates from an extracellular setting, by the activation of specific membrane receptors, to the nucleus, where these signals are transduced to modulated gene expression patterns. The vast

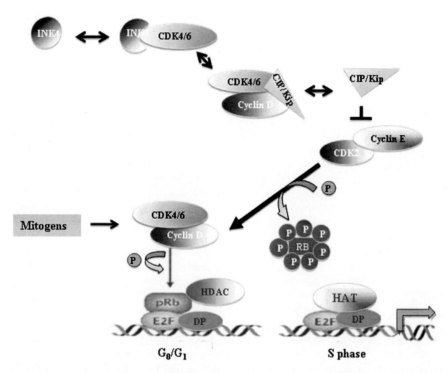

Fig. 5. Rb governs S phase entry. pRb functions as a negative cell growth regulator by binding to E2Fs transcription factor and thus repressing the transcription of genes required for S-phase entry. In G_0 and early G_1, hypophosphorylated Rb binds to E2F transcription factors and blocks their transcription domain. pRb represses transcription also by recruiting chromatin remodeling proteins on E2F-responsive elements such as HDAC that generate a transcriptional repressive state. In late Gl, Cyclin/CDK complexes phosphorylate Rb, which in its inactive hyperphosphorylated form dissociates from E2F, allowing the latter to transcribe E2F-responsive genes. In the absence of any associated pocket proteins, E2Fs can interact with transcription activating proteins such as HAT. This interaction generates a conformational transcriptionally active state that allows RNA polymerase to start the transcription of cell cycle E2F-dependent genes. Rb function is closely regulated by its phosphorylation status. Integrating positive and negative proliferation signals, cyclin/CDKs complexes and CDKIs coordinate Rb phosphorylation status and thus regulate the cell cycle progression.

Chapter 4 /Alterations in Cell Cycle Regulatory Genes in Breast Cancer

majority of mitogenic and antimitogenic signals influence pRB phosphorylation status, by activating or repressing cyclin D1 and cyclin E activity, respectively. The R point transition at late G1 represents a critical decision point in the life of a cell: however, once a cell has decided to trigger a proliferative destiny, passing the R point gateway, the remaining steps of the cell cycle proceed in a preprogrammed and automatic system *(27)*. The components that govern the G1/S transition are commonly deregulated in cancer cells, which by loosing cellular growth control acquire proliferative advantage. In addition to the molecules that control the G1/S transition, other proteins normally deregulated in cancer may be those involved in checkpoint in S and M phase. Their inactivation, however, does not seem to have direct consequence on uncontrolled cell proliferation, but may be ascribed to cancer cells' capacity to proliferate despite genetic abnormality. Cancer cells often gain the ability to proliferate abnormally despite genomic instability. Uncontrolled cancer cell growth may be attributable to the simultaneous inactivation of key components of apoptotic pathways and to the ability of damaged cells to bypass cell cycle control surveillance mechanisms *(28)*.

2. BREAST CANCER AND CELL CYCLE

2.1. *Cyclins D in Breast Cancer Pathogenesis*

Strong evidences designate *cyclin D1* amplification and overexpression as a driving force in human breast cancer. Cyclin D1 is the product of the *CCND1* gene located on chromosome 11q13, a region of the genome that is commonly amplified in a range of human carcinomas, including about 15% of breast cancers *(29)*. The further demonstration that cyclin D1 was overexpressed at the mRNA and protein level in up to 50% of primary breast cancers identified *cyclin D1* as one of the most commonly overexpressed oncogenes in breast cancer *(30)*. Since in many tumors this overexpression cannot be explined by an increase in gene copy numbers this suggests as the pathogenic activity of cyclin D1 can occur via additional mechanisms, including transcriptional and posttranscriptional deregulation due to primary activation of other oncogenic/mitogenic pathways. Deeper insight into the role of cyclins in mammary carcinomas has come from in vivo studies employing genetically manipulated mice. In Cyclin D1 transgenic mice mammary gland development is disturbed and it is followed by the formation of hyperplasia and adenocarcinoma. Tumors form in about 75% of the mice, but only after 18 months, suggesting that cyclin D1 is a relatively weak oncogene compared with activated c-neu, Ha-ras, and c-myc, which induce tumors at ~3, 6, and 11 months *(31)*. These observations suggest that additional events may be required so that cyclin D1 exerts its oncogenic potential. Furthermore, cyclin D1-deficent mice are resistant to mammary carcinomas induced by *c-neu/Her-2* and *ras* oncogenes, but not those induced by *c-myc* and *Wnt-1*, suggesting that cyclin D1 is implicated in the oncogenic actions of *c-neu/Her-2* and *ras*, while it is not necessary in *myc* and *Wnt-1*-induced mammary tumorigenesis *(32,33)*. Otherwise, cyclins D2 and D3 have been shown to be not required for normal mammary gland formation, while they are necessary as downstream targets of mammary oncogenes such as cmyc. Each of the three D-type cyclins is thus involved in the development of carcinoma, but each of them may be related to different cancer phenotypes. Overexpression of *cyclin D1* and D2 produces adenocarcinoma while cyclin D3 is predominantly linked to the squamous phenotype. Maybe these differences could be explained by assuming that the three D-type genes have similar effects on mammary epithelial cell proliferation but distinct effects on differentiation *(3)*. The oncogenic ability of cyclin D1 has been well documented by numerous studies. It has been shown that the induction of cyclin D1 in breast cancer cell lines shortens G1 and results in an increase in the number of cells processing through G1; consistently, entry into S phase is blocked by inhibiting *cyclin D1* expression *(34)*. It is widely accepted that cyclin D1 promotes cell proliferation essentially by the activation, as a regulatory subunit, of CDK4 and/or CDK6 and consequently by the phosphorylation of pRB. A noncatalytic function of cyclin D–CDK4/6 complexes lies in their ability to sequester CDK inhibitor proteins p21 and p27 from cyclin E–CDK2 complexes, working as additional mechanisms to promote cell progression. Since cyclin D1 acts as a key sensor and integrator of extracellular signals, its abundance is closely regulated in order to transduce pro- and antiproliferative stimuli in a growth response. Growth factors including EGF and IGF, hormones including estrogens, androgens, and retinoic acid, and different oncogenic signals including Ras, Src, ErbB2, and β-catenin induce cyclin D1 expression leading to the G1 transition trough cell cycle and cell proliferation *(33)*. On the contrary, TGFβ causes G1 arrest through the inhibition of *cyclin D1*. Alterations in each of these pathways lead to *cyclin D1* overexpression, providing a growth advantage to the tumor cells. Cyclin D1 plays a pivotal role in estrogen-induced breast cancer. The link between estrogen's mitogenic effect and cell cycle progression is well established, in particular at the G1/S transition where key effectors of estrogen action are c-Myc *(35)* and cyclin D1 *(36)*, which in turn converge in cyclin E–CDK2 complex activation and cell proliferation. While estrogen rapidly induces *cyclin D1* expression, antiestrogen has a converse inhibitory effect. Furthermore, abrogation of cyclin D1 activity by cyclin D1 antibodies or the CDK4 inhibitor p16INK4A blocks estrogen-induced G1-S phase progression, indicating that estrogen acts, at least in part, through upregulation of cyclin D1 expression. A well as c-Myc, cyclin D1 expression can mimic the effects of estrogen allowing cell cycle reentry in antiestrogen-arrested breast cancer cells *(37)*. Taken together, these data highlight the central role of cyclin D1 in breast cancer cell cycle control, and underline how its overexpression may provide a growth advantage to tumor cells and contribute toward resistance to endocrine therapy *(34)*.

Although *cyclin D1* overexpression might be expected to be associated with high proliferation rate, this is not the case in breast cancer, where cyclin overexpression is characteristic of slow-growing, more differentiated phenotypes. Since cyclin D1 is preferentially overexpressed in ER-positive cancer subgroups, it has given some directions to better understanding the CDK-pRB-independent oncogenic activity of this emblematic cyclin. Numerous experimental data have demonstrated that cyclin D1 neither correlates with Ki-67, a marker of cellular proliferation, nor with the levels of its downstream products. These records support the hypothesis of an alternative, CDK-independent mechanism by which *cyclin D1* contributes to breast cancer. Cyclin D1 can regulate the growth of estrogen-responsive tissues by activating the estrogen receptor (ER) in a ligand-independent fashion *(38)*. Cyclin D1 binds to the hormone-binding domain of ER and promotes association between ER and one of it coactivators, which in turn result in the upregulation of ER-mediated gene transcription *(39)*. Furthermore, the effect is not dependent on cyclin D1 cell cycle-associated function, given that this effect can be reproduced in cyclin D1 mutants unable to bind CDK4 or pRb. The finding that cyclin D1 can activate ER in a hormonally independent fashion may underline the oncogenic activity of cyclin D1 in breast cancer. In this way, cyclin D1 in a noncell cycle-associated fashion may drive all of the key mitogenic effects of estrogen in breast cancer epithelium. The ability of cyclin D1 to enhance the transcriptional activity of ER in a hormone-independent way is not inhibited by antiestrogens *(38)*. This suggests an additional mechanism by which *cyclin D1* overexpression could lead to persistent ER signaling and endocrine resistance. In recent years accumulating evidence suggests that cyclin D1 associates with and regulates the activity of several transcription factors (ER, androgen

Chapter 4 /Alterations in Cell Cycle Regulatory Genes in Breast Cancer

receptor, DMP1, Stat3) coactivators and corepressors that govern histone acetylation and chromatin remodeling proteins (C/EBPβ) *(33)*, strongly confirming the need to reevaluate the role of cyclin D1 in oncogenesis. The role of cyclin D1 as a phatogenetic breast cancer cornerstone may open the possibility for future anticyclin D1 therapies.

2.2. Cyclin E: A New Potential Prognostic Marker in Breast Cancer

Cyclin E together with cyclin D1 is the main activator of the G1/S transition. *Cyclin E* levels are strictly regulated during the cell cycle, with the level of proteins peaking during mid- to late-G1 phase, thus allowing the formation of active cyclin E–CDK2 complex. The accumulation of cyclin E and activation of cyclin E/CDK2 complex is a rate-limiting event for the G1/S transition. In addition to promoting S phase entry through pRB phosphorylation, cyclin E–CDK2 also phosphorylates a set of proteins more directly involved in DNA replication and components of prereplication complex *(40)*. Consistently with its critical role in normal cell homeostasis, cyclin E has been found deregulated in several malignancies, supporting its oncogenic properties. The oncogenic role of cyclin E has been suggested by studies on *cyclin E*-deficient cells, which are resistant to transformation induced by myc alone or in combination with ras, a dominant negative p53, or E1A, suggesting that cyclin E is a key component in oncogenic signaling *(41)*. *Cyclin E* overexpression induces premature S-phase entry *(42)* and genetic instability, a feature that leads the tumor to a more aggressive state. Cells unable to arrest in G1 potentially allow damaged cells to proceed into S-phase. These observations suggest that cyclin E deregulation may induce chromosomal instability by inappropriate initiation of DNA replication and centrosome duplication *(43)*. Although *cyclin E1* locus amplification is a relatively rare event in breast cancer, the protein product is overexpressed in ~40% of breast cancers as a series of isoforms ranging in size from 35 to 50 kDA *(44)*. Transgenic mouse models have allowed a better understanding of *cyclin E* role in normal mammary gland development and the consequence of its overexpression in breast cancer. *Cyclin E* overexpression in the mouse mammary gland results in adenocarcinoma formation in ~10% of female mice after 8–13 months, demonstrating that cyclin E as well as D-type cyclins are weak oncogenes in breast epithelium, able to induce carcinomas at low incidence and after long latency *(45)*. Constitutive overexpression of *cyclin E*, but not *cyclin D1* or *A*, in both immortalized rat embryo fibroblasts and human breast epithelial cells results in chromosome instability. Although *cyclin E*-overexpressing cells have normal centrosome numbers, they display an impaired S-phase progression, indicating that cyclin-E/CDK2 kinase activity in the G1/S-phase transition may be necessary for the maintenance of karyotypic stability *(46)*. Consistently with its role in cell cycle regulation, alterations in *cyclin E* expression are strongly related to loss of growth control in breast cancer, in which cyclin E level increases with increasing tumor stage and grade and appears to be associated with high proliferative rates in breast cancer *(3)*. Cyclin E, actually, is principally overexpressed in ER-negative breast cancer, representing a group of tumors poorly differentiated and with high histological grade. The association between *cyclin E* overexpression and proliferation markers suggests that the CDK-dependent function of cyclin E may be critical in mammary oncogenesis. In normal cells *cyclin E* expression is closely regulated: it is expressed when needed and then is rapidly degraded. In breast cancer, cyclin E deregulation may be just partially explained by *cyclin E* locus amplification. Moreover, alteration in protein degradation pathways *(47)* may perturb cyclin E periodicity, by increasing both protein stability and activity. Cyclin E activity can be deregulated indirectly by pRb inactivation, that cause premature induction of *cyclin E* transcription and thus an increase in the protein level *(48)*. The most significant cyclin E alteration is the posttranslational cleavage of the full-length cyclin E into low molecular weight (LMW) forms that are hyperactive compared to the full-length protein. Some breast cancer cell lines and human breast cancers express, in addition to the typical 50-kDa protein, a series of five LMW isoforms of cyclin E ranging in size from 49 to 34 kDa *(49)*. The LMW forms of cyclin E can phosphorylate substrates more effectively than normal cells, that only express the full-length form, and as a result tumor cells can progress through G1 and into S phase, bypassing the restriction point thus providing the tumor cells with an added growth advantage *(50)*. The LMW isoforms are unique to tumor cells and their expression strongly correlate with increasing stage and grade of breast cancer. These tumor-specific LMW forms of cyclin E predominantly derive from proteolytic processing of the full-length cyclin E. Two elastase-specific sites in the amino terminus of human cyclin E are cleaved to generate the LMW isoforms, holding an intact C-terminus domain. Porter and coworkers have exhaustively demonstrated that only tumors and not normally proliferating cells have the machinery to process cyclin E into its LMW forms. Firstly, this tumor-specific pattern cannot be explained as the result of overexpression or constitutive expression of *cyclin E*, since normal cells transfected with cyclin E under a strong constitutive promoter do not further process cyclin E into its LMW forms. Moreover, the proteolytic cleavage leading to LMW forms differs from the proteasome-dependent proteolysis of cyclin E. Although the destruction of cyclin E may be mediated through the ubiquitination-proteasome pathway, LMW forms of cyclin E do not seem to represent the intermediate proteolytic products of degradative machinery. Finally, the LMW forms of cyclin E are constitutively present in tumor cells and are not subject to cell cycle regulation *(50)*. The LMW forms of cyclin E keep pRb constitutively phosphorylated and are resistant to inhibition by p21 and p27. These events shorten G1 phase and, by increasing the rate of S-phase entry, increase tumorigenesis *(51)*. It has been postulated that the generation of cyclin E LMW forms may be due to an increase in elastase activity in tumors or in elastase inhibitor levels in normal. Therefore, it is possible to assume that inhibition of elastase in tumor cells may be a useful method for inhibit the effect of cyclin E and its LMW isoforms, without impacting normal cells. In fact, it has been demonstrated that specific elastase inhibitors not only repress the production of the LMW isoforms but also induce partial arrest of tumor cells in G1 phase without interfering with the cell cycle of normal breast epithelial cells. Given the well-accepted role of *elastase* in breast cancer metastasis *(52)*, the LMW forms of cyclin E could provide a novel target for metastatic breast cancer the treatment without harming normally proliferating cells in the body *(50)*.

2.3. Direct and Indirect Role of Rb in Breast Cancer

Cell cycle machinery is deregulated at multiple levels in breast cancer cells. The high incidence of abnormality in the RB pathway underscores how important the maintenance of cell cycle commitment is in tumor prevention. Cyclins, CDK inhibitors, and pRB are considered putative mammary oncogenes and tumor suppressor genes respectivelly, and their deregulation often impacts breast cancer clinical outcome and therapeutic response. RB is a key regulator of cell cycle and it is targeted for inactivation in the majority of human cancers. Multiple mechanisms can impact RB function compromising cell cycle checkpoints and contributing to tumor proliferation. Primary breast tumors negative for RB are commonly

Chapter 4 /Alterations in Cell Cycle Regulatory Genes in Breast Cancer 71

more proliferative and associated with poor disease outcome, suggesting that RB deficiency may impact with tumor progression and aggressiveness *(54)*. Loss of pRb function in mammary epithelium predisposes the tissue to malignant adenocarcinoma. However, analyzing of Rb inactivation performed on divergent mouse epithelial cell lines has demonstrated that alterations in Rb pathway is a common event in tumor initiation and progression but not a breast cancer exclusive feature. Despite the marked differences among divergent cell types, pRb inactivation causes a similar response, initially evoking increased proliferation and apoptosis and, ultimately, predisposing the tissue to tumorigenesis *(55)*. Given that RB function may be impared at different control levels it is not simple to evaluate the direct consequences of RB inactivation. RB exerts its tumor suppressive function mainly by inhibiting E2F-mediated transcription and its inactivation allows cells to commit itself in a replication cycle under nonproliferative conditions. Tumor samples lacking RB exhibit high levels of E2F downstream targets, among which there are several genes whose products have been independently correlated with poor outcome in breast cancer, including cyclin E and A, DNA replication factors, and chromatin remodeling enzyme *(54)*. RB functional status is directly and/or indirectly linked to breast cancer therapeutic response. Resistance to hormonal therapy in breast cancer is one of the major clinical problems and commonly involves alterations in the cell cycle regulatory components. Antiestrogen therapies antagonize the proliferative function of ER through a cascade of events that ultimately result in RB dephosphorylation and cell cycle arrest. Each condition that impairs RB function may be associated with resistance to antiestrogen therapy. RB knockdown cells not only fail to undergo cell cycle inhibition following hormone therapy but they also actively proliferate and become hormone independent. Conversely, in the context of DNA-damaging agents, RB deficiency results in increased sensitivity to these agents both in cell culture and xenograft models *(56)*. Loss of Rb protein produces a constitutive DNA replication signal that activate a p53-associated apoptotic response *(57)*. Moreover, DNA damage checkpoints are compromised in cells lacking RB, enabling DNA replication and cell cycle progression to proceed despite DNA lesions. RB deficiency may well sensitize cells to death following treatment with cytotoxic drugs, however may have the deleterious effect to simultaneously facilitate mutagenesis in a fraction of cells surviving such treatment *(54)*. In this scenario it is a reasonable wonder if the augmented drug sensitivity may represent a durable response or may be linked to a high risk for aggressive recurrence.

2.4. Alterations in CDK Inhibitor Pathways (Ckis): Several Strategies in Breast Cancer

As negative regulators of the cell cycle, both INK4 and Cip/Kip family members are potential tumor suppressor genes. Aberrant expression or altered activity of distinct CKIs results in cells escaping from cell cycle control leading to malignant transformation. The cyclin–CDK inhibitors of the Cip/Kip family p21, p27, and p57 halt the cell cycle in G_1 phase by binding to and inactivating cyclin–CDK complexes. In addition to regulate cell cycle progression, Cip/Kip proteins play an important role in apoptosis, transcriptional regulation, cell fate determination, cell migration, and cytoskeletal dynamics. A complex phosphorylation network modulates Cip/Kip proteins function by altering their subcellular localization, protein–protein interactions, and stability *(58)*. Alterations at each point of this network may impair the proteins' function and lead to uncontrolled cell proliferation. The majority of normal epithelial tissues, including breast, prostate, lung, and ovary, express high levels of nuclear p27 protein, especially in the terminally differentiated layers. In contrast, p27 is virtually undetectable in proliferating cells *(59)*. p27 null mice display an overall increased body size and multiple organ hyperplasia, revealing the importance of p27 in limiting growth *(60)*. A variable loss of p27 protein has been shown in many human tumors. Indeed, the loss of heterozygosity of 12p13 locus that encompass the *p27* gene is uncommon in human tumors, including breast cancer. However, p27 function is impaired in a majority of human cancers through accelerated proteolysis, sequestration by other proteins, and an imbalance in the mechanisms that regulate protein nuclear import and export. The important role of p27 as a mammary tumor suppressor gene has been confirmed by studies demonstrating that mice lacking p27 develop pituitary adenocarcinoma *(61)*. Human breast cancer cells often exhibit reduced p27 expression and or/and mislocalization of the protein to the cytosol, indicating that p27 function may be impaired both by enhancing protein degradation and keeping the protein away from its targets. p27 cytoplasmic mislocalization is seen in 41% of primary human breast cancers in conjunction with Akt activation and is correlated with a poor prognosis *(62)*. The p27 NLS contains a protein kinase B (PKB)/Akt-consensus site at threonine 157, and p27 phosphorylation by Akt impairs its nuclear import. Oncogenic activation of the PI3K/PKB pathway and the PKB-dependent phosphorylation of p27 is probably one of the mechanisms accountable for p27 cytoplasmic mislocalization of p27 in human breast cancers and can be coupled with an aggressive tumor phenotype *(63,64)*. Her2 overexpresson is observed in up to 30% of primary breast cancers and is associated with increased tumor invasiveness and a poor patient outcome. Since primary breast cancers overexpressing Her2 exhibit decreased p27 concentration. The oncogenic activity of Herb2 seems to rely on its ability to promote p27 degradation. It has been demonstrated that Her2/ErbB2 can activate p27 proteolysis in a MEK/MAPK-dependent manner *(65)*. *Her2/ErbB2* overexpression can also upregulate *c-Myc* and D-type cyclins, and this might facilitate p27 sequestration in cyclin D–CDK complexes and result in an increase in cyclin E–CDK2 activity *(66)*. Her2/ErbB2 promote cell cycle and tumor progression by hampering p27 activity both by enhancing its degradation and by reducing its ability to bind and inhibit its targets. The anti-Her2 antibody trastuzumab represents a frontline therapy for patient with metastatic breast cancer that overexpressed Her2. The induction of the p27 protein is one of the principal ways by which Her2-targeting antibodies operate. Anti-Her2 antibodies affect at least six pathways that work in concert to maximize the expression and the inhibitory effect of p27, which leads to cell cycle arrest and growth inhibition *(67)*, by antagonizing the Her2 proliferative signal. Interestingly, trastuzumab resistance may be associated with decreased p27 levels and may be susceptible to treatments that induce p27 expression *(68)*. p27 is also an independent predictor for responsiveness to endocrine therapy. In patients treated with tamoxifen, high levels of p27 expression strongly associate with improved overall and disease-free survival. An unfavorable outcome is conversely associated with low expression or improper cytoplasmatic localization of p27 *(69)*. p21 is implicated in the mechanisms of cell cycle arrest that allow DNA repair, cell differentiation, and apoptosis. p21 is a downstream effector of different tumor suppressors, including p53, BRCA1, WT1, and TGF-β. The main defined activity of p21 is in the p53 pathway, where it functions as a key mediator of p53-dependent cell cycle arrest. In response to DNA damaging agents, wild-type p53 induces p21 expression, which blocks cell cycle progression at the G1/S transition by inhibiting CDK2 and CDK4/6 activity. p21's ability to inhibit cell proliferation may contribute to its tumor suppressor function. Therefore, it is not surprising that in addition to p21 activation by several tumor suppressor genes, a number of oncogenes repress p21 leading to cell growth and tumorigenesis when upregulated. p21 abundance and functionality are controlled at transcriptional level as well as at posttranscriptional one through proteosomal degradation and protein subcellular localization.

Chapter 4 / Alterations in Cell Cycle Regulatory Genes in Breast Cancer

Although p21 does not have a direct role in breast cancer induction, it is able to strengthen the oncogenic potential of several mammary oncogenes in a cellular context-dependent manner. p21 null mice do not develop mammary cancers, although they display accelerated mammary tumor development after expression of Ras but not Myc. A p21-null background decreases the incidence of Myc-induced tumors, which is accompanied by decreased proliferation and reduced CDK activity; in contrast, p21 deficiency has opposite effects on Ras-induced tumors in which p21 increases cell proliferation and CDK activity. p21 can behave as a context-dependent inhibitor or promoter of the cell cycle in mammary epithelium (70).

The prognostic and predictive implication of p21 in breast cancer is not clear given its functional interaction with known prognostic factors, such as p53 and Her2, which may independently affect breast cancer outcome. The cellular localization of p21 has been proposed to be critical for the regulation of p21 function. The cell growth-inhibitory activity of p21 is strongly correlated with its nuclear localization. However, p21 can also localize in the cytoplasm, where it exhibits an important role in protecting cells from apoptosis by binding and inhibiting the apoptosis signal-regulating kinase 1 (17). The subcellular localization of p21, rather than overall expression levels, may be a better marker of therapeutic response and treatment outcome. In Her2-overexpressing breast cancer, p21 is transcriptionally upregulated and dislocated to the cytoplasm through a mechanism whereby Akt binds and phosphorylates p21 in its NLS. Cytoplasmic localization of p21 in combination with Her2 overexpression confers poor outcome. Xia and coworkers demonstrated that the 5-year survival rate of patients with low HER2/neu and negative/nuclear p21 was 79%, in contrast to only 16% in those patients with high HER2/neu and cytoplasmic p21. This novel combination not only provides a better prognostic prediction than any individual clinicopathological or biological marker, but also indicates that targeting only one molecule, such as HER2/neu, could be insufficient. Novel therapeutic agents that target phosphorylation/cytoplasmic localization of p21 may also contribute to optimal treatment of breast cancer patients (71).

The INK4/ARF locus encodes the p15(INK4B), p16(INK4A), and p14(ARF) tumor suppressor proteins whose loss of function is associated with the pathogenesis of many human cancers. Inactivation of INK4a/ARF may occur through mutation, gene silencing by promoter methylation and deletion. p16INK4a inhibits the G1 cyclin D-dependent kinases, CDK4 and CDK6, which phosphorylate pRb and facilitate entry into S phase.

The fact that p16INK4a can block G1-S-phase progression and that mutant p16INK4a proteins are nonfunctional in cell cycle arrest or CDK inhibition suggests that p16INK4a plays an important role in negative growth control. The p16INK4a knockout mouse model has provided clear and direct evidence that p16INK4a deficiency facilitates tumor development, confirming the tumor suppressive function of the gene (72).

p16Ink4a is deleted in almost 30% of breast cancer cell lines are deleted and p16Ink4a promoter methylation, occurs in 30% of human breast cancers. Unlike the situation in cancer cell lines, homozygous deletion and mutation in INK4a are very rarely observed in primary breast cancer, where p16 deregulation occurs frequently though overexpression of p16INK4a and de novo INK4a methylation. The reciprocal relation linking p16 and Rb complicates the possibility to assign a prognostic value for p16 expression. Numerous evidences suggest that p16INK4a and pRb expression is reciprocally counterbalanced. The absence of p16INK4a expression is seen predominantly in cells that retain wild-type RB(73); however, p16INK4a is overexpressed in cancer cell lines and tumors in which pRb is notfunctional (74).

Consistently with its tumor suppressive function, p16INK4a inactivation is associated with a more aggressive phenotype and worse prognosis in a wide range of neoplasms, in contrast with breast cancer in which high expression of p16 is associated with poor prognosis (75).

REFERENCES

1. Hall PA, Watt FM. Stem cells: the generation and maintenance of cellular diversity. Development 1989;106:619–633.
2. Morgan DO. Principles of CDK regulation. Nature 1995;374:131–134.
3. Sutherland RL, Musgrove EA. Cyclins and breast cancer. J Mammary Gland Biol Neoplasia 2004;9:95–104.
4. Miele L. The biology of cyclins and cyclin-dependent protein kinases: an introduction. Methods Mol Biol 2004;285:3–21.
5. Coqueret O. Linking cyclins to transcriptional control. Gene 2002;299:35–55.
6. Diehl JA, Cheng M, Roussel MF, Sherr CJ. Glycogen synthase kinase-3beta regulates cyclin D1 proteolysis and subcellular localization. Genes Dev 1998;12:3499–3511.
7. Diehl JA, Zindy F, Sherr CJ. Inhibition of cyclin D1 phosphorylation on threonine-286 prevents its rapid degradation via the ubiquitin-proteasome pathway. Genes Dev 1997;11:957–972.
8. Sherr CJ, Roberts JM. CDK inhibitors: positive and negative regulators of G1-phase progression. Genes Dev 1999;13:1501–1512.
9. Russo AA, Tong L, Lee J, Jeffrey PD, Pavletich NP. Structural basis for inhibition of the cyclin-dependent kinase Cdk6 by the tumour suppressor p16INK4a. Nature 1998;395:237–243.
10. Sherr CJ. The INK4a/ARF network in tumour suppression. Nat Rev Mol Cell Biol 2001;2: 731–737.
11. Reynisdottir I, Polyak K, Iavarone A, Massague J. Kip/Cip and Ink4 Cdk inhibitors cooperate to induce cell cycle arrest in response to TGF-$\beta\beta$. Genes Dev 1995;9:1831–1845.
12. Zindy F, Quelle DE, Roussel MF, Sherr CJ. Expression of the p16INK4a tumor suppressor versus other INK4 family members during mouse development and aging. Oncogene 1997;15:203–211.
13. Weinberg R. pRb and control of cell cycle. In: Weinberg RA, ed. The Biology of Cancer. Garland Science, Taylor and Francis Group, Abingdon, UK, 2007:255–306.
14. Li R, Waga S, Hannon GJ, Beach D, Stillman B. Differential effects by the p21 CDK inhibitor on PCNA-dependent DNA replication and repair. Nature 1994;371:534–537.
15. El-Deiry WS, Tokino T, Velculescu VE, Levy DB, Parsons R, Trent JM, Lin D, Mercer WE, Kinzler KW, Vogelstein B. *WAF1*, a potential mediator of p53 tumor suppression. Cell 1993;75:817–825.
16. Polyak K, Kato J, Solomon MJ, Sherr CJ, Massague J, Roberts JK, Koff A. p27Kip1, a cyclin-Cdk inhibitor, links transforming growth factor-beta and contact inhibition to cell cycle arrest. Genes Dev 1994;8:9–22.
17. Zafonte BT, Hulit J, Amanatullah DF, Albanese C, Wang C, Rosen E, Reutens A, Sparano JA, Lisanti MP, Pestell RG. Cell-cycle dysregulation in breast cancer: breast cancer therapies targeting the cell cycle. Front Biosci 2000;5:938–961.
18. Colozza M, Azambuja E, Cardoso F, Sotiriou C, Larsimont D, Piccart MJ. Proliferative markers as prognostic and predictive tools in early breast cancer: where are we now? Ann Oncol 2005;16:1723–1739.
19. Caldon CE, Daly RJ, Sutherland RL, Musgrove EA. Cell cycle control in breast cancer cells. J Cell Biochem 2006;97:261–274.
20. Matsuoka S, Edwards MC, Bai C, Parker S, Zhang P, Baldini A, Harper JW, Elledge SJ. p57KIP2, a structurally distinct member of the p21CIP1 Cdk inhibitor family, is a candidate tumor suppressor gene. Genes Dev 1995;9:650–662.
21. Tamrakar S, Rubin E, Ludlow JW. Role of pRB dephosphorylation in cell cycle regulation. Front Biosci 2000;5:121–137.
22. Claudio PP, Tonini T, Giordano A. The retinoblastoma family: twins or distant cousins? Genome Biol 2002;3:3012.1–3012.1.
23. Polager S, Kalma Y, Berkovich E, Ginsberg D. E2Fs up-regulate expression of genes involved in DNA replication, DNA repair and mitosis. Oncogene 2002;21:437–446.
24. Harbour JW, Dean DC. The Rb/E2F pathway: expanding roles and emerging paradigms. Genes Dev 2000;14:2393–2409.
25. Harbour JW, Dean DC. Rb function in cell-cycle regulation and apoptosis. Nat Cell Biol 2000;2:65–67.

Chapter 4 / Alterations in Cell Cycle Regulatory Genes in Breast Cancer

26. Harbour JW, Dean DC. Chromatin remodeling and Rb activity. Curr Opin Cell Biol 2000;12:685–689.
27. Pardee AB. G1 events and regulation of cell proliferation. Science 1989;246:603–608.
28. Malumbres M, Barbacid M. To cycle or not to cycle: a critical decision in cancer. Nat Rev Cancer 2001;1:222–231.
29. Ormandy CJ, Musgrove EA, Hui R, Daly RJ, Sutherland RL. Cyclin D1, EMS1 and 11q13 amplification in breast cancer. Breast Cancer Res Treat 2003;78:323–335.
30. Alle KM, Henshall SM, Field AS, Sutherland RL. Cyclin D1 protein is overexpressed in hyperplasia and intraductal carcinoma of the breast. Clin Cancer Res 1998;4:847–854.
31. Muller WJ, Sinn E, Pattengale PK, Wallace R, Leder P. Single-step induction of mammary adenocarcinoma in transgenic mice bearing the activated c-neu oncogene. Cell 1988;54:105–115.
32. Sinn E, Muller WJ, Pattengale PK, Tepler I, Wallace R, Leder P. Coexpression of *MMTV/v-Ha-ras* and *MMTV/c-myc* genes in transgenic mice: synergistic action of oncogenes in vivo. Cell 1987;49:465–475.
33. Fu M, Wang C, Li Z, Sakamaki T, Pestell RG. Cyclin D1: normal and abnormal functions. Endocrinology 2004;145:5439–5447.
34. Musgrove EA, Lee CS, Buckley MF, Sutherland RL. Cyclin D1 induction in breast cancer cells shortens G1 and is sufficient for cells arrested in G1 to complete the cell cycle. Proc Natl Acad Sci USA 1994;91:8022–8026.
35. Dubik D, Dembinski TC, Shiu RP. Stimulation of c-myc oncogene expression associated with estrogen-induced proliferation of human breast cancer cells. Cancer Res 1987;47:6517–6521.
36. Said TK, Conneely OM, Medina D, O'Malley BW, Lydon JP. Progesterone, in addition to estrogen, induces cyclin D1 expression in the murine mammary epithelial cell, in vivo. Endocrinology 1997;138:3933–3939.
37. Butt AJ, McNeil CM, Musgrove EA, Sutherland RL. Downstream targets of growth factor and oestrogen signalling and endocrine resistance: the potential roles of c-Myc, cyclin D1 and cyclin E. Endocr Relat Cancer 2005;12:S47–S59.
38. Zwijsen RML, Wientjens E, Klompmaker R, van der Sman J, Bernards R, Michalides RJ. CDK-independent activation of estrogen receptor by cyclin D1. Cell 1997;88:405–415.
39. Roy PG, Thompson AM. Cyclin D1 and breast cancer. Breast 2006;15:718–727.
40. Hwang HC, Clurman BE. Cyclin E in normal and neoplastic cell cycles. Oncogene 2005;24:2776–2786.
41. Geng Y, Yu Q, Sicinska E, Das M, Schneider JE, Bhattacharya S, Rideout WM, Bronson RT, Gardner H, Sicinski P. Cyclin E ablation in the mouse. Cell 2003;114:431–443.
42. Ohtsubo M, Theodoras AM, Schumacher J, Roberts JM, Pagano M. Human cyclin E, a nuclear protein essential for the G1-to-S phase transition. Mol Cell Biol 1995;15:2612–2624.
43. Berglund P, Landberg G. Cyclin E overexpression reduces infiltrative growth in breast cancer: yet another link between proliferation control and tumor invasion. Cell Cycle 2006;5:606–609.
44. Keyomarsi K, Conte D Jr, Toyofuku W, Fox MP. Deregulation of cyclin E in breast cancer. Oncogene 1995;11:941–950.
45. Bortner DM, Rosenberg MP. Induction of mammary gland hyperplasia and carcinomas in transgenic mice expressing human cyclin E. Mol Cell Biol 1997;17:453–459.
46. Spruck CH, Won KA, Reed SI. Deregulated cyclin E induces chromosome instability. Nature 1999;401:297–300.
47. Strohmaier H, Spruck CH, Kaiser P, Won K, Sangfelt O, Reed SI. Human F-box protein hCdc4 targets cyclin E for proteolysis and is mutated in a breast cancer cell line. Nature 2001;413:316–322.
48. Herrera RE, Sah VP, Williams BO, Mäkelä TP, Weinberg RA, Jacks T. Altered cell cycle kinetics, gene expression, and G1 restriction point regulation in Rb-deficient fibroblasts. Mol Cell Biol 1996;16:2402–2407.
49. Akli S, Keyomarsi K. Cyclin E and its low molecular weight forms in human cancer and as targets for cancer therapy. Cancer Biol Ther 2003;2:S38–S47.
50. Porter DC, Zhang N, Danes C, McGahren MJ, Harwell RM, Faruki S, Keyomarsi K. Tumor-specific proteolytic processing of cyclin E generates hyper-active lower-molecular-weight forms. Mol Cell Biol 2001;21:6254–6269.

51. Barton MC, Akli S, Keyomarsi K. Deregulation of Cyclin E meets dysfunction in p53: closing the escape hatch on breast cancer. J Cell Physiol 2006;209:686–694.
52. Yamahista JI, Ogawa M, Ikel S, Omachi H, Yamshita SI, Saishoji T, Nomura K, Sato H. Production of immunoreactive polymorphonuclear leucocyte elastase in the progression of human breast cancer. Br J Cancer 1994;69:72–76.
53. Pietiläinen T, Lipponen P, Aaltomaa S, Eskelinen M, Kosma VM, Syrjänen K. Expression of retinoblastoma gene protein (Rb) in breast cancer as related to established prognostic factors and survival. Eur J Cancer 1995;31:329–333.
54. Bosco E, Knudsen ES. RB in breast cancer: at the crossroads of tumorigenesis and treatment. Cell Cycle 2007;6:667–671.
55. Simin K, Wu H, Lu L, Pinkel D, Albertson D, Cardiff RD, Van Dyke T. pRb inactivation in mammary cells reveals common mechanisms for tumor initiation and progression in divergent epithelia. PLoS Biol 2004;2(2):E22.
56. Bosco EE, Wang Y, Xu H, Zilfou JT, Knudsen KE, Aronow BJ, Lowe SW, Knudsen ES. The retinoblastoma tumor suppressor modifies the therapeutic response of breast cancer. J Clin Invest 2007;117:218–228.
57. Almasan A, Yin Y, Kelly RE, Lee EY, Bradley A, Li W, Bertino JR, Wahl GM. Deficiency of retinoblastoma protein leads to inappropriate S-phase entry, activation of E2F-responsive genes, and apoptosis. Proc Natl Acad Sci USA 1995;92:5436–5440.
58. Besson A, Dowdy SF, Roberts JM. CDK inhibitors: cell cycle regulators and beyond. Dev Cell 2008;14:159–169.
59. Chiarle R, Pagano M, Inghirami G.The cyclin dependent kinase inhibitor p27 and its prognostic role in breast cancer. Breast Cancer Res 2001;3:91–94.
60. Fero ML, Rivkin M, Tasch M, Porter P, Carow CE, Firpo E, Polyak K, Tsai LH, Broudy V, Perlmutter RM, Kaushansky K, Roberts JM. A syndrome of multiorgan hyperplasia with features of gigantism, tumorigenesis, and female sterility in p27(Kip1)-deficient mice. Cell 1996;85:733–744.
61. Musgrove EA, Davison EA, Ormandy CJ. Role of the CDK inhibitor p27 (Kip1) in mammary development and carcinogenesis: insights from knockout mice. J Mammary Gland Biol Neoplasia 2004;9:55–66.
62. Alkarain A, Jordan R, Slingerland J. p27 deregulation in breast cancer: prognostic significance and implications for therapy. J Mammary Gland Biol Neoplasia 2004;9:67–80.
63. Liang J, Zubovitz J, Petrocelli T, Kotchetkov R, Connor MK, Han K, Lee JH, Ciarallo S, Catzavelos C, Beniston R, Franssen E, Slingerland JM. PKB/Akt phosphorylates p27, impairs nuclear import of p27 and opposes p27-mediated G1 arrest. Nat Med 2002;8:1153–1160.
64. Shin I, Yakes FM, Rojo F, Shin NY, Bakin AV, Baselga J, Arteaga CL. PKB/Akt mediates cell-cycle progression by phosphorylation of p27Kip1 at threonine 157 and modulation of its cellular localization. Nat Med 2002;8:1145–1152.
65. Lenferink AE, Busse D, Flanagan WM, Yakes FM, Arteaga CL. ErbB2/neu kinase modulates cellular p27Kip1 and cyclin D1 through multiple signaling pathways. Cancer Res 2001;61:6583–6591.
66. Lane HA, Beuvink I, Motoyama AB, Daly JM, Neve RM, Hynes NE. ErbB2 potentiates breast tumor proliferation through modulation of p27Kip1-Cdk2 complex formation receptor overexpression does not determine growth dependency. Mol Cell Biol 2000;20:3210–3223.
67. Le XF, Pruefer F, Bast RC Jr. HER2-targeting antibodies modulate the cyclin-dependent kinase inhibitor p27Kip1 via multiple signaling pathways. Cell Cycle 2005;4(1):87–95.
68. Esteva FJ, Sahin AA, Smith TL, Yang Y, Pusztai L, Nahta R, Buchholz TA, Buzdar AU, Hortobagyi GN, Bacus SS. Prognostic significance of phosphorylated P38 mitogen-activated protein kinase and HER-2 expression in lymph node-positive breast carcinoma. Cancer 2004;100:499–506.
69. Pohl G, Rudas M, Dietze O, Lax S, Markis E, Pirker R, Zielinski CC, Hausmaninger H, Kubista E, Samonigg H, Jakesz R, Filipits M. High p27Kip1 expression predicts superior relapse-free and overall survival for premenopausal women with early-stage breast cancer receiving adjuvant treatment with tamoxifen plus goserelin. J Clin Oncol 2003;21:3594–3600.
70. Bearss DJ, Lee RJ, Troyer DA, Pestell RG, Windle JJ. Differential effects of p21(WAF1/CIP1) deficiency on MMTV-ras and MMTV-myc mammary tumor properties. Cancer Res 2002;62:2077–2084.
71. Xia W, Chen JS, Zhou X, Sun PR, Lee DF, Liao Y, Zhou BP, Hung MC. Phosphorylation/cytoplasmic localization of p21Cip1/WAF1 is associated with HER2/neu overexpression and provides a novel

combination predictor for poor prognosis in breast cancer patients. Clin Cancer Res 2004;10:3815–3824.

72. D'Amico M, Wu K, Di Vizio D, Reutens AT, Stahl M, Fu M, Albanese C, Russell RG, Muller WJ, White M, Negassa A, Lee HW, DePinho RA, Pestell RG. The role of Ink4a/Arf in ErbB2 mammary gland tumorigenesis. Cancer Res 2003;63:3395–3402.

73. Otterson GA, Kratzke RA, Coxon A, Kim YW, Kaye FJ. Absence of p16INK4a protein is restricted to the subset of lung cancer lines that retains wild type RB. Oncogene 1994;9:3375–3378.

74. Parry D, Bates S, Mann DJ, Peters G. Lack of cyclin D–Cdk complexes in Rb-negative cells correlates with high levels of p16INK4/MTS1 tumour suppressor gene product. EMBO J 1995;14:503–511.

75. Hui R, Macmillan RD, Kenny FS, Musgrove EA, Blamey RW, Nicholson RI, Robertson JF, Sutherland RL. *INK4a* gene expression and methylation in primary breast cancer: overexpression of p16INK4a messenger RNA is a marker of poor prognosis. Clin Cancer Res 2000;6(7):2777–2787.

5 Neuregulins in the Nucleus

Carol M. McClelland and William J. Gullick

SUMMARY

The neuregulins are a subset of the ligands for the epidermal growth factor receptor family of receptors. They can bind to these receptors and evoke a range of cellular responses. Some of the neuregulins have however been found in the cell nucleus associated with nucleoli and intra-chromatin granules. This brief review summarises the data for nuclear expression obtained from observations on normal and malignant tissues and the various laboratory experiments conducted to explore the system. Finally, we discuss the possible functions that could result from intra-nuclear expression of these molecules.

Key Words: Neuregulin; Heregulin; NRG; Growth factor; Growth factor receptor; Breast cancer

1. INTRODUCTION

Cells need to both send and receive signals that instruct them or their neighbours in an organised tissue when to grow and to divide. One system involved in these processes is the peptide growth factors and their receptors, which possess ligand-regulated tyrosine kinase activity. A subclass of these is the epidermal growth factor (EGF) family of four receptors and their 11 ligands. In the conventional signalling pathway membrane bound or secreted ligands interact with the extracellular domain of the appropriate growth factor receptor(s) on the plasma cell membrane, causing receptor dimerisation (and oligomerisation), thereby inducing increased receptor phosphorylation and transducing signals to the nucleus (and other sites such as the cytoskeleton) via a cascade of second messengers. This results in transcription factors mediating altered gene expression leading to many diverse events including differentiation, proliferation, cell migration, or apoptosis.

From: *Current Clinical Oncology: Breast Cancer in the Post-Genomic Era,*
Edited by: A. Giordano and N. Normanno, DOI: 10.1007/978-1-60327-945-1_5,
© Humana Press, a part of Springer Science + Business Media, LLC 2009

There is now, however, much evidence that some of the ligands are present unexpectedly within the nucleus of cells in tissues. This evidence involves not just the members of the EGF family of related ligands but many others from a variety of signalling systems. Perhaps the best studied are the fibroblast growth factors (FGFs), which have been extensively investigated by Olsnes and coworkers for many years. Excellent reviews covering this large body of work have appeared (1–3). Other molecules from different families with growth regulatory activity reported in the nucleus are platelet derived growth factor (4), interferon γ, vascular endothelial growth factor, parathyroid hormone-related protein, prolactin, growth hormone (5,6), hepatoma growth factor and several of the cytokines (1).

All proteins are synthesised on ribosomes and so originate in the cytoplasm. Some leave this compartment by exocytosis and are released into the interstitial space as soluble proteins while others are membrane incorporated molecules, which, following transport to the plasma cell membrane, can be released by regulated proteolytic cleavage (7). When these released ligands bind to receptors at the cell surface they may be internalised, and in some cases escape the alternatives of degradation or recycling to the cell exterior by exiting from these pathways and gaining access to the cytoplasm. The pathway undertaken by the FGFs involves receptor binding and internalisation in endosomes but, as these become acidified, the ligands apparently unfold and traverse the endosomal membrane reaching the cytoplasmic compartment (1,2). Others synthesised in the cytoplasm may simply remain there. The two alternatives are therefore very distinct and involve quite different systems and interactions.

This review concerns the intranuclear localisation of (at least) one of the splice variants of the *NRG1* gene and some less extensive observations on the *NRG2, 3* and *4* gene products. The EGF family consists of the four receptors (EGFR/HER1/ErbB1, HER2/ErbB2, HER3/ErbB3 and HER4/ErbB4) and the 11 known ligands (EGF, TGF alpha, heparin binding-EGF, Amphiregulin, Betacellulin, Epiregulin, Epigen and the four NRG genes). Several of these ligands have been reported to be found, on occasions, inside the nucleus including EGF itself (3), Betacellulin (8) and both the human Amphiregulin protein (9) and its rat equivalent called Schwannoma derived growth factor (10,11). They could be bound to membrane-associated proteins or be present complexed with intranuclear protein ensembles such as nucleoli and the variety of, to date rather poorly molecularly characterised, systems such as splicosomes, and various intranuclear entities such as PML bodies (see https://npd.hgu.mrc. ac.uk/index.html for the Nuclear Protein Database) or, finally, they may be genuinely soluble in the nucleoplasm.

2. OBSERVATIONS ON NRG IN THE NUCLEUS

The neuregulins are ligands for the HER3/ErbB3 and HER4/ErbB4 receptors, which, when present extracellularly, may bind to these receptors and elicit a number of intracellular activities (12). Four members of the family have so far been identified definitively: these are NRG 1, 2, 3 and 4. Other candidate ligands such a Neuroglycan C (13) or the Tomoregulins (14) have not, as yet, been studied in great detail and more data on their behaviour is required before they can be accepted as bona fide members of the NRG family. NRGs 1–4 are signalling proteins involved in many organ systems in normal tissues including the breast, heart and nervous system. Each gene produces multiple splice variants of a considerable variety of structures (for NRG 1 reviewed by (12) and for NRG 2, 3 and 4 (7)). Signalling by NRGs leads to cell responses including migration, differentiation, stimulation or inhibition of proliferation, apoptosis and adhesion. Neuregulins are also expressed in many forms of cancer including breast, colon, head and neck, lung, ovarian, skin and prostate (15).

Some of the neuregulins have been found in cell nuclei. The first observation reported in the literature was that radioactively labelled NRG1, when administered to cultured breast cancer cells, was taken up and shown to accumulate within the nucleus where it was reported to promote induction of expression and nuclear translocation of the proto-oncogene *c-myc* *(16)*. Other evidence supporting this finding has since accumulated using immunohistochemical staining. The neuregulin precursor was shown to localise to the nucleus in papillary thyroid carcinoma but not in normal thyroid tissue *(17)*. Human endometrial stromal cells have been shown to occasionally display staining in the nucleus with antibodies against NRG1α and β *(8)*. Immunohistochemical staining of DCIS of the breast showed rather dramatic nuclear expression of NRG1α, NRG1β and NRG3 in 40–50% of the cases examined *(18)* (Fig. 1a). It should be noted, however, that immunohistochemical staining of invasive breast cancers using the same antibodies for NRG1α and β, NRG2α and β, NRG3 and NRG4 gave little evidence of nuclear staining *(19)*. An antibody specific to the A1 isoform of NRG4 showed intense staining of the nucleus in rat salivary gland tissue *(20)* but NRG4 did not show nuclear staining in prostate cancer cases studied *(20)*. Clearly these results are fragmentary and a systematic study of the subcellular localisation of the main isoforms of the products of the four NRG genes should be undertaken in both normal and malignant human tissue to fully catalogue the incidence of intranuclear expression. Not only will this complete the data but it may generate hypotheses as to why some tissue types show intranuclear expression and others do not.

3. NRG EXPERIMENTS

While observations of NRGs in the nucleus have been made in normal and malignant tissues what experimental evidence is available to confirm these observations? And does any of this information give insight into why NRGs are found in the nucleus and what possible consequences might this have in diseases such as breast cancer? This information may be of some practical value as soluble NRG1 has, for instance, been shown to be associated with breast cancer progression *(21)* and is a key promoter of breast cancer tumorigenicity and metastasis independently of erbB-2 overexpression *(22)*. Indeed blocking the expression of NRG1 suppresses the aggressive phenotype of a breast cancer cell line and *in vivo* reduces tumour formation, size and halts metastasis *(22)*.

NRG1β3 one of at least 15 different isoforms of NRG1, which lacks a transmembrane domain, is not secreted from the cell but has a putative nuclear localization sequence (NLS) at its N-terminus *(23)*. Immunohistochemical staining in DCIS of the breast using antibodies specific for NRG1β showed nuclear localisation *(18)* but this technique cannot resolve which structures in the nucleus NRG1 could be co-localising to. Digital fluorescent microscopy has higher resolution and, in addition, experiments can be performed with mutated or truncated NRG forms. NRG1β3 tagged with GFP (either at the C or N terminus) was transfected into a variety of cell types (including fibroblasts or epithelial cells and using cells from human, monkey, rodents or dog) and the localisation of the expression of the protein was visualised using low-light wide-field or confocal digital microscopy. When expressed in each of these cell types this isoform showed localisation to nucleoli alone, localisation to SC35-positive nuclear speckles alone or a combination of both patterns in one cell *(23)* (Fig. 1b).

Two lines of evidence demonstrate that this localisation is receptor-independent *(23)*. NRG1β3 localisation using NR6 cells, which lack all the EGFR family receptors, was indistinguishable from other cell types and second, deletion of the EGF domain had no effect on nucleolar or SC35 spliceosome localisation *(23)*. The observation of two patterns was resolved by filming individual cell nuclei where the patterns could be seen to interconvert over a period of about 90 min. It is not yet known if this occurs at a particular phase of the

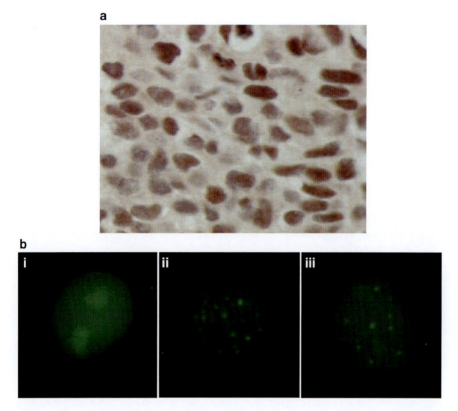

Fig. 1. (a) Immunohistochemical staining of a breast adenocarcinoma treated with a NRG1β antibody displaying strong, nuclear staining in the epithelial cells (hp × 400). (b) The distribution of NRG1β3-GFP within the nucleus of African green monkey kidney (Cos7) cells using low-light digital microscopy. These pictures show three different patterns of distribution that occur: (1) nucleoli localisation, (2) localisation to SC35-positive speckles and (3) an intermediate pattern containing speckles and nucleoli.

cell cycle nor if the NRG molecules move from one location to the other (or are degraded and resynthesised) but experiments are underway to answer these issues. Deletion analysis by Golding et al. *(23)* and by Breuleux et al. *(24)* showed that the N-terminal 21 amino acids of NRG1β3 were required for intranuclear accumulation and localisation to nucleoli and that residues within the IgG domain (which lies N-terminal to the EGF motif) are required for localisation to spliceosomes.

4. NRG FUNCTIONS IN THE NUCLEUS

Two basic alternative mechanisms of action (if any occurs) in the nucleus can be hypothesised, receptor-mediated and non-receptor mediated (clearly these are not exclusive). While it has been shown that nuclear localisation does not require the presence of a member

Chapter 5 / Neuregulins in the Nucleus

of the EGF receptor family, nor the presence of an EGF domain in the NRG, this does not resolve the issue as to whether a receptor-mediated function could occur once the molecule has reached the nucleus.

The evidence for members of the EGF family of growth factor *receptors* in the nucleus mostly comes from the use of directly labelled proteins (using reporters such as radioactive isotopes or GFP tagging) or indirectly by the use of antibodies for immunogold labelling and electron microscopy, immunofluorescence and immunostaining. These latter methods are progressively less precise in their ability to reliably determine subcellular localisation. Immuno-staining cannot (at least in most hands) conclusively differentiate between peri-nuclear and genuine nuclear localisation. On the other hand immunogold labelling is known to be subject to occasional artifactual positive results and is rarely accepted on its own as sufficient proof of nuclear expression. Immunofluorescence can also be prone to error unless carefully performed and controlled.

In a recent review by Bryant and Stow *(3)* the authors discuss 'the continuing conundrum' of the assumption of full length transmembrane growth factor receptors 'moving out of membranes and existing as matrix-associated proteins in cell nuclei'. The authors readily acknowledge that this 'remains a prickly concept'. Many would agree when considering a typical transmembrane growth factor receptor such as the EGFR, which has about 500 amino acids 'extracellular' that are folded into a highly organised structure, stabilised with 25 disulphide bonds and decorated with about 60 KDa of complex sugars. In this hypothesis it is assumed that this structure unfolds, the disulphide bonds break and the (essentially) linear sequence of the protein, presumably together with the 11 or so complex carbohydrate chains, cross the membrane of (for instance) an intracellular vesicle. Then the protein refolds (in its glycosylated form) and its 25 disulphide bonds all reform in the correct arrangement in the cytoplasm (which is a non-oxidising environment due to the ratio of glutathione and reduced glutathione) *(25)* such that it can resume its cellular functions as a soluble protein. Currently there is no evidence that this can occur for any transmembrane protein, and thermodynamic as well as many other considerations make the possibility remote.

An alternative hypothesis is that growth factor receptors are indeed found associated with nuclei but in the nuclear membrane, not in a full-length soluble form in the nucleoplasm. Evidence in support of this concept includes that receptors will be synthesised by nuclear membrane associated ribosomes (as the nuclear membrane is contiguous with the ER). The nuclear membrane is not a simple balloon surrounding the nucleus but has multiple intranuclear invaginations and pores *(26)*. Thus nascent receptors will be found in the outer leaflet of the nuclear envelope, and in any intranuclear invaginations of this, but it is arguable if these are functional as they are yet to be glycosylated, a fate which awaits them in the Golgi apparatus. Of course, it has been well known that growth factor receptors, after ligand activation, migrate in vesicles to the peri-nuclear tubulovesicular membrane structures where they are easily seen using experiments such as GFP tagging. Whether these can fuse with membranes contiguous with the nuclear membrane remains a possibility.

How could the view that intranucleoplasmic localisation of full-length growth factor receptors occurs have arisen? A typical (non-polarised) cultured cell is remarkably flat with an aspect ratio often exceeding 10:1 (similar to a dinner plate). Thus, in such a flat cell the nucleus is much like the ham in a sandwich of (from the top) plasma membrane, endoplas-mic reticulum, various vesicular structures and then the double nuclear membrane (with nuclear invaginations) and the same set of membranes present in the reverse order below the nucleoplasmic compartment. In each of these membrane layers growth factor receptors will be found according to current thinking regarding their site of synthesis and subsequent movements and destinations. It is not surprising that using wide-field microscopy, and even perhaps confocal microscopy, that distinguishing the ham from the sandwich requires rather careful experiments.

The exception to this is the HER4/ErbB4 receptor, which is subject to regulated proteolysis, which results in a soluble intracellular fragment that clearly does traffic to the nucleus and enters the nucleoplasm *(27)*. In this case, however, the fragment lacks all of the ligand binding sites and could not interact with, nor be activated by a neuregulin ligand. Thus, it is perhaps best to view the issue of genuinely nucleoplasmic, full-length, soluble growth factor receptors as open. Finally, it has been very recently reported that addition of an inhibitor of the EGF receptor, Gefitinib, causes alterations in the intranuclear location of NRG1 but this drug is now known to inhibit up to 37 kinases *(28)* and to have further off-target effects so whether this is indicative of the involvement of the specific receptors, other kinases or simply a response to cell stress remains to be shown *(29)*.

If there are no relevant members of the EGF receptor family in the nucleus what could NRG1 be doing there? The only clues come from the sub-nuclear localisation to nucleoli and to interchromatin granules. Even more intriguing is the apparent transition from one location to another, although it is yet to be shown that the molecules move rather than being degraded and re-synthesised. Several proteins share this behaviour of being sequestered in the nucleolus and then being released, notably Cdc14, which is a cell cycle regulator *(30)*. Thus, it will be important to determine if the nuclear NRG is released and re-localises, and whether this is associated with a particular phase of the cell cycle. Possible functions in these sub-compartments are regulating ribosome synthesis and pre-mRNA splicing. Some evidence for an involvement in the latter comes from the use of a yeast two hybrid system and co-immunoprecipitation where interactions with nuclear proteins involved in transcriptional control were detected *(24)*. The receptor-mediated effects of NRGs are to stimulate quiescent cells to enter the cell cycle, and to decrease the time of the cycle, thereby increasing cell numbers. In parallel the cell has to increase its rate of molecular synthesis, an event linked to the number (and efficiency) of ribosomes. It is not inconceivable that NRG may have a dual role in promoting transit through the cell cycle and cell growth but this is currently speculation. Experimental approaches to the problem may be based on 'candidate' effects such as the level of ribosomal RNA or splicing efficiency or discovery approaches such as transcriptomics or proteomics.

When first observed, perhaps mainly because it did not fit with current paradigms of cellular signalling, nuclear growth factors were considered an artefact. With the large body of observations and experiments this now seems unlikely. The main unresolved question remains what are the functions of these molecules in this compartment. When this is determined much of the other aspects of the system may fall into place.

REFERENCES

1. Olsnes S, Klingenberg O, Wiedłocha A. Transport of exogenous growth factors and cytokines to the cytosol and to the nucleus. Physiol Rev 2003;83(1):163–182.
2. Johnson HM, Subramaniam PS, Olsnes S, Jans DA. Trafficking and signaling pathways of nuclear localizing protein ligands and their receptors. Bioessays 2004;26(9):993–1004.
3. Bryant DM, Stow JL. Nuclear translocation of cell-surface receptors: lessons from fibroblast growth factor. Traffic 2005;6:947–954.
4. Jans DA, Hassan G. Nuclear targeting by growth factors, cytokines and their receptors: a role in signalling? Bioessays 1998;20:400–411.
5. Lobie PE, Wood TJJ, Chen CM, Waters MJ, Norstedt G. Nuclear translocation and anchorage of the growth hormone receptor. J Biol Chem 1994;269(50):31735–31746.
6. Lobie PE, Mertani H, Morel G, Morales-Bustos O, Norstedt G, Waters MJ. Receptor-mediated nuclear translocation of growth hormone. J Biol Chem 1994;269(33):21330–21339.

Chapter 5 / Neuregulins in the Nucleus

7. Hayes N, Gullick WJ. The neuregulin family of genes and their multiple splice variants in breast cancer. J Mammary Gland Biol Neoplasia 2008;2:205–214.
8. Srinivasan R, Benton E, McCormick F, Thomas H, Gullick WJ. Expression of the c-erbB-3/HER3 and c-erbB-4 growth factor receptors and their ligands, neuregulin-1 alpha, neuregulin-1 beta, and betacellulin, in normal endometrium and endometrial cancer. Clin Cancer Res 1999;5:2877–2883.
9. Johnson GR, Saeki T, Auersperg N, Gordon AW, Shoyab M, Salomon DS, Stromberg K. Response to and expression of amphiregulin by ovarian carcinoma and normal ovarian surface epithelial cells: nuclear localization of endogenous amphiregulin. Biochem Biophys Res Commun 1991;180(2):481–488.
10. Kimura H. Schwannoma-derived growth factor must be transported into the nucleus to exert its mitogenic activity. Proc Natl Acad Sci USA 1993;90(6):2165–2169.
11. Arnoys EJ, Wang JL. Dual localization: proteins in extracellular and intracellular compartments. Acta Histochem 2007;109(2):89–110.
12. Falls D. Neuregulins: functions, forms and signalling strategies. Exp Cell Res 2003;284:14–30.
13. Kinugasa Y, Ishiguro H, Tokita Y, Oohira A, Ohmoto H, Higashiyama S. Neuroglycan C, a novel member of the neuregulin family. Biochem Biophys Res Commun 2004;321:1045–1049.
14. Uchida T, Wada K, Akamatsu T, Yonezawa M, Noguchi H, Mizoguchi A, Kasuga M, Sakamoto C. A novel epidermal growth factor-like molecule containing two follistatin modules stimulates tyrosine phosphorylation of erbB-4 in MKN28 gastric cancer cells. Biochem Biophys Res Commun 1999;266(2):593–602.
15. Stove C, Bracke M. Roles for neuregulins in human cancer. Clin Exp Met 2004;21:665–684.
16. Li W, Park JW, Nuijens A, Sliwkowski MX, Keller GA. Heregulin is rapidly translocated to the nucleus and its transport is correlated with c-myc induction in breast cancer cells. Oncogene 1996;12:2473–2477.
17. Fluge O, Akslen LA, Haugen DR, Varhaug JE, Lillehaug JR. Expression of heregulins and associations with the ErbB family of tyrosine kinase receptors in papillary thyroid carcinomas. Int J Cancer 2000;87(6):763–770.
18. Marshall C, Blackburn E, Clark M, Humphreys S, Gullick WJ. Neuregulins 1–4 are expressed in the cytoplasm or nuclei of ductal carcinoma (in situ) of the human breast. Breast Cancer Res Treat 2006;96(2):163–168.
19. Dunn M, Sinha P, Campbell R, Blackburn E, Levinson N, Rampaul R, Bates T, Humphreys S, Gullick WJ. Co-expression of neuregulins 1,2,3 and 4 in human breast cancer. J Pathology 2004;203(2):672–680.
20. Hayes NVL, Blackburn E, Smart LV, Boyle MM, Russell GA, Frost TM, Morgan BJ, Baines AJ, Gullick WJ. Identification and characterization of novel spliced variants of neuregulin 4 in prostate cancer. Clin Cancer Res 2007;13(11):3147–3155.
21. Atlas E, Bojanowski K, Mehmi I, Lupa RA. A deletion mutant of heregulin increases the sensitivity of breast cancer cells to chemotherapy without promoting tumorigenicity. Oncogene 2003;22:3441–3451.
22. Tsai MS, Shamon-Taylor LA, Mehmi I, Tang CK, Lupu R. Blockage of heregulin expression inhibits tumorigenicity and metastasis of breast cancer. Oncogene 2003;22(5):761–768.
23. Golding M, Ruhrberg C, Sandle J, Gullick WJ. Mapping nucleolar and spliceosome localization sequences of neuregulin 1-β3. Exp Cell Res 2004;299:110–118.
24. Breuleux M, Schoumacher F, Rehn D, Küng W, Mueller H, Eppenberger U. Heregulins implicated in cellular functions other than receptor activation. Mol Cancer Res 2006;4(1):27–37.
25. Hwang C, Sinskey AJ, Lodish HF. Oxidized redox state of glutathione in the endoplasmic reticulum. Science 1992;11;257(5076):1496–1502.
26. Fricker M, Hollinshead M, White N, Vaux D. Interphase nuclei of many mammalian cell types contain deep, dynamic, tubular membrane-bound invaginations of the nuclear envelope. J Cell Biol 1997:10;136(3):531–544.
27. Jones FE. HER4 intracellular domain (4ICD) activity in the developing mammary gland and breast cancer. J Mammary Gland Biol Neoplasia 2008;13(2):247–258.
28. Brehmer D, Greff Z, Godl K, Blencke S, Kurtenbach A, Weber M, Müller S, Klebl B, Cotten M, Kéri G, Wissing J, Daub H. Cellular targets of gefitinib. Cancer Res 2005;65(2):379–382.
29. Ferrer-Soler L, Vazquez-Martin A, Brunet J, Menendez JA, De Llorens R, Colomer R. An update of the mechanisms of resistance to EGFR-tyrosine kinase inhibitors in breast cancer: Gefitinib

(Iressa)-induced changes in the expression and nucleo-cytoplasmic trafficking of HER-ligands (Review). Int J Mol Med 2007;20(1):3–10.
30. Visintin R, Hwang ES, Amon A. Cfi1 prevents premature exit from mitosis by anchoring Cdc14 phosphatase in the nucleolus. Nature 1999;398(6730):818–823.

6

Role of the EGF-CFC Family in Mammary Gland Development and Neoplasia

Luigi Strizzi, Kazuhide Watanabe, Mario Mancino, David S. Salomon, and Caterina Bianco

SUMMARY

Members of the Epidermal Growth Factor-Cripto-1/FRL-1/Cryptic (EGF-CFC) family, such as human Cripto-1, are important mediators of crucial events that take place during embryonic pattern formation. New evidences from gene expression and transgenic mouse studies have also shown that perturbation of Cripto-1 signaling may lead to cell transformation and tumor formation *in vivo*. In addition, Cripto-1 is expressed at high levels in a wide variety of human carcinomas including early and late breast cancers. Despite the clear correlation between Cripto-1 overexpression and human and mouse tumors, the exact molecular mechanism of Cripto-1 contribution to the cell transformation process is not clear. Cripto-1 has been shown to activate multiple signaling pathways to promote either differentiation during embryogenesis or cancer growth. In this review we will discuss the multifunction properties of the EGF-CFC family of proteins and the complex network of signaling molecules activated by Cripto-1 focusing in particular on the mammary gland. A better understanding of the intracellular signaling pathways that mediate Cripto-1 activity in human tumors might identify novel points of intervention to target Cripto-1 in human malignancies.

Key Words: Cripto-1, TGFβ signaling; Human breast cancer; Serological markers for cancer; Epithelial to mesenchymal transition; Transgenic mouse models

From: *Current Clinical Oncology: Breast Cancer in the Post-Genomic Era,*
Edited by: A. Giordano and N. Normanno, DOI: 10.1007/978-1-60327-945-1_6,
© Humana Press, a part of Springer Science + Business Media, LLC 2009

1. EGF-CFC PROTEIN FAMILY: STRUCTURE AND POSTTRANSLATIONAL MODIFICATIONS

Human and mouse Cripto-1 (CR-1/Cr-1) are GPI-anchored membrane glycoproteins, which have been shown to play an important role in vertebrate development and in tumor progression *(1,2)*. CR-1/Cr-1 belongs to the *Epidermal Growth Factor-Cripto-1/FRL-1/ Cryptic (EGF-CFC)* gene family *(1)*. This conserved family of genes includes three *Xenopus Cripto* homologs *(XCR-1/FRL-1, XCR-2, XCR-3) (3)*, zebrafish *one-eye pinhead* (*oep*) *(4)*, chicken *cryptic (5,6)*, mouse *Cr-1 (7)* and *cryptic (cfc*1*) (8)*, human *CR-1 (9)* and *Cryptic (CFC1) (10)*. To date, *EGF-CFC* family genes have been identified in vertebrates but not in invertebrates. However, since *Nodal* and *Lefty* genes, which require EGF-CFC proteins to induce cellular signaling, have been identified and characterized from cephalochordates, tunicates, and echinoderms *(11,12)*, EGF-CFC-related genes might possibly exist also in invertebrates. Although the overall primary sequence identity is relatively low (22–32%, Fig. 1a), the *EGF-CFC* gene family shares well-conserved structural modules such as exon-intron organization, suggesting that these genes are evolutionarily related and probably arose from a common ancestor gene *(5,13)*. In addition, several human and mouse *Cripto-1*-related intronless pseudogenes have been identified and the human *Cripto-3 (CR-3)* pseudogene has been reported to be expressed as a transcript in undifferentiated embryonal carcinoma cells *(14)*. Mouse and human Cripto-1 proteins consist of 188 and 177 amino acids, respectively, and exhibit a unique structural profile highly conserved among EGF-CFC family members, containing an NH2-terminal signal peptide, a variant EGF-like motif, a Cripto-FRL1-Cryptic (CFC) motif, and a short hydrophobic COOH-terminal segment, which functions as a glycosylphosphatidylinositol (GPI) cleavage and attachment signal *(1)* (Fig. 1a, d). Structural analysis of EGF-CFC family members has elucidated unique biochemical features of these proteins *(13,15–20)*. The EGF-CFC domain contains 12 highly conserved cysteine residues, six in the EGF-like motif and six in the CFC motif (Fig. 1a–c). Unlike the canonical EGF motif that contains three disulfide loops (A, B, and C), the variant EGF-like domain in EGF-CFC proteins completely lacks the A-loop and possess a truncated B-loop and a complete C-loop (Fig. 1b) *(15)*. The CFC domain of CR-1/Cr-1 has been shown to exhibit C1-C4, C2-C6, and C3-C5 disulfide pattern *(17–19)* (Fig. 1c). Even though CFC motifs are exclusively found in the EGF-CFC protein family, this motif may be considered as a truncated form of the von-Willebrand Factor C-like domain from homology analysis and the disulfide binding pattern *(18)*. In addition to its primary structure, CR-1/Cr-1 is known to be processed posttranslationally as a GPI-anchored glycoprotein *(20–25)*. The expected molecular weight (MW) of the mature human CR-1 protein after removal of the NH2-terminal signal peptide and COOH-terminal GPI-signal peptide is 14.7 kD, while endogenous CR-1 protein is observed as multiple species with a MW ranging from 14 to 36 kD. Biochemical characterization by peptide mapping, mass spectrometric analysis, and glycosidase treatment of a COOH-terminally deleted, soluble form of human CR-1 protein revealed several glycosyl modifications including O-linked glycosylation at Ser40 and Ser161 (which is lately identified as a ω-site for GPI-attachment), N-linked glycosylation at Asn79, and O-linked single fucosylation at Thr88. Among them, the O-linked fucose modification is relatively rare and exclusively found within the EGF-like modules of extracellular proteins, including urinary-type plasminogen activator (uPA), coagulation factor VII and IX, and Notch receptors and their ligands *(21,26)* (Fig. 1). A consensus site for O-linked fucosylation has been identified as C_2XXGGS/TC_3 where the site is located between the second and third cysteines of the EGF module. This consensus site is present in all EGF-CFC family proteins *(1)*, while the other glycosylation sites such as O-linkage at Ser40 or N-linkage at Asn79 are not well conserved among the EGF-CFC proteins (Fig. 1a). O-fucosylation has been reported to affect protein function.

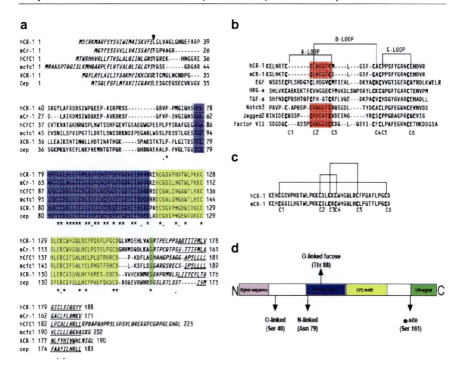

Fig. 1. (a) Multiple amino acid sequence alignment of EGF-CFC family proteins. hCR-1 human Cripto-1, mCr-1 mouse Cripto-1, hCFC1 human Cryptic, mcfc1 mouse cryptic. * and – indicate amino acid identity among 6/6 and 4–5/6 proteins, respectively. EGF-like domains of the various EGF-CFC proteins are highlighted in blue and the CFC motifs are marked in yellow. NH2-terminal signal sequences and COOH-terminal GPI signals are italicized. Arrowhead indicates the signal sequence cleavage sites. Potential ω-sites for GPI attachment are marked in *green*. Hydrophobic COOH-terminus domains are underlined. (b) Disulfide pattern and sequence homologies of EGF-like motif of human and mouse Cripto-1 with other EGF-related motif containing proteins. EGF, human EGF; HRGα, human heregulin α; TGF-α, human transforming growth factor α; Notch3, human Nocth3; Jagged2, human Jagged2; Factor VII, human coagulation factor VII. O-fucosylation consensus sites are marked in *red*. (c) Disulfide pattern of CFC motif of human and mouse Cripto-1. (d) Schematic of posttranslational modifications of human Cripto-1 protein.

For example, uPA lacking *O*-fucose loses its mitogenic activity *(27)* and the human disease CADASIL is caused by a mutation in Notch 3, which disrupts the *O*-linked fucosylation site *(28)*. *O*-linked fucosylation of EGF-CFC proteins has been shown to be necessary for activity of human and mouse Cripto-1 proteins in a Nodal-dependent signaling pathway *(20,22)*. For istance, substitution of the threonine residue to alanine (Thr88Ala in human CR-1 and Thr72Ala in mouse Cr-1, respectively) completely abrogated the activity of these proteins with respect to induction of Nodal-Smad-2-dependent signaling *(20–22)*. However, a recent report demonstrated that addition of fucose to this consensus site is not required for the ability of Cr-1 to activate a Nodal-dependent signaling pathway, but the threonine residue itself is important for this Cr-1 function *(21)*. In this respect, Cr-1 can induce Nodal signaling in fucosylation-deficient embryonic stem cells and a Thr72Ser mutant of mouse Cr-1, which still can be fucosylated on the serine residue, fails to induce Nodal signaling *(21)*. Another important posttranslational modification in EGF-CFC proteins is the GPI modification. Most of the EGF-CFC proteins have been experimentally demonstrated or have been predicted to possess the GPI-anchor signal in their COOH-terminus *(1,23,24)*. Ser161 of human CR-1 has been identified as a ω-site for the cleavage and GPI-attachment *(24,25)* (Fig. 1d). GPI-anchoring determines membrane localization of CR-1/Cr-1 in lipid raft microdomains and within caveolae *(24,29)*. Human and mouse Cripto-1 proteins can be released from the cell membrane following treatment with bacterial phosphatidylinositol-phospholipase C (PI-PLC) *(23,24)* and by the activity of the endogenous enzyme GPI-phospholipase D (GPI-PLD) *(24)*. This controlled release mechanism may define the activity of CR-1 as a membrane-associated coreceptor or as a soluble ligand. GPI-anchoring of CR-1 is required for optimal activity of CR-1 to induce Nodal signaling *(25)*, although several studies have shown that a COOH-terminally truncated, soluble form of mouse or human Cripto-1 protein is still able to activate a Nodal/Smad signaling pathway *(13,20,30)*, In addition, GPI-anchoring of CR-1/Cr-1 should be important in Nodal-independent, c-src/MAPK/Akt-dependent signaling, since some essential factors in this Nodal-independent pathway, such as Glypican-1 and Caveolin-1 (Cav-1), are also prone to localize in lipid raft microdomains *(29,31)*.

2. SIGNALING PATHWAYS ACTIVATED OR INHIBITED BY CRIPTO-1

Although Cripto-1 was initially identified as a member of the EGF family of peptides, the variant EGF-like motif of Cripto-1 is unable to bind directly to any of the four erbB type I tyrosine kinase receptors (erbB-1/EGFR, erbB-2, erbB-3, erbB-4) since the conserved amino acids within the A loop of canonical EGF-related peptides are essential for binding to *erb*B tyrosine kinase receptors *(32)*. To date several proteins have been shown to directly bind to Cripto-1 through interaction with the EGF-like motif or CFC domain. Two are the major signaling pathways that are activated by Cripto-1: a Nodal/Alk4/Alk7/Smad-2 signaling pathway and a Glypican-1/c-src/MAPK/Akt signaling pathway (Table 1).

Table 1
Cripto-1 binding partners

Proteins	Binding domain	Function	References
Nodal	EGF-like	Nodal-Smad signaling (coreceptor)	*(22,37)*
GDF1, GDF3	EGF-like	GDF-Smad signaling (coreceptor)	*(34–36)*
Glypican-1	EGF-like (?)	Glypican-1/c-src/MAPK/Akt signaling (ligand)	*(2,31,57)*
Activin/TGFβ	EGF-like/CFC	TGFβ-Smad signaling (antagonist)	*(42,48,49)*
Lefty1, 2	EGF-like (?)	Nodal signaling (inhibition)	*(44,46,47)*
wnt 11	EGF-like	Canonical wnt signaling (coreceptor?)	*(62)*
Alk-4/7	CFC	Nodal-Smad signaling (coreceptor)	*(17–19,37)*
Tomoregulin-1	CFC	Nodal singaling (inhibition)	*(43)*
GRP78	CFC	TGFβ-Smad signaling (synergistic inhibition)	*(51)*
Caveolin-1	Unknown	Glypican-1/c-src/MAPK/Akt signaling (inhibition)	*(29)*

3. NODAL/ALK4/ALK7/SMAD-2 SIGNALING PATHWAY

Extracellular-membrane attached EGF-CFC proteins act as coreceptors with the type I Activin serine-threonine kinase receptor Alk4 or Alk7 for the transforming growth factor β-related peptides Nodal and Growth and Differentiation factor 1 and 3 (GDF1 and GDF3) (33–36). Nodal and EGF-CFC proteins are inactive independently and together function through activation of an Activin type II (ActRIIA or ActRIIB) and type IB (Alk4/ActRIB or Alk7) receptor complex (37). Activation of Alk4/ActRIB can in turn phosphorylate Smad-2 and Smad-3 signaling factors, which bind to Smad-4 and then interact with FoxH1 (FAST1) to enhance transcription of target genes (38–40). EGF-CFC proteins can also mediate Nodal signaling via the type I Alk7 receptor (41). However, the mechanism by which Nodal activates the Alk4 and Alk7 type I receptors is different. In fact, Nodal signaling through Alk4 is fully dependent upon EGF-CFC proteins. In contrast, Nodal can bind directly to Alk7 and can signal in the absence of CR-1. Nevertheless, CR-1 is still able to significantly potentiate the responsiveness of the Alk7/ActRIIB receptor complex to Nodal, indicating that both Alk7 and Alk4 collaborate with CR-1 (41,42). Unlike Nodal, Activin also utilizes the same receptors (Alk4 and ActRIIB), but does not require EGF-CFC coreceptors for binding to the type I Alk4 receptor. Therefore, a critical function of EGF-CFC proteins during development is to render Alk4 competent for activation by Nodal or GDF1 and GDF3 and to enhance the ability of Alk7 to respond to Nodal. Site-directed mutagenesis experiments have demonstrated that the CFC domain is responsible for interaction with Alk4, while the EGF-like domain is important for binding to Nodal, GDF1, GDF3, Activin and TGFβ1 (37,42). In addition, Tomoregulin-1, Lefty/Antivin can antagonize Nodal signaling through binding to the EGF-CFC coreceptors (43,44). Tomoregulin-1 is a transmembrane protein that contains two follistatin domains and an EGF-motif in the extracellular domain and a short cytoplasmic tail and that can activate the type I EGF receptor tyrosine kinase erbB4 (45). In this respect, CR-1 has been shown to indirectly enhance the tyrosine phosphorylation of erbB4 but whether this response is modulated by binding to Tomoregulin-1 is not known (32). Tomoregulin-1 and Alk4 both interact with CR-1 through its CFC-domain (43). It is therefore possible that both proteins compete for binding to CR-1, and the interaction of Tomoregulin-1 with CR-1 might exclude binding of CR-1 to Alk4, leading to inhibition of Nodal signaling. The Lefty/Antivin subfamily of TGFβ proteins is another example of extracellular antagonists of Nodal signaling (33). Genetic and biochemical studies have shown that Lefty 1 and Lefty 2 function as antagonists of the EGF-CFC coreceptors, by directly binding to CR-1 and to Nodal thereby sequestering them from binding to Alk4 (46). Therefore, the competitive binding of Lefty to EGF-CFC coreceptors enables Lefty to antagonize Nodal signaling preventing its interaction with type I and type II Activin receptors. Furthermore, Lefty can also directly interact with Nodal in solution, preventing Nodal from binding its receptor complex (47). CR-1 can also act as an inhibitor of Activin and TGF-β1 signaling (42,48,49). In this respect, CR-1 binds directly to Activin B, through the CFC domain, or Activin A and TGF-β1, through the EGF-like domain, disrupting the ability of these signaling molecules to bind and to activate a functional type I/type II receptor complex. Since Activin A and B and TGF-β1 are potent inhibitors of cell growth in different cell lines, antagonism of Activin A and B and TGF-β1 signaling might represent one of the mechanisms by which CR-1 regulates and promotes tumorigenesis. Moreover, a recent study provides evidence of a differential modulation of CR-1 expression in human embryonal and colon carcinoma cell lines by two distinct members of the TGF-β family: BMP-4 and TGF-β1 (50). In this regard, while TGF-β1 enhances CR-1 mRNA and protein expression in colon cancer LS172-T cells and embryonal carcinoma NTERA2 cells, BMP-4 strongly downregulates CR-1 expression in the same cell lines, suggesting that growth factors differentially modulate CR-1 expression in cancer cells.

Finally, a recent study has identified an additional CR-1 binding partner: GRP78 *(51)*. GRP78 is a multifunctional regulator of endoplasmic reticulum homeostasis that regulates the degradation of misfolded proteins through the poteosomic-ubiquitin pathway *(52)*. GRP78, which can also be expressed on the cell membrane of cancer cells, binds directly to CR-1, thereby inhibiting TGFβ signaling and therefore enhancing cell growth *(53)*. In fact, GRP78 expression has been shown to correlate with drug resistance in breast cancer *(54)*.

4. GLYPICAN-1/C-SRC/MAPK/AKT SIGNALING PATHWAY

In addition to functioning as a coreceptor for Nodal, CR-1 can also function as a ligand for Glypican-1, which is a GPI-anchored heparan sulfate proteoglycan (HSPG) tethered to the plasma membrane in lipid rafts. Binding of CR-1 to Glypican-1 activates the c-src/MAPK/phophatidylinositol 3'-kinase (PI3K)/Akt signaling pathway that regulates cell proliferation, cell motility, and survival *(31,55,56)*. Activation of these two signaling pathways is mediated by direct binding of CR-1 to the GPI-linked HSPG, Glypican-1, which can then activate the cytoplasmic tyrosine kinase c-src triggering activation of MAPK and PI3K/Akt *(31)*. Although the domain within CR-1 protein that binds to Glypican-1 has not been identified yet, it is possible that the EGF-like domain might be responsible for interaction with Glypican-1, since a synthetic peptide corresponding to the EGF-like motif can activate MAPK/Akt signaling pathway and promote cellular proliferation in mammalian cells *(57)*. Moreover, Glypican-1 and c-src are required by CR-1 to stimulate MAPK and Akt phosphorylation in mammary epithelial cells *(31)*. Reciprocally, CR-1 can enhance Smad-2 phosphorylation in mammary epithelial cells independently of Glypican-1 and c-src, suggesting that these two distinct pathways can be independently activated by CR-1 in mammalian cells *(58)*. Finally, an intact c-src kinase is required by CR-1 to induce *in vitro* transformation and to enhance migration in mammary epithelial cells, suggesting that inappropriate activation of c-src by CR-1 in a Nodal and ALK4-independent manner may play a key role in promoting cellular transformation *(31)*. Recently, the membrane protein Cav-1 has been shown to function as a negative modulator of the Glypican-1/c-src/MAPK pathway activated by Cripto-1 *(29)*. In fact, Cav-1 can interact with CR-1 within lipid rafts microdomains and impairs CR-1 ability to activate downstream signaling molecules, such as c-src and MAPK. This strongly interferes with the ability of CR-1 to stimulate migration, invasion, and proliferation in mammary epithelial cells *(29)*.

5. CRIPTO-1 AND THE WNT SIGNALING PATHWAY

A potential interaction between the canonical wnt/β-catenin/Tcf pathway and the Nodal/Cripto-1 signaling pathways has been demonstrated by microarray analysis where Cripto-1 was identified as a primary target gene in the wnt/β-catenin signaling pathway during early mouse embryonic development and in human colon carcinoma cells *(59)*. Moreover, a recent study has demonstrated the ability of the canonical wnt/β-catenin/Tcf pathway to regulate the expression of the short form of human CR-1 in human colon carcinoma cells and in hepatoma cells *(60)*. This cross-talk between the wnt/β-catenin and Cripto-1 signaling pathways might be functionally significant since activation of β-catenin signaling in cells might lead to Cripto-1 overexpression, thereby facilitating cell proliferation and transformation such as in colonic epithelial cells where an activated wnt/β-catenin pathway contributes to the pathogenesis of colon cancer *(61)*. Moreover, wnt11, which is in most cases identified as an activator of noncanonical wnt signaling pathway, has been shown to induce canonical wnt signaling

Chapter 6 / Role of the EGF-CFC Family in Mammary Gland Development   93

by binding to the EGF-like motifs of XCR-1 or Cr-1 *(62)*. Finally, in *Xenopus* and in the mouse, Nodal expression can be regulated by both a canonical wnt/β-catenin pathway and/ or by activation of a canonical Notch 1 pathway *(63,64)*.

6. FUNCTION AND EXPRESSION OF EGF-CFC PROTEIN FAMILY DURING EMBRYONIC DEVELOPMENT

During early mouse embryogenesis, Cr-1 mRNA expression is found in the embryonic ectoderm following implantation of the blastocyst. On day 6.5 of gestation Cr-1 is detected at increasing levels in the epiblast cells undergoing epithelial to mesenchymal transition (EMT) as they migrate through the nascent primitive streak and in the developing mesoderm cells *(7,65–67)*. By day 7 Cr-1 is detected mostly in the truncus arteriosus of the developing heart. With the exception of the developing heart, little if any expression of Cr-1 mRNA can be detected in the remainder of the embryo after day 8 *(23,65)*. Cripto-1 null mice *(Cr-1$^{-/-}$)* die at day 7.5 due to their inability to gastrulate and form appropriate germ layers *(7)*. Fibroblasts that were derived from Cr-1$^{-/-}$ embryos were impaired in their ability to migrate toward either fibronectin or type 1 collagen as compared to embryonic fibroblasts from wild-type embryos *(67)*. In zebrafish, the *Cr-1* ortholog *oep* with the two *Nodal*-related genes *squint* (*sqt*) and *Cyclops* (*cyc*) is necessary for initiating mesoderm, endoderm, and A/P axis formation *(4,68,69)*. Mutations in *oep* result in cyclopia, absence of head and trunk meso-derm, loss of prechordal plate and ventral neuroectoderm, impairment of gastrulation move-ments, loss of A/P axis patterning and positioning, and L/R laterality defects *(4,68)*. Rescue of the *oep* mutant phenotype can be achieved by expression of either full-length or secreted COOH-terminal truncated forms of the oep protein suggesting that oep can function under certain conditions as a paracrine effector. Ectopic expression of *Xenopus* FRL-1 or mouse Cr-1, overexpression of Activin, or activation of downstream components in an Activin-like signaling pathway such as the Alk4 receptor (TARAM-A) or Smad-2 can also rescue *oep* inactivating mutations *(68)*. Oep, like mouse Cr-1, is absolutely required for the migration of mesendoderm cells through the primitive streak *(70)*. The Nodal/cryptic signaling path-way is also involved in the establishment of the L/R embryonic axis, demonstrating that the same signaling molecules are utilized in multiple developmental pathways *(69)*. However, at this developmental stage with the exception of oep, cryptic replaces the function of Cripto-1 as the coreceptor for Nodal. Nodal signaling in zebrafish during L/R asymmetry develop-ment also requires a functional *oep* gene *(71–73)*. Mutation and partial rescue of *oep* in the zebrafish or targeted disruption of *cryptic in* mice (*Cfc1*) and humans (*CFC1*) results in laterality defects including atrial-ventricular septal defects, pulmonary right isomerization, inverted positioning of abdominal organs (situs inversus), and holoprosencephaly *(74,75)*. Germline deletion of cryptic eventually leads to postnatal death at approximately 2 weeks because of severe cardiac malfunction *(71,73)*.

7. EGF-CFC PROTEINS IN MAMMARY GLAND DEVELOPMENT

Expression of Cr-1 has been detected during different stages of postnatal mammary gland development in the mouse. In fact, Cr-1 protein was detected in 4–12-week old virgin, mid-pregnant and lactating FVB/N mouse mammary glands *(76,77)*. A recent study also detected biologically active CR-1 in human milk demonstrating that CR-1 is a secretory component of the mammary gland and suggests that this secreted form of CR-1 may play a role in the regulation of proliferation and differentiation of milk producing cells *(78)*. Further support for CR-1 regulation of mammary epithelial function comes from data, which show increased ability of mouse mammary epithelial cells to respond to the lactogenic hormones, dexamethasone, insulin, and prolactin (DIP) when pretreated with CR-1 and inhibition of β-casein expression, via a p21*ras*- and PI3K-dependent pathway, when these cells were simultaneously treated with both CR-1 and DIP *(55)*.

8. CRIPTO-1 IN TRANSFORMATION AND TUMORIGENESIS OF MAMMARY EPITHELIUM

Experiments involving overexpression of CR-1 cDNA in normal mouse mammary epithelial cells induced these cells to grow in soft agar and increased growth rates in different human breast cancer cells *(9,79,80)*. Insertion of Elvax pellets containing the EGF-like motif of CR-1 protein into the mammary gland of ovariectomized virgin mice produced dramatic increases in DNA synthesis in mammary epithelial cells immediately adjacent to the pellets *(81)*. Human estrogen receptor positive MCF-7 breast cancer cells that overexpress CR-1 (MCF7 CR-1) fail to grow in the absence of estrogen but do have increased proliferation rates, form increased numbers of colonies in soft agar, have increased resistance to apoptosis when grown in anchorage-independent conditions, and show increased propensity to invade and migrate through matrix-coated membranes *(82)*. Biochemical changes such as reduced expression of E-cadherin or increased expression of vimentin that characterize epithelial to mesenchymal transition (EMT) *(83)* were observed in mammary gland hyperplasias and tumors from mice, engineered to express human CR-1 using the MMTV LTR promoter *(84)*, and in the mouse mammary epithelial cell line, HC-11 overexpressing CR-1 (HC-11/CR-1) *(85)*. E-cadherin expression was significantly decreased in tissue extracts from the mammary tumors that express the human CR-1 transgene and in extracts from HC-11/CR-1 cells. These extracts also showed significant increases in the expression of N-cadherin, vimentin, and integrins α-3, α-v, β-1, β-3, and β-4 as well as an increase in the phosphorylated forms of signaling molecules such as c-src, focal adhesion kinase (FAK), and Akt, which are also known to be activated during EMT and which probably play a role in increasing tumor cell invasion *(85,86)*. Also, in the CR-1 transgenic mammary gland tumors and HC-11/CR-1 cells, the zinc-finger repressor transcription factor, Snail, which is known to downregulate or interfere with the normal expression of E-cadherin, was detected by RT-PCR and by western blot analysis at significantly higher levels as compared to control non-tumorigenic mammary tissue suggesting for the first time a possible link between CR-1 expression and Snail activity *(85)*. In addition, both the MMTV-CR-1 transgenic mammary tumors and the HC-11/CR-1 cells were found to express the non-phosphorylated or active form of β-catenin. Continuous turnover of the intercellular adhesion components may lead to cytoplasmic accumulation of β-catenin but this is normally prevented by GSK-3β-dependent phosphorylation of β-catenin, leading to proteosome ubiquitination and degradation of the phosphorylated β-catenin *(87)*. It is interesting to note that in a second transgenic mouse model overexpressing CR-1 *(88)*, this time using the whey acidic promoter (WAP) to drive transgene expression, the mammary gland tumors that arose in the multiparous WAP-CR-1 transgenic mice were morphologically distinct from the mammary gland tumors that formed in the multiparous MMTV-CR-1 transgenic mice. While the mammary gland tumors in the MMTV-CR-1 transgenic mice were predominantly papillary adenocarcinomas, the mammary tumors found in the WAP-CR-1 transgenic mice showed, in addition to papillary adenocarcinomas similar to those detected in the MMTV-CR-1 transgenic mammary glands, also areas with microglandular, solid, and myoepithelial morphology along with focal areas of squamous metaplasia that were similar to the mammary tumors with mixed histotype described in MMTV-*wnt*1 mice or in mammary tumors that develop in mice expressing stabilized mutant forms of β-catenin *(89,90)*.

Chapter 6 / Role of the EGF-CFC Family in Mammary Gland Development

During wnt signaling, non-phosphorylated β-catenin translocates to the nucleus in a complex with Tcf/Lef-1 and functions as a transcription factor activating genes such as c-myc and cyclin-D1, shown to be involved in increased cell survival, proliferation, and migration *(91)*. Cr-1 has been shown to be a target gene during canonical wnt/β-catenin signaling *(59)*, and the association between CR-1 overexpression and accumulation of active β-catenin in WAP-CR-1 transgenic mammary tumors and in HC-11/CR-1 cells strongly suggests a possible link between CR-1 and a canonical wnt signaling pathway and their potential role during cellular transformation and tumorigenesis. A recent study shows that mammary tumors that arise in MMTV-CR-1 transgenic mice have a dramatic reduction in Cav-1 expression in the epithelial compartment of the tumor *(29)*. That same study demonstrates how Cav-1 can function as an inhibitor of CR-1 function in the context of the mammary gland and suggests that during the process of mammary transformation CR-1 may evade the inhibitory function of Cav-1, possibly by downregulating Cav-1 expression *(29)*.

9. EXPRESSION OF CR-1 IN HUMAN BREAST CARCINOMAS

Several studies have demonstrated that CR-1 is overexpressed in primary human breast carcinomas. CR-1 mRNA and/or immunoreactive protein can be detected in ~80% of primary human infiltrating breast carcinomas, in 47% of ductal carcinoma in situ (DCIS), in 13% of uninvolved adjacent breast tissue samples, and in ~6% of normal breast specimens *(92–95)*. In these studies, no significant correlations were observed between CR-1 mRNA expression or immunoreactivity and various clinicopathological parameters such as tumor stage, estrogen receptor status, lymph node involvement, histologic grade, proliferative index as assessed by Ki-67 staining, or loss of heterozygosity (LOH) on chromosome 17p *(92–95)*. More recently, a cohort of 120 patients with operable breast cancer was analyzed for expression of CR-1 by using tissue arrays *(96,97)*. Expression of CR-1 was detected in 47.5% of patients. Interestingly, a significant association was found between CR-1 immunostaining and several clinicopathological features of the tumors. In particular, expression of CR-1 was more frequent in patients with poor prognosis according to the Nottingham Prognostic Index, histological grade 3 tumors as compared with grade 1 lesions, and high cell proliferation Ki-67 index as compared with low index. A long follow-up was available for these patients (median 125 months). Univariate analysis revealed a significant correlation between overexpression of CR-1 and poor prognosis. Multivariate analysis confirmed that CR-1 expression is an independent prognostic factor in breast cancer patients. Finally, in human primary breast carcinomas, CR-1 is frequently coexpressed with other EGF-related peptides, such as TGFα, AR, and heregulin, implying that different growth factors might cooperate in supporting the autonomous proliferation of breast cancer cells *(93,95)*. A positive correlation between nuclear erbB-4 expression and CR-1 expression in primary human breast carcinomas has also been described *(98)*. This finding is interesting because it has been shown that CR-1 can indirectly enhance the tyrosine phosphorylation of erbB-4 *(32)*. In addition to being expressed in breast cancer tissues, soluble CR-1 can also be detected in the plasma of breast cancer patients. In this regard, using a highly sensitive and specific sandwich-type enzyme-linked immunosorbent assay (ELISA) for CR-1, a statistically significant increase in the plasma levels of CR-1 was found in breast cancer patients (2.97 ng/ml) when compared with a control group of healthy volunteers (0.32 ng/ml) *(99)*. At a cut-off level of 0.7 ng/ml the ELISA test had 100% sensitivity (all cancer patients were positive to the test) and 95% specificity (only 1 out of 21 controls was positive in the ELISA test). High CR-1 plasma levels were detected also in breast cancer patients at an early stage, suggesting that CR-1 might be useful in the early diagnosis of this disease. No significant correlation between CR-1 levels in the plasma of breast cancer patients and various clinicopathologic parameters, such as tumor size, lymph node involvement, proliferative index, estrogen and progesterone receptor status or *er*B-2 status was found probably due to the small sample size analyzed in that study. Moderate levels of CR-1 were also found in the plasma of 21 women with benign breast lesions, including hyperplasia and atypical ductal hyperplasia *(99)*. In fact, the mean CR-1 levels in the plasma of patients with benign breast lesions (1.7 ng/ml) were significantly lower that the mean CR-1 plasma levels detected in patients with breast carcinomas (2.97 ng/ml). Within the benign breast lesions, CR-1 plasma levels were higher in lesions characterized by the presence of sclerosis and in fibroadenomas, a lesion characterized by the presence of epithelial hyperplasia and fibrosis. Because pathological fibrosis, including renal, lung, and liver fibrosis, has been associated with morphological and functional modification of epithelial cells that acquire a fibroblastic-mesenchymal phenotype through EMT, it is possible that CR-1 might have a role in inducing EMT in mammary epithelial cells of nonmalignant breast lesions *(100–102)*. In fact, interference with Cr-1-regulated EMT by exogenous soluble Netrin-1 recombinant protein can significantly inhibit migration, invasion, and colony formation in matrigel of EpH4/Cr-1 cells and allometric outgrowth of mammary gland ducts in MMTV-CR-1 transgenic mice *(103)*.

Because of the high levels of CR-1 expression in human carcinomas, as compared to normal tissues, CR-1 represents a potential target for therapeutic intervention *(1,2)*. Different approaches have been used to block CR-1 expression and/or activity, such as antisense oligonucleotides that reduce CR-1 expression or neutralizing antibodies that block the activity of the CR-1 protein *(48,104,105)*. Sequence-specific antisense (AS) oligonucleotides or AS expression vectors, which block expression of specific proteins by binding to the corresponding mRNA and therefore preventing translation, have been successfully used to impair CR-1 expression in several different types of human carcinoma cells including breast cancer cell lines *(106,107)*. In particular, inhibition of CR-1 expression in human MDA-MB-468 and SK-BR-3 breast cancer cells by using a CR-1 AS phosphorothioate oligonucleotide resulted in a significant growth inhibition in vitro *(106)*. An additive effect was observed on reducing the growth of MDA-MB-468 cells in vitro when a CR-1 AS oligonucleotide was combined with TGFα AS and AR AS oligonucleotides, suggesting that different growth factors contribute to regulate the proliferation of breast cancer cells *(106,107)*. Anti-CR-1 second generation antisense oligonucleotides, containing phosphorothioate backbone and a segment of 2'-*O*-methylribonucleosides modified at both the 5' and 3' ends of the oligonucleotide (MBOs), were able to block the in vitro growth of carcinoma cell lines derived from different carcinoma types, including colon and breast cancer *(108,109)*. Treatment of carcinoma cells with CR-1 AS oligonucleotides resulted in a significant reduction in the levels of expression of CR-1 mRNA and protein. More recently, monoclonal blocking antibodies directed against CR-1 have been developed. In particular, Adkins et al. *(48)* have generated mouse monoclonal antibodies (mAbs) that were able to prevent the binding of CR-1 to Activin B and, therefore, to reverse the CR-1 blockade of Activin B-induced growth suppression in human breast carcinoma cells in vitro. The anti-CR-1 antibodies were also able to inhibit tumor cell growth in vivo up to 70% in two xenograft models of testicular and colon cancers and showed antiangiogenic activity in a Directed In Vivo Angiogenic Assay (DIVAA) *(110)*. Finally, rat monoclonal antibodies directed against the EGF-like domain of the CR-1 peptide produced a significant inhibition of the in vitro growth of different carcinoma cell lines *(105)*. The anti-CR-1 mAbs also prevented tumor development in vivo and inhibited the growth of established xenograft tumors of LS174T colon cancer cells and multidrug-resistant CEM/A7R leukaemia cells in immunocompromised mice *(111,112)*. Treatment with the anti-CR-1 mAbs produced a significant reduction in the levels of activation of AKT, activation of c-Jun-NH2-terminal kinase and p38 kinase signaling pathways, and ultimately apoptosis in cancer cells.

10. CONCLUSIONS

Cripto-1 was initially identified as a GPI-linked cell surface glycoprotein that functions as an obligatory functional coreceptor for Nodal and GDF1 and GDF3 to activate a Smad2 and Smad3 intracellular signaling pathway during different stages of early vertebrate embryogenesis. Subsequent studies demonstrated that Cripto-1 is expressed at levels that exceed expression levels in most normal adult tissues in a wide spectrum of human carcinomas including early and late stage breast cancers. This property of Cripto-1 as a pantumor/oncofetal antigen has been exploited to selectively target human carcinomas with blocking and toxin-conjugated humanized monoclonal antibodies. In addition, the presence of discriminatory levels of Cripto-1 in the plasma of cancer patients suggests a potential diagnostic and/or prognostic role for this protein. Since *Cripto-1* is the founding member of a larger family of orthologous genes, these different *EGF-CFC* genes probably perform multiple functions in a cell context-specific manner as several signaling pathways have been identified which Cripto-1 activates and which are either Nodal/Alk4-dependent or -independent. In addition, Cripto-1 can function as a direct antagonist for TGFβ1 and Activin A and B by sequestering these growth factors from their respective receptors, which may mitigate the antiproliferative effects of these growth factors on the early stages of tumor cell proliferation. Expression of Cripto-1 has been detected in normal mouse and human breast tissues. During postnatal development of the mouse mammary gland, Cripto-1 expression parallels the pattern of Nodal expression suggesting that in this tissue these two proteins may be functioning through an Alk4 and Smad2/3 signaling pathway to regulate growth and differentiation. However, the in vitro transforming activity of Cripto-1 and the ability of Cripto-1 to stimulate EMT, migration, invasion and endothelial cell functions may be restricted to a Nodal-independent signaling pathway that predominantly depends upon the activation of c-src and PI3K, although a role for Nodal involvement *in vivo* in these biological responses cannot yet be formally excluded. This is certainly possible with respect to the ability of Cripto-1 to induce hyperplastic lesions and frank carcinomas in the mouse mammary gland following overexpression due to the long latency periods that are observed before tumors arise in the mammary gland and the prometastatic and invasive effects that have been demonstrated for Nodal in human melanomas *(113)*. Further delineation of the intracellular signaling pathways that mediate Cripto-1 activity in human tumors, identifying novel binding partners for Cripto-1 and elucidating epigenetic and genetic pathways that regulate Cripto-1 expression and/or activity will further our knowledge on the role of this gene in cancer pathogenesis.

REFERENCES

1. Salomon DS, Bianco C, Ebert AD, et al. The EGF-CFC family: novel epidermal growth factor-related proteins in development and cancer. Endocr Relat Cancer 2000;7(4):199–226.
2. Bianco C, Strizzi L, Normanno N, Khan N, Salomon DS. Cripto-1: an oncofetal gene with many faces. Curr Top Dev Biol 2005;67:85–133.
3. Dorey K, Hill CS. A novel Cripto-related protein reveals an essential role for EGF-CFCs in Nodal signalling in Xenopus embryos. Dev Biol 2006;292(2):303–16.
4. Zhang J, Talbot WS, Schier AF. Positional cloning identifies zebrafish one-eyed pinhead as a permissive EGF-related ligand required during gastrulation. Cell 1998;92(2):241–51.
5. Colas JF, Schoenwolf GC. Subtractive hybridization identifies chick-cripto, a novel EGF-CFC ortholog expressed during gastrulation, neurulation and early cardiogenesis. Gene 2000; 255(2):205–17.
6. Schlange T, Schnipkoweit I, Andree B, et al. Chick CFC controls Lefty1 expression in the embryonic midline and nodal expression in the lateral plate. Dev Biol 2001;234(2):376–89.

7. Ding J, Yang L, Yan YT, et al. Cripto is required for correct orientation of the anterior-posterior axis in the mouse embryo. Nature 1998;395(6703):702–7.
8. Shen MM, Wang H, Leder P. A differential display strategy identifies Cryptic, a novel EGF-related gene expressed in the axial and lateral mesoderm during mouse gastrulation. Development 1997;124(2):429–42.
9. Ciccodicola A, Dono R, Obici S, Simeone A, Zollo M, Persico MG. Molecular characterization of a gene of the 'EGF family' expressed in undifferentiated human NTERA2 teratocarcinoma cells. EMBO J 1989;8(7):1987–91.
10. Bamford RN, Roessler E, Burdine RD, et al. Loss-of-function mutations in the EGF-CFC gene *CFC1* are associated with human left-right laterality defects. Nat Genet 2000;26(3):365–9.
11. Shen MM. Nodal signaling: developmental roles and regulation. Development 2007; 134(6):1023–34.
12. Duboc V, Rottinger E, Besnardeau L, Lepage T. Nodal and BMP2/4 signaling organizes the oral-aboral axis of the sea urchin embryo. Dev Cell 2004;6(3):397–410.
13. Minchiotti G, Manco G, Parisi S, Lago CT, Rosa F, Persico MG. Structure–function analysis of the EGF-CFC family member Cripto identifies residues essential for nodal signalling. Development 2001;128(22):4501–10.
14. Hentschke M, Kurth I, Borgmeyer U, Hubner CA. Germ cell nuclear factor is a repressor of CRIPTO-1 and CRIPTO-3. J Biol Chem 2006;281(44):33497–504.
15. Lohmeyer M, Harrison PM, Kannan S, et al. Chemical synthesis, structural modeling, and biological activity of the epidermal growth factor-like domain of human cripto. Biochemistry 1997;36(13):3837–45.
16. Seno M, DeSantis M, Kannan S, et al. Purification and characterization of a recombinant human cripto-1 protein. Growth Factors 1998;15(3):215–29.
17. Marasco D, Saporito A, Ponticelli S, et al. Chemical synthesis of mouse cripto CFC variants. Proteins 2006;64(3):779–88.
18. Foley SF, van Vlijmen HW, Boynton RE, et al. The CRIPTO/FRL-1/CRYPTIC (CFC) domain of human Cripto Functional and structural insights through disulfide structure analysis. Eur J Biochem 2003;270(17):3610–18.
19. Calvanese L, Saporito A, Marasco D, et al. Solution structure of mouse Cripto CFC domain and its inactive variant Trp107Ala. J Med Chem 2006;49(24):7054–62.
20. Schiffer SG, Foley S, Kaffashan A, et al. Fucosylation of Cripto is required for its ability to facilitate nodal signaling. J Biol Chem 2001;276(41):37769–78.
21. Shi S, Ge C, Luo Y, Hou X, Haltiwanger RS, Stanley P. The threonine that carries fucose, but not fucose, is required for Cripto to facilitate Nodal signaling. J Biol Chem 2007;282(28):20133–41.
22. Yan YT, Liu JJ, Luo Y, et al. Dual roles of Cripto as a ligand and coreceptor in the nodal signaling pathway. Mol Cell Biol 2002;22(13):4439–49.
23. Minchiotti G, Parisi S, Liguori G, et al. Membrane-anchorage of Cripto protein by glycosylphosphatidylinositol and its distribution during early mouse development. Mech Dev 2000;90(2):133–42.
24. Watanabe K, Bianco C, Strizzi L, et al. Growth factor induction of cripto-1 shedding by GPI-phospholipase D and enhancement of endothelial cell migration. J Biol Chem 2007;282(43):31643–55.
25. Watanabe K, Hamada S, Bianco C, et al. Requirement of glycosylphosphatidylinositol anchor of cripto-1 for 'trans' activity as a nodal co-receptor. J Biol Chem 2007;282(49):35772–86.
26. Rampal R, Luther KB, Haltiwanger RS. Notch signaling in normal and disease States: possible therapies related to glycosylation. Curr Mol Med 2007;7(4):427–45.
27. Rabbani SA, Mazar AP, Bernier SM, et al. Structural requirements for the growth factor activity of the amino-terminal domain of urokinase. J Biol Chem 1992;267(20):14151–6.
28. Joutel A, Corpechot C, Ducros A, et al. Notch3 mutations in CADASIL, a hereditary adult-onset condition causing stroke and dementia. Nature 1996;383(6602):707–10.
29. Bianco C, Strizzi L, Mancino M, et al. Regulation of Cripto-1 signaling and biological activity by Caveolin-1 in mammary epithelial cells. Am J Pathol 2008;172:345–357.
30. Parisi S, D'Andrea D, Lago CT, Adamson ED, Persico MG, Minchiotti G. Nodal-dependent Cripto signaling promotes cardiomyogenesis and redirects the neural fate of embryonic stem cells. J Cell Biol 2003;163(2):303–14.

Chapter 6 / Role of the EGF-CFC Family in Mammary Gland Development

31. Bianco C, Strizzi L, Rehman A, et al. A Nodal- and ALK4-independent signaling pathway activated by Cripto-1 through Glypican-1 and c-Src. Cancer Res 2003;63(6):1192–7.
32. Bianco C, Kannan S, De Santis M, et al. Cripto-1 indirectly stimulates the tyrosine phosphorylation of erb B-4 through a novel receptor. J Biol Chem 1999;274(13):8624–9.
33. Schier AF. Nodal signaling in vertebrate development. Annu Rev Cell Dev Biol 2003;19:589–621.
34. Cheng SK, Olale F, Bennett JT, Brivanlou AH, Schier AF. EGF-CFC proteins are essential coreceptors for the TGF-beta signals Vg1 and GDF1. Genes Dev 2003;17(1):31–6.
35. Chen C, Ware SM, Sato A, et al. The Vg1-related protein Gdf3 acts in a Nodal signaling pathway in the pre-gastrulation mouse embryo. Development 2006;133(2):319–29.
36. Andersson O, Bertolino P, Ibanez CF. Distinct and cooperative roles of mammalian Vg1 homologs GDF1 and GDF3 during early embryonic development. Dev Biol 2007;311(2):500–11.
37. Yeo C, Whitman M. Nodal signals to Smads through Cripto-dependent and Cripto-independent mechanisms. Mol Cell 2001;7(5):949–57.
38. Attisano L, Silvestri C, Izzi L, Labbe E. The transcriptional role of Smads and FAST (FoxH1) in TGFbeta and activin signalling. Mol Cell Endocrinol 2001;180(1–2):3–11.
39. Yamamoto M, Mine N, Mochida K, et al. Nodal signaling induces the midline barrier by activating Nodal expression in the lateral plate. Development 2003;130(9):1795–804.
40. Shen MM, Schier AF. The EGF-CFC gene family in vertebrate development. Trends Genet 2000;16(7):303–9.
41. Reissmann E, Jornvall H, Blokzijl A, et al. The orphan receptor ALK7 and the Activin receptor ALK4 mediate signaling by Nodal proteins during vertebrate development. Genes Dev 2001;15(15):2010–22.
42. Gray PC, Shani G, Aung K, Kelber J, Vale W. Cripto binds transforming growth factor beta (TGF-beta) and inhibits TGF-beta signaling. Mol Cell Biol 2006;26(24):9268–78.
43. Harms PW, Chang C. Tomoregulin-1 (TMEFF1) inhibits nodal signaling through direct binding to the nodal coreceptor Cripto. Genes Dev 2003;17(21):2624–9.
44. Tanegashima K, Haramoto Y, Yokota C, Takahashi S, Asashima M. Xantivin suppresses the activity of EGF-CFC genes to regulate nodal signaling. Int J Dev Biol 2004;48(4):275–83.
45. Uchida T, Wada K, Akamatsu T, et al. A novel epidermal growth factor-like molecule containing two follistatin modules stimulates tyrosine phosphorylation of erbB-4 in MKN28 gastric cancer cells. Biochem Biophys Res Commun 1999;266(2):593–602.
46. Cheng SK, Olale F, Brivanlou AH, Schier AF. Lefty blocks a subset of TGFbeta signals by antagonizing EGF-CFC coreceptors. PLoS Biol 2004;2(2):E30.
47. Chen C, Shen MM. Two modes by which Lefty proteins inhibit nodal signaling. Curr Biol 2004;14(7):618–24.
48. Adkins HB, Bianco C, Schiffer SG, et al. Antibody blockade of the Cripto CFC domain suppresses tumor cell growth in vivo. J Clin Invest 2003;112(4):575–87.
49. Gray PC, Harrison CA, Vale W. Cripto forms a complex with activin and type II activin receptors and can block activin signaling. Proc Natl Acad Sci USA 2003;100(9):5193–8.
50. Mancino M, Strizzi L, Wechselberger C, et al. Regulation of human cripto-1 gene expression by TGF-beta1 and BMP-4 in embryonal and colon cancer cells. J Cell Physiol 2008;215:192–203.
51. Shani G, Fischer WH, Justice NJ, Kelber JA, Vale W, Gray PC. GRP78 and Cripto form a complex at the cell surface and collaborate to inhibit TGF-β signaling and enhance cell growth. Mol Cell Biol 2008;28:666–677.
52. Li J, Lee AS. Stress induction of GRP78/BiP and its role in cancer. Curr Mol Med 2006;6(1):45–54.
53. Lee AS. GRP78 induction in cancer: therapeutic and prognostic implications. Cancer Res 2007;67(8):3496–9.
54. Lee E, Nichols P, Spicer D, Groshen S, Yu MC, Lee AS. GRP78 as a novel predictor of responsiveness to chemotherapy in breast cancer. Cancer Res 2006;66(16):7849–53.
55. De Santis ML, Kannan S, Smith GH, et al. Cripto-1 inhibits beta-casein expression in mammary epithelial cells through a p21ras-and phosphatidylinositol 3'-kinase-dependent pathway. Cell Growth Differ 1997;8(12):1257–66.

56. Ebert AD, Wechselberger C, Frank S, et al. Cripto-1 induces phosphatidylinositol 3′-kinase-dependent phosphorylation of AKT and glycogen synthase kinase 3beta in human cervical carcinoma cells. Cancer Res 1999;59(18):4502–5.
57. Bianco C, Normanno N, De Luca A, et al. Detection and localization of Cripto-1 binding in mouse mammary epithelial cells and in the mouse mammary gland using an immunoglobulin-cripto-1 fusion protein. J Cell Physiol 2002;190(1):74–82.
58. Bianco C, Adkins HB, Wechselberger C, et al. Cripto-1 activates nodal- and ALK4-dependent and -independent signaling pathways in mammary epithelial Cells. Mol Cell Biol 2002;22(8):2586–97.
59. Morkel M, Huelsken J, Wakamiya M, et al. Beta-catenin regulates Cripto- and Wnt3-dependent gene expression programs in mouse axis and mesoderm formation. Development 2003;130(25):6283–94.
60. Hamada S, Watanabe K, Hirota M, et al. beta-Catenin/TCF/LEF regulate expression of the short form human Cripto-1. Biochem Biophys Res Commun 2007;355(1):240–4.
61. Segditsas S, Tomlinson I. Colorectal cancer and genetic alterations in the Wnt pathway. Oncogene 2006;25(57):7531–7.
62. Tao Q, Yokota C, Puck H, et al. Maternal wnt11 activates the canonical wnt signaling pathway required for axis formation in Xenopus embryos. Cell 2005;120(6):857–71.
63. Zamparini AL, Watts T, Gardner CE, Tomlinson SR, Johnston GI, Brickman JM. Hex acts with beta-catenin to regulate anteroposterior patterning via a Groucho-related co-repressor and Nodal. Development 2006;133(18):3709–22.
64. Krebs LT, Iwai N, Nonaka S, et al. Notch signaling regulates left-right asymmetry determination by inducing Nodal expression. Genes Dev 2003;17(10):1207–12.
65. Dono R, Scalera L, Pacifico F, Acampora D, Persico MG, Simeone A. The murine cripto gene: expression during mesoderm induction and early heart morphogenesis. Development 1993;118(4):1157–68.
66. Johnson SE, Rothstein JL, Knowles BB. Expression of epidermal growth factor family gene members in early mouse development. Dev Dyn 1994;201(3):216–26.
67. Xu C, Liguori G, Persico MG, Adamson ED. Abrogation of the Cripto gene in mouse leads to failure of postgastrulation morphogenesis and lack of differentiation of cardiomyocytes. Development 1999;126(3):483–94.
68. Gritsman K, Zhang J, Cheng S, Heckscher E, Talbot WS, Schier AF. The EGF-CFC protein one-eyed pinhead is essential for nodal signaling. Cell 1999;97(1):121–32.
69. Schier AF, Shen MM. Nodal signalling in vertebrate development. Nature 2000;403(6768):385–9.
70. Warga RM, Kane DA. One-eyed pinhead regulates cell motility independent of Squint/Cyclops signaling. Dev Biol 2003;261(2):391–411.
71. Yan YT, Gritsman K, Ding J, et al. Conserved requirement for EGF-CFC genes in vertebrate left-right axis formation. Genes Dev 1999;13(19):2527–37.
72. Saijoh Y, Adachi H, Sakuma R, et al. Left-right asymmetric expression of lefty2 and nodal is induced by a signaling pathway that includes the transcription factor FAST2. Mol Cell 2000;5(1):35–47.
73. Gaio U, Schweickert A, Fischer A, et al. A role of the cryptic gene in the correct establishment of the left-right axis. Curr Biol 1999;9(22):1339–42.
74. Schier AF, Talbot WS. Nodal signaling and the zebrafish organizer. Int J Dev Biol 2001;45(1):289–97.
75. de la Cruz JM, Bamford RN, Burdine RD, et al. A loss-of-function mutation in the CFC domain of TDGF1 is associated with human forebrain defects. Hum Genet 2002;110(5):422–8.
76. Kenney NJ, Huang RP, Johnson GR, et al. Detection and location of amphiregulin and Cripto-1 expression in the developing postnatal mouse mammary gland. Mol Reprod Dev 1995;41(3):277–86.
77. Kenney NJ, Adkins HB, Sanicola M. Nodal and cripto-1: embryonic pattern formation genes involved in mammary gland development and tumorigenesis. J Mammary Gland Biol Neoplasia 2004;9(2):133–44.
78. Bianco C, Wechselberger C, Ebert A, Khan NI, Sun Y, Salomon DS. Identification of Cripto-1 in human milk. Breast Cancer Res Treat 2001;66(1):1–7.
79. Brandt R, Normanno N, Gullick WJ, et al. Identification and biological characterization of an epidermal growth factor-related protein: cripto-1. J Biol Chem 1994;269(25):17320–8.
80. Ciardiello F, Dono R, Kim N, Persico MG, Salomon DS. Expression of cripto, a novel gene of the epidermal growth factor gene family, leads to in vitro transformation of a normal mouse mammary epithelial cell line. Cancer Res 1991;51(3):1051–4.

Chapter 6 / Role of the EGF-CFC Family in Mammary Gland Development 101

81. Kenney N, Smith G, Johnson M, Rosemberg K, Salomon DS, Dickson R. Cripto-1 activity in the intact and ovariectomized virgin mouse mammary gland. Pathogenesis 1997;1:57–71.

82. Normanno N, De Luca A, Bianco C, et al. Cripto-1 overexpression leads to enhanced invasiveness and resistance to anoikis in human MCF-7 breast cancer cells. J Cell Physiol 2004;198(1):31–9.

83. Thiery JP, Chopin D. Epithelial cell plasticity in development and tumor progression. Cancer Metastasis Rev 1999;18(1):31–42.

84. Wechselberger C, Strizzi L, Kenney N, et al. Human Cripto-1 overexpression in the mouse mammary gland results in the development of hyperplasia and adenocarcinoma. Oncogene 2005;24(25):4094–105.

85. Strizzi L, Bianco C, Normanno N, et al. Epithelial mesenchymal transition is a characteristic of hyperplasias and tumors in mammary gland from MMTV-Cripto-1 transgenic mice. J Cell Physiol 2004;201(2):266–76.

86. Thiery JP. Epithelial-mesenchymal transitions in tumour progression. Nat Rev Cancer 2002;2(6):442–54.

87. Henderson BR, Fagotto F. The ins and outs of APC and beta-catenin nuclear transport. EMBO Rep 2002;3(9):834–9.

88. Sun Y, Strizzi L, Raafat A, et al. Overexpression of human Cripto-1 in transgenic mice delays mammary gland development and differentiation and induces mammary tumorigenesis. Am J Pathol 2005;167(2):585–97.

89. Miyoshi K, Rosner A, Nozawa M, et al. Activation of different Wnt/beta-catenin signaling components in mammary epithelium induces transdifferentiation and the formation of pilar tumors. Oncogene 2002;21(36):5548–56.

90. Miyoshi K, Shillingford JM, Le Provost F, et al. Activation of beta-catenin signaling in differentiated mammary secretory cells induces transdifferentiation into epidermis and squamous metaplasias. Proc Natl Acad Sci USA 2002;99(1):219–24.

91. Polakis P. Wnt signaling and cancer. Genes Dev 2000;14(15):1837–51.

92. Normanno N, Kim N, Wen D, et al. Expression of messenger RNA for amphiregulin, heregulin, and cripto-1, three new members of the epidermal growth factor family, in human breast carcinomas. Breast Cancer Res Treat 1995;35(3):293–7.

93. Dublin EA, Bobrow LG, Barnes DM, Gullick WJ. Amphiregulin and cripto-1 overexpression in breast cancer: relationship with prognosis and clinical and molecular variables. Int J Oncol 1995;7:617–22.

94. Panico L, D'Antonio A, Salvatore G, et al. Differential immunohistochemical detection of transforming growth factor alpha, amphiregulin and CRIPTO in human normal and malignant breast tissues. Int J Cancer 1996;65(1):51–6.

95. Qi CF, Liscia DS, Normanno N, et al. Expression of transforming growth factor alpha, amphiregulin and cripto-1 in human breast carcinomas. Br J Cancer 1994;69(5):903–10.

96. Gong YP, Yarrow PM, Carmalt HL, et al. Overexpression of Cripto and its prognostic significance in breast cancer: a study with long-term survival. Eur J Surg Oncol 2007;33(4):438–43.

97. Carmalt HL, Gong YP, Yarrow PM, Lin BP, Xing PX, Gillett DJ. Bs10 the prognostic significance of the overexpression of the growth factor cripto in patients with breast cancer. ANZ J Surg 2007;77 Suppl 1:A3.

98. Srinivasan R, Gillett CE, Barnes DM, Gullick WJ. Nuclear expression of the c-erbB-4/HER-4 growth factor receptor in invasive breast cancers. Cancer Res 2000;60(6):1483–7.

99. Bianco C, Strizzi L, Mancino M, et al. Identification of cripto-1 as a novel serologic marker for breast and colon cancer. Clin Cancer Res 2006;12(17):5158–64.

100. Zeisberg M, Kalluri R. The role of epithelial-to-mesenchymal transition in renal fibrosis. J Mol Med 2004;82(3):175–81.

101. Willis BC, Liebler JM, Luby-Phelps K, et al. Induction of epithelial-mesenchymal transition in alveolar epithelial cells by transforming growth factor-beta1: potential role in idiopathic pulmonary fibrosis. Am J Pathol 2005;166(5):1321–32.

102. Liu Y. Epithelial to mesenchymal transition in renal fibrogenesis: pathologic significance, molecular mechanism, and therapeutic intervention. J Am Soc Nephrol 2004;15(1):1–12.

103. Strizzi L, Bianco C, Raafat A, et al. Netrin-1 regulates invasion and migration of mouse mammary epithelial cells overexpressing Cripto-1 in vitro and in vivo. J Cell Sci 2005;118 (Part 20):4633–43.

104. Normanno N, Bianco C, Damiano V, et al. Growth inhibition of human colon carcinoma cells by combinations of anti-epidermal growth factor-related growth factor antisense oligonucleotides. Clin Cancer Res 1996;2(3):601–9.
105. Hu XF, Xing PX. Cripto as a target for cancer immunotherapy. Expert Opin Ther Targets 2005;9(2):383–94.
106. De Luca A, Casamassimi A, Selvam MP, et al. EGF-related peptides are involved in the proliferation and survival of MDA-MB-468 human breast carcinoma cells. Int J Cancer 1999;80(4):589–94.
107. Casamassimi A, De Luca A, Agrawal S, Stromberg K, Salomon DS, Normanno N. EGF-related antisense oligonucleotides inhibit the proliferation of human ovarian carcinoma cells. Ann Oncol 2000;11(3):319–25.
108. De Luca A, Arra C, D'Antonio A, et al. Simultaneous blockage of different EGF-like growth factors results in efficient growth inhibition of human colon carcinoma xenografts. Oncogene 2000;19(51):5863–71.
109. Normanno N, De Luca A, Maiello MR, Bianco C, Mancino M, Strizzi L, Arra C, Ciardiello F, Agrawal S, Salomon DS. Cripto-1: a novel target for therapeutic intervention in human carcinoma. Int J Oncol 2004;25(4):1013–20.
110. Bianco C, Strizzi L, Ebert A, Chang C, Rehman A, Normanno N, Guedez L, Salloum R, Ginsburg E, Sun Y, Khan N, Hirota M, Wallace-Jones B, Wechselberger C, Vonderhaar BK, Tosato G, Stetler-Stevenson WG, Sanicola M, Salomon DS. Role of human cripto-1 in tumor angiogenesis. J Natl Cancer Inst 2005;97(2):132–41.
111. Xing PX, Hu XF, Pietersz GA, Hosick HL, McKenzie IF. Cripto: a novel target for antibody-based cancer immunotherapy. Cancer Res 2004;64(11):4018–23.
112. Hu XF, Li J, Yang E, Vandervalk S, Xing PX. Anti-Cripto Mab inhibit tumour growth and overcome MDR in a human leukaemia MDR cell line by inhibition of Akt and activation of JNK/SAPK and bad death pathways. Br J Cancer 2007;96(6):918–27.
113. Topczewska JM, Postovit LM, Margaryan NV, Sam A, Hess AR, Wheaton WW, Nickoloff BJ, Topczewski J, Hendrix MJ. Embryonic and tumorigenic pathways converge via Nodal signaling: role in melanoma aggressiveness. Nat Med 2006;12(8):925–32.

7

Modeling Human Breast Cancer: The Use of Transgenic Mice

Rachelle L. Dillon and
William J. Muller

SUMMARY

The advances in genomic technologies have made it possible to examine the effects of altered gene expression in the context of specific cellular compartments within the whole organism. As such, transgenic mice have proven to be an invaluable tool to investigate genes involved in many human diseases, including genes implicated in the induction and progression of breast cancer. Human breast cancer is heterogeneous and no single mouse model recapitulates all aspects of the disease. In this regard, various mouse models are necessary to investigate specific characteristics of human breast cancer. In this chapter, we discuss various transgenic mouse strains that have been developed for the purpose of modeling breast cancer and will address their relevance to observations made in human breast tumors.

Breast cancer is the most commonly diagnosed form of cancer and it is estimated that one in eight women will develop breast cancer in her lifetime. Once initiated, cancer progresses as a result of an accumulation of genetic abnormalities within cells, the most frequently observed lesions of which can be divided into two categories: (a) DNA amplification and/or overexpression of genes responsible for the generation of proliferative and survival signals, and (b) loss of heterozygosity (LOH), in genes involved in preventing unrestrained cell growth.

Genetically modified animals generated by transgenic and gene-targeting knockout technology have contributed immensely to our understanding of gene function and regulation at the molecular level in the context of the whole organism. Since the first transgenic mouse model describing mammary tumors in 1984 *(1)*, a wealth of transgenic mice for modeling breast cancer have been reported. Transgenic models encompassing a wide array of targets including growth factors, receptors, cell cycle regulators, oncogenes, and tumor suppressor genes have been generated for use in breast cancer research. In addition to conventional transgenic overexpression and germline knockouts, the advent of increasingly complex technology has allowed for the generation of more elaborate mouse models including conditional knockouts, conditional activating mutations, and

From: *Current Clinical Oncology: Breast Cancer in the Post-Genomic Era,*
Edited by: A. Giordano and N. Normanno, DOI: 10.1007/978-1-60327-945-1_7,
© Humana Press, a part of Springer Science + Business Media, LLC 2009

inducible oncogenes or knockouts. Studies of the pathology of mammary carcinomas in genetically modified mice have demonstrated neoplasms that are morphologically similar to human breast cancer *(2)*. While this chapter will describe a variety of genetically engineered mouse models of human breast cancer, it is by no means comprehensive and will not cover the entire spectrum of transgenic mouse models generated to date.

Key Words: Breast cancer; Transgenic mice; Oncogenes; Growth factors; Growth factor receptors

1. PROMOTERS

A number of different promoters have been used to drive transgene expression for the purpose of modeling breast cancer. The mouse mammary tumor virus long terminal repeat (MMTV-LTR) has been most extensively used for targeting transgene expression specifically to the mammary epithelium. The MMTV-LTR has some promotional activity during murine embryogenesis and significantly greater promotional activity in the mammary gland during pregnancy and lactation as a result of stimulation of the MMTV-LTR by progesterone, prolactin, and glucocorticoids. The MMTV promoter drives expression in both the ductal and alveolar epithelial cells of the mammary gland. An extension of the MMTV-driven oncogene system employing a somatic gene transfer method has been described *(3)*. For this, transgenic mice expressing the avian subgroup A receptor gene *tva* by means of the MMTV promoter have been developed allowing retroviral delivery of oncogenes via intraductal injection of replication-competent avian sarcoma-leukosis virus *(3)*.

Other commonly used promoters driving mammary-specific gene expression are the whey acidic protein (WAP) and β-lactoglobulin (BLG) promoters. These promoters target primarily the alveolar epithelium and thus induce phenotypes in alveolar cells. Given that these promoter are derived from milk-specific genes, they drive the highest levels of gene expression during pregnancy and lactation *(4)*. Other less commonly used promoters for mammary tumorigenesis studies include the 5' flanking sequence of the rat C3(1) prostate steroid binding protein gene and the metallothionein (MT) promoter. Recently, transgenic mouse strains have been developed using tetracycline-responsive promoters, allowing for temporal control of transgene expression. In addition, the use of the native promoter of an oncogene *(5)* or hormonally non-responsive promoters *(6)* have been utilized in order to circumvent pregnancy-induced oncogene expression. It is interesting to note that some of these new strains develop neoplasias that are ERα-positive *(6)*, which has proven to be an infrequent observation in mouse models of breast cancer.

2. ONCOGENES

2.1. Growth Factors

2.1.1. TGFα

The expression of Transforming Growth Factor α (TGFα) is upregulated in 30–70% of breast cancers. TGFα shares a high degree of homology with epidermal growth factor (EGF) and acts in a similar manner as an EGF receptor ligand *(7)*. TGFα was originally discovered based on its ability to transform fibroblasts following retroviral infection *(8)*; however, it has subsequently been identified in a variety of cell types, including a wide range of normal cells *(9–11)*.

Chapter 7 / Modeling Human Breast Cancer: The Use of Transgenic Mice 105

A number of mouse models have been generated to examine the role of TGFα in mammary tumorigenesis and have validated the importance of TGFα in the early stages of neoplastic transformation of the mammary gland. In an early study using the MT promoter which induced weak expression of human TGFα in the mammary epithelium, the mice displayed increased cellular proliferation and delayed ductal outgrowth into the mammary fat pad *(12)*. A subsequent study in which the MT promoter was used to direct rat TGFα expression demonstrated that females developed hyperplastic nodules and mammary epithelial dysplasia following multiple pregnancies *(13)*. Specific targeting of TGFα to the mammary epithelium by use of the MMTV or WAP promoters led to more striking effects than the weak expression induced by the MT promoter. In this regard, MMTV-TGFα mice displayed hyperproliferation, precocious lobulo-alveolar development, and hyperplasias in the mature virgin mammary gland *(14)*. Following multiple pregnancies, the animals went on to develop hyperplastic and dysplastic lesions. Upon further examination of the MMTV-TGFα mice, 40% of multiparous and 30% of virgin females were observed to develop mammary tumors by 16 months of age *(15)*. The use of the WAP promoter to direct mammary epithelial-specific expression of the rat TGFα resulted in an even more dramatic phenotype. WAP-TGFα mice displayed a similar proliferative phenotype to the MT- and MMTV-based mouse models; however, the WAP-TGFα mice developed mammary tumors at an increased incidence and reduced latency *(16)*. However, tumor development in the WAP-TGFα mice still required multiple rounds of pregnancy to initiate tumor development. This observation, along with the involution defect in these mice, led the investigators to suggest that the non-regressed epithelial cells may contribute to an expanded target cell population that is predisposed to transformation *(16)*.

2.1.2. FIBROBLAST GROWTH FACTORS

Fibroblast growth factors (FGFs) are secreted peptide growth factors that bind to FGF receptors and heparin sulfate forming a ternary signaling complex *(17)*. The FGF receptors are tyrosine kinases, that upon activation through ligand binding, transmit intracellular signals that affect a number of cellular processes including cell growth and differentiation *(18,19)*. *Fgf-3* was identified as the gene transactivated by MMTV provirus insertion at the *int-2* locus in mammary tumors of MMTV-infected mice *(20)*. Further analysis of other proviral integration sites has led to the identification of two other *Fgf* family members, *Fgf-4/hst-1* and *Fgf-8* as genes transactivated in mammary tumors *(21,22)*.

Following the implication of Fgf-3 in mammary tumorigenesis by proviral insertion mutagenesis, the Leder and Dickson laboratories directly addressed the transforming potential of Fgf-3 overexpression in the mammary glands of transgenic mice *(23–25)*. The ectopic expression of Fgf-3 resulted in epithelial hyperplasia in multiparous females. A later study using an inducible mouse model directing Fgf-3 expression to the mammary epithelium similarly observed mammary gland hyperplasia that was dependent on the length and levels of Fgf-3 expression *(26)*. Overexpression of Fgf-7 by use of the MMTV promoter resulted in the development of mammary hyperplasias that progressed to metastatic mammary adenocarcinomas *(27)*. Similarly, MMTV-Fgf-8 females developed mammary tumors after multiple pregnancies with a latency of about 8 months *(28)*. In the virgin females, 4 out of 23 MMTV-Fgf-8 mice developed mammary tumors at less than 4 months of age; however, the remainder of the mice did not develop tumors by 1 year of age.

The transgenic mouse models overexpressing various FGFs suggest that these growth factors may play an important role in mammary tumorigenesis. The relevance of these observations to human breast cancer however is unclear. Analysis of human breast tumors has provided conflicting results in terms of Fgf-2 expression in tumors as well as the association with prognosis [reviewed in *(29)*]. *Fgf-3* and *Fgf-4* are closely located on mouse chromosome

7 in a region that is syntenic to human chromosome 10q13. About 15% of breast cancers show somatic amplification at the *Fgf-3/Fgf-4* locus; however, RNA analysis revealed that *Fgf-3* and *Fgf-4* were not transcribed in the vast majority of these tumors. Subsequently, the *CCND1* gene encoding Cyclin D1 was found to be closely linked to *Fgf-3/Fgf-4* and present in the same amplicon, and it is now believed that *CCND1* is the important oncogene in this chromosomal region in breast cancer [reviewed in *(30)*]. In contrast, elevated levels of Fgf-8 expression has been associated with a small subset of malignant human breast cancers *(31,32)*. Furthermore, some breast cancers show amplification of FGF receptor genes, including *Fgf1R (~20%)* and *Fgfr4 (~30%) (33–35)*.

2.2. Growth Factor Receptors

2.2.1. ERBB2

The ErbB2/neu/Her2 receptor tyrosine kinase is a member of the Epidermal Growth Factor Receptor family. The *erbB2* gene is located at a region of chromosomal amplification in human breast cancers. Indeed, *20–30%* of human breast cancers express elevated ErbB2 levels as a result of genomic amplification of the *erbB2* gene *(36,37)*. ErbB2 amplification and overexpression has been shown to correlate with poor prognostic outcome in both lymph node-positive and lymph node-negative breast cancer patients *(38–41)*. The rat c-*neu* was originally described as a dominantly transforming oncogene from a chemically induced neuroblastoma *(42)*. The oncogenic form of neu was found to contain a valine to glutamic acid substitution in the transmembrane domain of the receptor *(43–45)* that leads to constitutive receptor dimerization. This activated neu and human Her-2 with the corresponding mutation have been demonstrated to induce mammary tumor formation when expressed in the mammary epithelium of transgenic mice, thus confirming a direct role for ErbB2 in mammary tumorigenesis *(46–49)*. Furthermore, the expression of wild-type neu in the mammary epithelium using the MMTV promoter also led to the development of mammary tumors. These tumors were focal in nature and of a comedoadenocarcinoma morphology which developed after an average latency of 7 months *(50)*. Interestingly, further examination of the tumors in this model revealed that the tumor tissue, but not the normal adjacent mammary epithelium, contained sporadic mutations in *neu* leading to constitutive activation of the receptor *(51)*. The observed mutations consisted of in-frame deletions, insertions, or point mutations in the cysteine-rich extracellular domain of the receptor and resulted in increased transforming ability due to the ability to form intermolecular disulfide bonds *(52)*. To directly assess the impact of the activating mutations in mammary tumorigenesis, transgenic mice expressing the mutated receptors in the mammary epithelium were generated. Similar to the point activated neu, mice expressing the mutated *neu* transgenes developed multifocal mammary tumors in all female carriers and the tumors frequently metastasized to the lung *(53)*. Although similar transmembrane domain mutations have not been noted in human breast cancers, an alternatively spliced form of Her2 has been detected in human breast cancers and breast cancer-derived cell lines *(53,54)*. The splice isoform contains a deletion of 16 amino acids in the juxtatransmembrane domain of the receptor and similar to the neu deletion mutants this leads to increased transforming ability as a result of constitutive dimerization.

One of the drawbacks of using the strong viral MMTV promoter is that expression is hormonally regulated. In order to circumvent this difficulty mice conditionally expressing an activated *neu* from the endogenous *erbB2* promoter have recently been generated *(5)*. Mice expressing this activated *neu* developed focal mammary tumors after a long latency period. Similar to what is observed in human breast cancer, tumor progression in this strain was

Chapter 7 / Modeling Human Breast Cancer: The Use of Transgenic Mice 107

associated with selective genomic amplification of the activated *neu* allele *(5)*. Collectively, the results of these experiments provide strong evidence that ErbB2 is a potent oncogene in the mammary epithelium.

2.2.2. EGFR

The epidermal growth factor receptor (EGFR) is a receptor tyrosine kinase that is stimulated upon binding of ligands such as EGF, TGFα, and amphiregulin. Studies of EGFR expression in human breast cancer have reported that EGFR overexpression is correlated with poor prognosis *(55–57)* and in particular, when in combination with ErbB2 expression *(58)*. To address the importance of EGFR in mammary tumorigenesis, transgenic mice expressing EGFR from both the MMTV and BLG promoters were reported in 2000 *(59)*. Both the MMTV- and BLG-driven EGFR expressing virgin mice showed defects in normal mammary gland development. Furthermore, these mice developed mammary epithelial hyperplasias, which progressed to dysplasias after multiple pregnancies. Adenocarcinomas were noted at a very low frequency in multiparous females in both strains. A second report of MMTV-EGFR transgenic mice supports the weak transforming ability of EGFR in the mouse mammary epithelium. In this study, 55% of MMTV-EGFR transgenic mice developed epithelial hyperplasias and slight dysplasia by 2 years of age though no overt tumors were noted *(60)*. The results of these studies suggest that EGFR can contribute to cellular transformation, although it is insufficient for complete malignant transformation of the epithelium.

2.2.3. CSF-1

The macrophage colony stimulating factor (CSF-1) was first identified as a hematopoietic growth factor capable of stimulating proliferation, differentiation, and survival of monocytes, macrophages, and their bone marrow progenitors [reviewed in *(61)]*. CSF-1 binds to a cell surface receptor, CSF-1R, encoded by the c-*fms* protooncogene, the cellular homolog of the retroviral v-*fms* oncogene *(62)*. Abnormal CSF-1R expression, with or without CSF-1 expression, has been observed in a number of human carcinomas and their derived cell lines including carcinomas of the breast *(63–66)*. Immunohistochemical analyses of primary human breast cancers demonstrated CSF-1R expression in 58% of all breast cancers and 85% of invasive breast cancers, with CSF-1R expression localized to neoplastic epithelial cells as well as stromal macrophages *(66)*. Furthermore, about half of CSF-1R-positive breast cancers express activated receptor *(67)*. Additionally, significant levels of CSF-1 have been observed in the serum and ascites of patients with breast cancer and this has been correlated with metastatic disease *(68–70)*. The importance of CSF-1 and its receptor in mammary tumorigenesis has been evaluated through the generation of separate strains of transgenic mice. MMTV-CSF-1 and MMTV-c-fms mice displayed increased ductal branching and lobulo-alveolar growth in virgins of 6 to 8 months of age *(71)*. In animals of over 1 year of age, ductal hyperplasia and glandular dysplasia was observed in all MMTV-CSF-1 and MMTV-c-fms animals and about half of the females displayed microscopic mammary tumors of adenocarcinoma and papillary carcinoma pathologies *(71)*. Interestingly, the CSF-1 expressing mammary tissue showed increased infiltration of macrophages, which further supports the hypothesis that CSF-1 expression may serve to recruit macrophages to breast tumor tissues. A study using mice homozygous for a null mutation in the *Csf-1* gene (*Csf-1op*), in the context of the Polyoma virus middle T antigen (PyVmT) mammary tumor background resulted in a reduction of primary tumor progression to malignancy and metastasis *(71)*. To further validate the importance of CSF-1 in this process, the conditional overexpression of CFS-1 in the mammary epithelium in both the PyVmT and PyVmT/CFS-1op/op transgenic mice led to an acceleration of tumor progression and an increase in pulmonary metastases *(71)*. CSF-1 overexpression was also associated with increased macrophage infiltration in the primary mammary tumor *(71)*. In this regard, it is interesting to note that it has recently been demonstrated that tumor-associated macrophages are important in the angiogenic process and thus help contribute to the progression to malignancy *(72)*. Furthermore, multiphoton microscopic visualization of mammary tumors in transgenic mice has demonstrated that perivascular macrophages of the tumor are associated with the intravasation of tumor cells into the hematogenous system *(73)*.

2.2.4. The Met Receptor Tyrosine Kinase Family

Met is a receptor tyrosine kinase that is activated upon binding of its ligand hepatocyte growth factor/scatter factor (HGF-SF). An oncogenic form of c-met (tpr-met) was originally identified in a chemically treated human osteosarcoma cell line *(74–76)*. The *tpr-met* fusion gene is a result of chromosomal rearrangement resulting in a translocation involving chromosomes 1 and 7. The end consequence is a tpr-met fusion protein which due to the presence of a leucine zipper encoded by the open reading frame of the *tpr* sequence results in dimerization and thus constitutive activation of the Met tyrosine kinase domain, ultimately leading to transforming ability *in vitro (77)*. Met is frequently amplified in various transformed cell lines and human tumors *(78,79)*. Of particular relevance, elevated expression of Met and its ligand HGF, has been reported by a number of groups in invasive ductal carcinomas from human breast cancers that have been associated with poor prognosis *(80–85)*.

A number of mouse models have been developed in order to directly assess the importance of Met and HGF in mammary tumorigenesis. The first study utilized mice expressing Tpr-Met from the MT promoter and noted that the majority of multiparous mice displayed mammary hyperplastic alveolar nodules and several had foci of microscopic carcinoma *(86)*. As the predominant phenotype of the MT-Trp-Met mice was a breast cancer phenotype, it was suggested that the mammary epithelium may be intrinsically susceptible to transformation by this oncogene. Another study used the MT promoter to drive expression of mutationally activated Met receptors *(87)* that were identified as missense mutations in human papillary renal carcinomas that lead to increased enzymatic activity of the receptor *(88,89)*. Although the incidence of tumor formation in these mice was quite low, with only one mouse developing mammary adenocarcinomas in each transgenic line, the tumors in these mice were metastatic (to the lung in both strains, and also to the lymph node, kidney, and heart in one line). Transgenic mice expressing the Met ligand, HGF, have also been generated and examined for a role in mammary tumorigenesis. The first study expressed HGF by use of the MT promoter. Along with a diverse spectrum of neoplasms including tumors of epithelial and mesenchymal origin, both virgin and parous transgenic mice expressing HGF were found to develop mammary tumors *(90)*. Mammary tumors were detected in 41% of transgenic females and the tumors were categorized as adenocarcinomas and adenosquamous carcinomas *(90)*. Another study implicating the HGF/Met pathway in mammary tumorigenesis was reported for mice expressing HGF from the WAP promoter. Virgin female mice displayed hyperplastic ductal trees with a thick layer of fibroblasts surrounding the mammary epithelium and 20% of the virgin mice developed mammary tumors by 1 year of age *(91)*. Furthermore, almost all multiparous females developed mammary carcinomas by 10 months of age and lung metastases were observed in about 20% of tumor bearing mice. The tumors developed displayed a glandular and squamous pattern with extensive necrosis and showed characteristics of breast tumors with an aggressive phenotype.

Another member of the Met family, the Ron receptor tyrosine kinase which is activated by binding of its ligand, macrophage-stimulating protein (MSP), has been implicated in breast cancer. Overexpression and constitutive activation of Ron has been observed in

Chapter 7 / Modeling Human Breast Cancer: The Use of Transgenic Mice

about 50% of primary human breast cancers *(92)* and increased Ron expression has been correlated with a more aggressive phenotype in node-negative breast cancers *(93)*. Transgenic mouse studies using both the wild-type Ron and an active form of Ron demonstrated a direct role for Ron in the initiation of breast cancer. Separate strains of mice expressing either the wild-type or activated *Ron* cDNA from the MMTV promoter developed metastatic mammary tumors at 100% penetrance with a latency of about 6 months *(94)*. The tumors were primarily/an of adenocarcinoma morphology with varying degrees of desmoplastic epithelial malignancy and the vast majority of tumor bearing mice had metastases to both the lung and liver *(94)*.

2.2.5. WNT FAMILY

Genes of the *Wnt* family encode secreted proteins that bind to two families of cell surface receptors, members of the frizzled family and members of the LDL receptor-related proteins. The Wnt ligands activate intracellular pathways that are classified into two categories; the canonical Wnt signaling pathway (involving stabilization of β-catenin) and the noncanonical Wnt signaling pathway. Early studies with MMTV insertion sites revealed frequent proviral activation of the *Wnt1* (formerly *int-1*) gene in virus-induced carcinomas *(95)*. Studies with transgenic mice confirmed the oncogenic potential of Wnt1, whereby MMTV-*Wnt1* mice rapidly develop lobulo-alveolar hyperplasias leading to focal carcinomas later in life *(96)*.

2.3. Signal Transduction

2.3.1. POLYOMAVIRUS MIDDLE T ANTIGEN

The Polyomavirus middle T antigen (PyVmT) is a membrane attached protein that is encoded by the small DNA Polyoma virus. Although PyVmT is a virally encoded protein that is not present in humans, it has proven very useful in studying breast cancer. The middle T antigen is a potent oncogene as it strongly activates a number signal transduction pathways including the Ras and phosphatidyl-inositol-3 kinase (PI3K) pathways and the Src family of kinases and thus effectively transforms the mammary epithelium. The development of MMTV-PyVmT transgenic mice established the potent transformation potential of PyVmT in the mouse mammary epithelium *(97)*. Separate lines of MMTV-PyVmT mice developed multifocal metastatic mammary tumors in all female transgene carriers after a short latency *(97)*.

A detailed characterization of the MMTV-PyVmT mouse model has recently been described by Lin et al. *(98)*. Tumor progression was described as occurring in four stages in accordance with the recommendations of the mouse mammary tumor pathology panel *(2,98)*. By 10 weeks of age about 50% of the MMTV-PyVmT primary mammary tumors have progressed to a late carcinoma stage *(98)*. Due to this rapid nature of tumor onset and the aggressive phenotype of the tumors, the MMTV-PyVmT model is frequently employed to investigate the potential of candidate tumor suppressors and to study the progression of metastatic disease.

The examination of transgenic mice expressing mutant forms of PyVmT that are unable to recruit either PI3K or Shc have implicated these signaling molecules in PyVmT-mediated transformation. Compared to the wild type MMTV-PyVmT mice, the abrogation of PI3K or Shc binding led to a delay in tumor formation in both strains of mice *(99)*. Interestingly, a small proportion of the tumors derived from mice expressing the PyVmT incapable of recruiting Shc displayed somatic mutations in the transgene that restored a functional Shc binding site *(99)*.

2.4. Cell Cycle

2.4.1. D-TYPE CYCLINS

The human genome encodes for three different D-type cyclins, Cyclin D1, Cyclin D2, and Cyclin D3. The D-type cyclins are maximally expressed during mid-G_1 phase at which point they form functional complexes with cdk4 or cdk6 *(100,101)*, a critical step in progression through the G_1 phase of the cell cycle. The *CCND1* gene encoding Cyclin D1 is found within the chromosome 11q13 region, which has been found to be amplified in a variety of human cancers, including about 15% of primary breast cancers *(102)*. Furthermore, Cyclin D1 is overexpressed at the mRNA and protein level in up to 50% of primary breast cancers and is one of the most commonly overexpressed oncogenes in breast cancer *(103–106)*. MMTV-driven expression of *Cyclin D1* in the mammary epithelium resulted in abnormalities including increased proliferation and precocious lobulo-alveolar development *(107)*. Furthermore, about 75% of transgenic mice developed focal mammary adenocarcinomas at a latency of 18 months *(107)*. The incomplete penetrance and long latency suggest that additional genetic events are required for the development of mammary tumorigenesis.

In addition to Cyclin D1, Cyclin D3 is also frequently overexpressed in several cancer types *(108)* and its expression is associated with high-grade breast tumors *(109)*. To establish a role for Cyclin D3 in mammary tumorigenesis, transgenic mice expressing Cyclin D3 in the mammary epithelium have been generated. Pirkmaier et al. demonstrated that MMTV-driven expression of Cyclin D3 leads to the development of mammary tumors in 73% of female transgene carriers following multiple pregnancies *(110)*. Tumors arose after an extended latency and most were small and detected only by wholemount analysis; however, about 10% of tumor bearing mice developed palpable mammary tumors. In contrast to the development of mainly adenocarcinomas in the MMTV-Cyclin D1 transgenic mice *(107)*, the MMTV-Cyclin D3 mice developed squamous cell carcinomas *(110)*.

2.5. Transcription Factors

2.5.1. C-MYC

The *c-myc* protooncogene was identified as the mammalian homolog of *v-myc*, the viral transforming oncogene responsible for avian myelocytomatosis *(111)*. Genomic amplification and increased RNA levels of c-*myc* were first observed in a study of primary human breast cancers in 1986 *(112)*. Further analyses have identified alteration of the c-*myc* locus as a recurring genetic lesion in human breast cancer using fluorescent *in situ* hybridization (FISH), comparative genomic hybridization (CGH), and spectral karyotyping (SKY) *(113–115)*. Since the original description of MMTV-c-*myc* mice from the Leder laboratory in 1984 *(1)*, three other independent groups have generated transgenic mice expressing c-*myc* in the mammary epithelium *(16,116,117)*. The expression of c-myc from the MMTV promoter led to mammary tumor development with complete penetrance after multiple pregnancies, whereas tumors arose in about half of the virgin females after a latency of 7–14 months *(1,118–120)*. MMTV-c-*myc* mammary tumors were originally described as moderately well-differentiated adenocarcinomas *(1)* but have more recently been characterized as aggressive, high-grade, cribiform glandular adenocarcinomas with significant cellular atypia *(2)*.

The ability of c-*myc* to transform the mammary epithelium is further supported by transgenic mice expressing c-*myc* from the WAP promoter. Almost all multiparous WAP-c-*myc* transgenic mice developed mammary tumors; however, tumors were not noted in virgin females *(16,116)*. Interestingly, following involution c-*myc* expression was observed

Chapter 7 / Modeling Human Breast Cancer: The Use of Transgenic Mice

in the mammary tumors, but not in the normal mammary epithelium, suggesting a loss of the requirement of lactogenic hormone stimulation of the WAP promoter following cellular transformation *(116)*.

Cytogenic analyses of MMTV-c-*myc* mammary tumors have revealed similar patterns of chromosomal aberrations in independent MMTV-c-*myc* animals *(121)*, suggesting that specific genetic lesions cooperate with dysregulated c-*myc* expression. Furthermore, the patterns of chromosomal abnormalities found in the MMTV-c-*myc* mammary tumors showed synteny to aberrations identified in human breast tumors *(121)*.

An additional model for examining c-*myc*-induced mammary tumorigenesis was reported by D'Cruz et al. *(117)* and comprised of a tetracycline-inducible model of c-*myc* expression in the mammary epithelium. Almost all c-*myc* expressing induced animals developed mammary tumors that were described as invasive mammary adenocarcinomas, similar to those described for MMTV-c-*myc* transgenic mice *(122,123)*. Following deinduction of c-*myc* expression by doxycycline withdrawal, a proportion of the mammary tumors fully regressed, whereas a subset of tumors either continued growing or resumed growing after a brief decrease in size *(117)*. Interestingly, the non-regressed tumors contained secondary mutations in *ras*, particularly in the *Kras2* gene *(117)*. Furthermore, *Kras2* mutations were shown to occur at a similar frequency in MMTV-c-*myc*-induced mammary tumors *(117)*.

2.6. Hormones

2.6.1. Estrogen Receptor α

The development and function of the mammary gland occurs in response to ovarian hormones, with estrogen being one of the predominant hormones involved. The importance of estrogen receptor α (ERα) in mammary gland development is highlighted in mice homozygous for a null allele. ERα knockout mice show dramatic defects in pubertal mammary gland development, with only a rudimentary ductal structure observed *(124)*. A role for ERα in the promotion of mammary gland abnormalities was demonstrated using a tetracycline-inducible system in which ERα expression was deregulated in the mammary epithelium of transgenic mice *(125)*. Lobular hyperplasia was observed in 52%, ductal hyperplasia in 36%, and ductal carcinoma in situ in 21% of 4-month-old mice induced to express ERα in the mammary epithelium *(125)*.

Although the estrogen receptor β (ERβ) knockout mice were originally reported to have no defects in mammary gland development *(126)*, a subsequent detailed analysis of these mammary glands showed a decrease in ductal branching in the virgin animals and a decrease in lobulo-alveolar development in lactating mice *(127)*.

2.6.2. Amplified in Breast Cancer 1

Amplified in breast cancer 1 (*AIB1*) was originally identified as a gene on human chromosome 20q, a region that is frequently amplified in breast cancer *(128)*. Indeed, it has been reported that *AIB1* is amplified in 5–10% of primary human breast cancers, and mRNA and protein overexpression has been noted in about 30–60% of breast cancer cases *(129–134)*. AIB1 has been shown to interact with ER in breast cancer cells *(135)* and as a coactivator, functions to enhance ER-dependent gene transcription *(129,136)*. A function for AIB1 in normal mammary gland function was demonstrated in mice null for AIB1, whereby the knockout mice displayed less mammary ductal arborization and very limited alveolar development *(137)*.

Mammary epithelial-specific overexpression of AIB1 using the MMTV promoter has demonstrated a direct role for AIB1 in the development of mammary tumors. As early as

5 months of age, numerous hyperplastic lesions were observed in the MMTV-AIB1 mice and by 20 months of age, 50% of the mice displayed adenocarcinomas of several subtypes including acinar, ductal, solid comedotype, and papillary carcinomas *(138)*. Tumor incidence was similar in virgin and parous animals and the majority of tumors were invasive and showed metastases to the lung, bones, and kidney *(138)*. Interestingly, 85% of the tumors were ERα-positive and may therefore be a useful model to study hormone-responsive breast cancer. Another study using the MMTV promoter in which AIB1 was only moderately over-expressed in the mammary epithelium noted that AIB1 transgenic mice exhibited increased proliferation and branching of the mammary ducts *(139)*. However, no mammary tumors were noted in these transgenic mice by 2 years of age *(139)*, suggesting that a threshold of AIB1 expression is required for full transformation of the mammary epithelium.

In addition to the full-length AIB1 isoform an N-terminally truncated AIB1 (AIB1Δ3), occurring naturally as a result of alternative splicing, has been observed and functions as a more potent coactivator of ERα *(140,141)*. AIB1Δ3 has also been shown to be overexpressed in human breast tumor tissue *(140)*. Overexpression of the AIB1Δ3 isoform in transgenic mice using the human cytomegalovirus immediate early gene 1 (hCMVIE1) promoter led to an increase in mammary gland size and weight and was associated with an increase in mammary epithelial cell proliferation *(142)*. Furthermore, 40% of hCMVIE1-AIB1Δ3 transgenic mice developed ductal ectasia by 13 months of age *(142)*. Given the more dramatic phenotype observed in the MMTV-AIB1 high expressing transgenic mice, it would be interesting to examine the effects of expressing the AIB1Δ3 isoform using a similar mammary epithelial-specific promoter and with higher levels of transgene expression.

2.6.3. AROMATASE

A common MMTV insertion site was originally described in chemically induced hyperplastic alveolar nodules, referred to as the *int-5* locus [formerly *int-H (143)*], and was subsequently demonstrated to correspond to the aromatase gene *(144)*. Aromatase catalyzes the conversion of androgens to estrogens, the rate-limiting step in estrogen biosynthesis. *In situ* estradiol synthesis is a mechanism to increase the local estrogen levels and one of these pathways, the conversion of androstenedione to estrone, is catalyzed by aromatase *(145,146)*. The expression of aromatase in breast tumors was first described in 1974 *(147)*, and later studies have corroborated this observation *(145,148)*. Aromatase mRNA levels and activity have been demonstrated to be elevated in tumor-bearing quadrants when compared to normal quadrants of breast tissue *(149,150)*. Furthermore, immunohistochemical localization has revealed increased aromatase protein expression in breast tumor tissues when compared to normal areas of the breast *(151)*. Elevated expression/of aromatase leading to augmented estrogen content has been observed in breast tumors of postmenopausal women, despite reduced estradiol plasma levels *(152)*. The role of aromatase in mammary tumorigenesis has been evaluated through the use of transgenic mice. Overexpression of aromatase in the mammary epithelium by use of the MMTV promoter led to a variety of abnormalities. In young virgin animals, the MMTV-aromatase mice displayed enlarged ducts, hyperplastic and dysplastic lesions at various frequencies and about 15% of the ducts were characterized as fibroadenomas *(153)*. Following 8 weeks of involution some of the mice displayed hyperplastic alveolar nodules and atypical ductal and glandular hyperplasia, *(153)*. Further characterization of the MMTV-aromatase mice revealed that the preneoplastic and neoplastic changes were present even in the absence of circulating ovarian-derived estrogen *(154)*. In addition, the neoplastic and biochemical changes observed in the MMTV-aromatase transgenic mice could be reversed by treatment with the aromatase inhibitor, letrozole *(155,156)*, providing direct evidence for the involvement of aromatase activity in inducing the changes in the mammary glands of these mice.

3. CONCLUSIONS

Although various transgenic mouse models for the study of breast cancer have been illustrated above, we have not described the various combinations of bitransgenics that have been generated. Undoubtedly, the coexpression of multiple oncogenes and/or combinations of oncogenes in parallel with tumor suppressor deletions mimic the multiple genetic events that are observed in human breast cancer and serve as invaluable tools for modeling the human disease.

Based on the expression of keratins in breast cancers it is generally accepted that luminal epithelial cells are the main contributors to neoplastic transformation in the human breast *(157–159)*. Indeed, the observations in many mouse models for breast cancer are consistent in this regard *(2)*. While transgenic mouse models have identified a number of proteins that are involved in mammary tumorigenesis, there are aspects of these models that do not fully recapitulate the human disease.

The tumor microenvironment has emerged as an important participant in the progression of malignancy and it supports epithelial cells with local growth factors. In turn, epithelial cells signal back to the stroma, which then becomes competent to support epithelial proliferation and differentiation. In this regard, it is important to note that the stromal compartment of the mouse and human breast is not identical. While the mouse mammary stroma largely consists of adipose tissue, the human stroma contains a relatively high amount of fibrous cells surrounding the epithelial compartment. Tumor fibroblasts have been shown to have an active phenotype different to that of resting tissue fibroblasts, and reports have suggested that cancer stromal alterations precede the malignant conversion of tumor cells *(160)*. Indeed, microdissection of the epithelial and mesenchymal components of breast tumors has revealed genetic aberrations in the mesenchymal cells, including LOH at several loci exclusive to the stromal cells *(160)*. To further our knowledge of breast cancer it will be important to develop methods that allow investigators to address the contribution of stromal components in mouse models. It would be invaluable to identify promoters that will allow targeting gene expression to the different cell types of the stroma including fibroblasts and adipose cells in order to accurately address the cross-talk between the cells present within the tumor.

Another important component of human breast cancer that is lacking in transgenic mouse models is the hormone receptor status. While approximately half of all human breast cancers are ER-positive, the majority of lesions observed in the mouse models are ER-negative. Although a few recent transgenic models have demonstrated to some extent to develop ER-positive mammary tumors, additional models will be important to fully dissect the role of hormones in breast cancer and for testing therapeutic agents that target this feature of breast cancer.

In addition, the majority of existing cancer models do not reproduce aspects of advanced human breast cancers especially in terms of the frequency and location of metastases. Breast cancer in humans typically spreads lymphatically starting with local lymph glands, followed by distant metastases to predominantly the bone, brain, adrenal gland, liver, and lung. In contrast, mouse mammary cancers metastasize almost exclusively to the lung via the hematogenous route. The establishment of mouse models that metastasize analogous to human breast cancer is an important aim that needs to be addressed in order to appropriately investigate mechanisms of metastasis and to evaluate anticancer therapies that interfere with metastatic pathways.

Through the increased analysis and further development of strains of transgenic mice modeling breast cancer, it is hopeful that novel targets for the treatment of breast cancer can be identified and hopefully mouse models that recapitulate the human disease will prove useful in the testing of therapeutic agents.

REFERENCES

1. Stewart TA, Pattengale PK, Leder P. Spontaneous mammary adenocarcinomas in transgenic mice that carry and express MMTV/myc fusion genes. Cell 1984;38(3):627–37.
2. Cardiff RD, Anver MR, Gusterson BA, et al. The mammary pathology of genetically engineered mice: the consensus report and recommendations from the Annapolis meeting. Oncogene 2000;19(8):968–88.
3. Du Z, Podsypanina K, Huang S, et al. Introduction of oncogenes into mammary glands in vivo with an avian retroviral vector initiates and promotes carcinogenesis in mouse models. Proc Natl Acad Sci U S A 2006;103(46):17396–401.
4. Amundadottir LT, Merlino G, Dickson RB. Transgenic mouse models of breast cancer. Breast Cancer Res Treat 1996;39(1):119–35.
5. Andrechek ER, Hardy WR, Siegel PM, Rudnicki MA, Cardiff RD, Muller WJ. Amplification of the neu/erbB-2 oncogene in a novel mouse model of mammary tumorigenesis. Proc Natl Acad Sci U S A 2000;97(7):3444–9.
6. Rose-Hellekant TA, Arendt LM, Schroeder MD, Gilchrist K, Sandgren EP, Schuler LA. Prolactin induces ERα-positive and ERα-negative mammary cancer in transgenic mice. Oncogene 2003;22(30):4664–74.
7. Todaro GJ, Fryling C, de Larco JE. Transforming growth factors produced by certain human tumor cells: polypeptides that interact with epidermal growth factor receptors. Proc Natl Acad Sci U S A 1980;77(9):5258–62.
8. de Larco JE, Todaro GJ. Growth factors from murine sarcoma virus-transformed cells. Proc Natl Acad Sci U S A 1978;75(8):4001–5.
9. Coffey RJJ, Derynck R, Wilcox JN, et al. Production and auto-induction of transforming growth factor-α in human keratinocytes. Nature 1987;328(6133):817–20.
10. Derynck R. Transforming growth factor-α. Mol Reprod Dev 1990;27(1):3–9.
11. Driman DK, Kobrin MS, Kudlow JE, Asa SL. Transforming growth factor-α in normal and neoplastic human endocrine tissues. Hum Pathol 1992;23(12):1360–5.
12. Jhappan C, Stahle C, Harkins RN, Fausto N, Smith GH, Merlino GT. TGFα overexpression in transgenic mice induces liver neoplasia and abnormal development of the mammary gland and pancreas. Cell 1990;61(6):1137–46.
13. Sandgren EP, Luetteke NC, Palmiter RD, Brinster RL, Lee DC. Overexpression of TGFα in transgenic mice: induction of epithelial hyperplasia, pancreatic metaplasia, and carcinoma of the breast. Cell 1990;61(6):1121–35.
14. Matsui Y, Halter SA, Holt JT, Hogan BL, Coffey RJ. Development of mammary hyperplasia and neoplasia in MMTV-TGFα transgenic mice. Cell 1990;61(6):1147–55.
15. Halter SA, Dempsey P, Matsui Y, et al. Distinctive patterns of hyperplasia in transgenic mice with mouse mammary tumor virus transforming growth factor-α: Characterization of mammary gland and skin proliferations. Am J Pathol 1992;140(5):1131–46.
16. Sandgren EP, Schroeder JA, Qui TH, Palmiter RD, Brinster RL, Lee DC. Inhibition of mammary gland involution is associated with transforming growth factor a but not c-myc-induced mammary tumorigenesis in mice. Cancer Res 1995;55(17):3915–27.
17. Klagsbrun M, Baird A. A dual receptor system is required for basic fibroblast growth factor activity. Cell 1991;67(2):229–31.
18. Basilico C, Moscatelli D. The FGF family of growth factors and oncogenes. Adv Cancer Res 1992;59:115–65.
19. Ornitz DM, Xu J, Colvin JS, et al. Receptor specificity of the fibroblast growth factor family. J Biol Chem 1996;271(25):15292–7.
20. Peters G, Brookes S, Smith R, Dickson C. Tumorigenesis by mouse mammary tumor virus: evidence for a common region for provirus integration in mammary tumors. Cell 1983;33(2):369–77.
21. Peters G, Brookes S, Smith R, Placzek M, Dickson C. The mouse homolog of the *hst/k-FGF* gene is adjacent to *int-2* and is activated by proviral insertion in some virally induced mammary tumors. Proc Natl Acad Sci U S A 1989;86(15):5678–82.
22. MacArthur CA, Shankar DB, Shackleford GM. *Fgf-8*, activated by proviral insertion, cooperates with the *Wnt-1* transgene in murine mammary tumorigenesis. J Virol 1995;69(4):2501–7.

Chapter 7 / Modeling Human Breast Cancer: The Use of Transgenic Mice 115

23. Muller WJ, Lee FS, Dickson C, Peters G, Pattengale P, Leder P. The *int-2* gene product acts as an epithelial growth factor in transgenic mice. EMBO J 1990;9(3):907–13.

24. Ornitz DM, Moreadith RW, Leder P. Binary system for regulating transgene expression in mice: targeting int-2 gene expression with yeast *GAL4/UAS* control elements. Proc Natl Acad Sci U S A 1991;88(3):698–702.

25. Stamp G, Fantl V, Poulsom R, et al. Nonuniform expression of a mouse mammary tumor virus-driven *int-2*/Fgf-3 transgene in pregnancy-responsive breast tumors. Cell Growth Differ 1992;3(12):929–38.

26. Ngan ES, Ma ZQ, Chua SS, DeMayo FJ, Tsai SY. Inducible expression of FGF-3 in mouse mammary gland. Proc Natl Acad Sci U S A 2002;99(17):11187–92.

27. Kitsberg DI, Leder A. Keratinocyte growth factor induces mammary and prostatic hyperplasia and mammary adenocarcinoma in transgenic mice. Oncogene 1996;13(12):2507–15.

28. Daphna-Iken D, Shankar DB, Lawshe A, Ornitz DM, Shackleford GM, MacArthur CA. MMTV-*Fgf8* transgenic mice develop mammary and salivary gland neoplasia and ovarian stromal hyperplasia. Oncogene 1998;17(21):2711–7.

29. Dickson C, Spencer-Dene B, Dillon C, Fantl V. Tyrosine kinase signalling in breast cancer: fibroblast growth factors and their receptors. Breast Cancer Res 2000;2(3):191–6.

30. Lammie GA, Peters G. Chromosome 11q13 abnormalities in breast cancer. Cancer Cells 1991;3(11):413–20.

31. Marsh SK, Bansal GS, Zammit C, et al. Increased expression of fibroblast growth factor 8 in human breast cancer. Oncogene 1999;18(4):1053–60.

32. Tanaka A, Furuya A, Yamasaki M, et al. High frequency of fibroblast growth factor (FGF) 8 expression in clinical prostate cancers and breast tissues, immunohistochemically demonstrated by a newly established neutralizing monoclonal antibody against FGF-8. Cancer Res 1998;58(10):2053–6.

33. Penault-Llorca F, Bertucci F, Adelaide J, et al. Expression of FGF and FGF receptor genes in human breast cancer. Int J Cancer 1995;61(2):170–6.

34. Theillet C, Adelaide J, Louason G, et al. FGFR1 and PLAT genes and DNA amplification at 8p12 in breast and ovarian cancers. Genes Chromosomes Cancer 1993;7(4):219–26.

35. Adnane J, Gaudray P, Dionne CA, et al. BEK and FLG, two receptors to members of the FGF family, are amplified in subsets of human breast cancers. Oncogene 1991;6(4):659–63.

36. Slamon DJ, Clark GM, Wong SG, Levin WJ, Ullrich A, McGuire WL. Human breast cancer: correlation of relapse with amplification of the *HER-2/neu* oncogene. Science 1987;235(4785):177–82.

37. Slamon DJ, Godolphin W, Jones LA, et al. Studies of the *HER-2/neu* proto-oncogene in human breast and ovarian cancer. Science 1989;244(4905):707–12.

38. Hynes NE, Stern DF. The biology of erbB-2/neu/Her-2 and its role in cancer. Biochim Biophys Acta 1994;1198(2-3):165–84.

39. Mansour EG, Ravdin PM, Dressler L. Prognostic factors in early breast carcinoma. Cancer 1994;74(Suppl):381–400.

40. Ravdin PM, Chamness GC. The c-erbB-2 proto-oncogene as a prognostic and predictive marker in breast cancer: a paradigm for the development of other macromolecular markers- A review. Gene 1995;159(1):19–27.

41. Andrulis IL, Bull SB, Blackstein ME, et al. *neu/erbB-2* amplification identifies a poor-prognosis group of women with node-negative breast cancer. Toronto Breast Cancer Study Group. J Clin Oncol 1998;16(4):1340–9.

42. Shih C, Padhy LC, Murray M, Weinberg RA. Transforming genes of carcinomas and neuroblastomas introduced into mouse fibroblasts. Nature 1981;290(5803):261–4.

43. Schechter AL, Stern DF, Vaidyanathan L, et al. The *neu* oncogene: an *erb-B*-related gene encoding a 185,000-Mr tumour antigen. Nature 1984;312(5994):513–6.

44. Bargmann CI, Hung MC, Weinberg RA. The *neu* oncogene encodes an epidermal growth factor receptor-related protein. Nature 1986;319(6050):226–30.

45. Bargmann CI, Hung MC, Weinberg RA. Multiple independent activations of the neu oncogene by a point mutation altering the transmembrane domain of p185. Cell 1986;45(5):649–57.

46. Muller WJ, Sinn E, Pattengale PK, Wallace R, Leder P. Single-step induction of mammary adenocarcinoma in transgenic mice bearing the activated c-neu oncogene. Cell 1988;54(1):105–15.

47. Bouchard L, Lamarre L, Tremblay PJ, Jolicoeur P. Stochastic appearance of mammary tumors in transgenic mice carrying the MMTV/c-neu oncogene. Cell 1989;57(6):931–6.
48. Stocklin E, Botteri F, Groner B. An activated allele of the c-erbB-2 oncogene impairs kidney and lung function and causes early death of transgenic mice. J Cell Biol 1993;122(1):199–208.
49. Guy CT, Cardiff RD, Muller WJ. Activated *neu* induces rapid tumor progression. J Biol Chem 1996;271(13):7673–8.
50. Guy CT, Webster MA, Schaller M, Parsons TJ, Cardiff RD, Muller WJ. Expression of the *neu* protooncogene in the mammary epithelium of transgenic mice induces metastatic disease. Proc Natl Acad Sci U S A 1992;89(22):10578–82.
51. Siegel PM, Dankort DL, Hardy WR, Muller WJ. Novel activating mutations in the neu proto-oncogene involved in the induction of mammary tumors. Mol Cell Biol 1994;14(11):7068–77.
52. Siegel PM, Muller WJ. Mutations affecting conserved cysteine residues within the extracellular domain of Neu promote receptor dimerization and activation. Proc Natl Acad Sci U S A 1996;93(17):8878–83.
53. Siegel PM, Ryan ED, Cardiff RD, Muller WJ. Elevated expression of activated forms of Neu/ErbB-2 and ErbB-3 are involved in the induction of mammary tumors in transgenic mice: Implications for human breast cancer. EMBO J 1999;18(8):2149–64.
54. Kwong KY, Hung MC. A novel splice variant of *HER2* with increased transformation activity. Mol Carcinog 1998;23(2):62–8.
55. Sainsbury JR, Malcolm AJ, Appleton DR, Farndon JR, Harris AL. Presence of epidermal growth factor receptor as an indicator of poor prognosis in patients with breast cancer. J Clin Pathol 1985;38(11):1225–8.
56. Harris AL, Nicholson S, Sainsbury JR, Farndon J, Wright C. Epidermal growth factor receptors in breast cancer: association with early relapse and death, poor response to hormones and interaction with neu. J Steroid Biochem 1989;34(1–6):123–31.
57. Klijn JG, Berns PM, Schmitz PI, Foekens JA. The clinical significance of epidermal growth factor receptor (EGF-R) in human breast cancer: a review on 5232 patients. Endocr Rev 1992;13(1):3–17.
58. Nieto Y, Nawaz F, Jones RB, Shpall EJ, Nawaz S. Prognostic significance of overexpression and phosphoryla(66)tion of epidermal growth factor receptor (EGFR) and the presence of truncated EGFRvIII in locoregionally advanced breast cancer. J Clin Oncol 2007;25(28):4405–13.
59. Brandt R, Eisenbrandt R, Leenders F, et al. Mammary gland specific hEGF receptor transgene expression induces neoplasia and inhibits differentiation. Oncogene 2000;19(17):2129–37.
60. Marozkina NV, Stiefel SM, Frierson Jr. HF, Parsons SJ. MMTV-EGF receptor transgene promotes preneoplastic conversion of multiple steroid hormone-responsive tissues. J Cell Biochem 2007;Epub Oct 24.
61. Stanley ER, Berg KL, Einstein DB, et al. Biology and action of colony-stimulating factor-1. Mol Reprod Dev 1997;46(1):4–10.
62. Heisterkamp N, Groffen J, Stephenson JR. Isolation of v-*fms* and its human cellular homolog. Virology 1983;126(1):248–58.
63. Slamon DJ, deKernion JB, Verma IM, Cline MJ. Expression of cellular oncogenes in human malignancies. Science 1984;224(4646):256–62.
64. Horiguchi J, Sherman ML, Sampson-Johannes A, Weber BL, Kufe DW. CSF-1 and C-FMS gene expression in human carcinoma cell lines. Biochem Biophys Res Commun 1988;157(1):395–401.
65. Ramakrishnan S, Xu FJ, Brandt SJ, Niedel JE, Bast Jr RC, Brown EL. Constitutive production of macrophage colony-stimulating factor by human ovarian and breast cancer cell lines. J Clin Invest 1989;83(3):921–6.
66. Tang R, Beuvon F, Ojeda M, Mosseri V, Pouillart P, Scholl S. M-CSF (monocyte colony stimulating factor) and M-CSF receptor expression by breast tumour cells: M-CSF mediated recruitment of tumour infiltrating monocytes? J Cell Biochem 1992;50(4):350–6.
67. Flick MB, Sapi E, Perrotta PL, et al. Recognition of activated CSF-1 receptor in breast carcinomas by a tyrosine 723 phosphospecific antibody. Oncogene 1997;14(21):2553–61.
68. Tang RP, Kacinski B, Validire P, et al. Oncogene amplification correlates with dense lymphocyte infiltration in human breast cancers: a role for hematopoietic growth factor release by tumor cells? J Cell Biochem 1990;44(3):189–98.

Chapter 7 / Modeling Human Breast Cancer: The Use of Transgenic Mice

69. Scholl SM, Mosseri V, Tang R, et al. Expression of colony-stimulating factor-1 and its receptor (the protein product of c-*fms*) in invasive breast tumor cells. Induction of urokinase production via this pathway? Ann N Y Acad Sci 1993;698:131–5.

70. Scholl SM, Crocker P, Tang R, Pouillart P, Pollard JW. Is colony-stimulating factor-1 a key mediator of breast cancer invasion and metastasis? Mol Carcinog 1993;7(4):207–11.

71. Kirma N, Luthra R, Jones J, et al. Overexpression of the colony-stimulating factor (CSF-1) and/or its receptor c-fms in mammary glands of transgenic mice results in hyperplasia and tumor formation. Cancer Res 2004;64(12):4162–70.

72. Lin EY, Li JF, Gnatovskiy L, et al. Macrophages regulate the angiogenic switch in a mouse model of breast cancer. Cancer Res 2006;66(23):11238–46.

73. Wyckoff JB, Wang Y, Lin EY, et al. Direct visualization of macrophage-assisted tumor cell intravasation in mammary tumors. Cancer Res 2007;67(6):2649–56.

74. Park M, Dean M, Cooper CS, et al. Mechanism of met oncogene activation. Cell 1986;45(6):895–904.

75. Chan AM, King HW, Tempest PR, Deakin EA, Cooper CS, Brookes P. Primary structure of the met protein tyrosine kinase domain. Oncogene 1987;1(2):229–33.

76. Park M, Dean M, Kaul K, Braun MJ, Gonda MA, Vande Woude GF. Sequence of *MET* protooncogene cDNA has features characteristic of the tyrosine kinase family of growth-factor receptors. Proc Natl Acad Sci U S A 1987;84(18):6379–83.

77. Rodrigues GA, Park M. Autophosphorylation modulates the kinase activity and oncogenic potential of the Met receptor tyrosine kinase. Oncogene 1994;9(7):2019–27.

78. Di Renzo MF, Narsimhan RP, Olivero M, et al. Expression of the Met/HGF receptor in normal and neoplastic human tissues. Oncogene 1991;6(11):1997–2003.

79. Rong S, Jeffers M, Resau JH, Tsarfaty I, Oskarsson M, Vande Woude GF. Met expression and sarcoma tumorigenicity. Cancer Res 1993;53(22):5355–60.

80. Jin L, Fuchs A, Schnitt SJ, et al. Expression of scatter factor and c-met receptor in benign and malignant breast tissues. Cancer 1997;79(4):749–60.

81. Ghoussoub RA, Dillon DA, D'Aquila T, Rimm EB, Fearon ER, Rimm DL. Expression of c-met is a strong independent prognostic factor in breast carcinoma. Cancer 1998;82(8):1513–20.

82. Camp RL, Rimm EB, Rimm DL. Met expression is associated with poor outcome in patients with axillary lymph node negative breast cancer. Cancer 1999;86(11):2259–65.

83. Edakuni G, Sasatomi E, Satoh T, Tokunaga O, Miyazaki K. Expression of the hepatocyte growth factor/c-Met pathway is increased at the cancer front in breast carcinoma. Pathol Int 2001;51(3):172–8.

84. Kang JY, Dolled-Filhart M, Ocal IT, et al. Tissue microarray analysis of hepatocyte growth factor/Met pathway components reveals a role for Met, matriptase, and hepatocyte growth factor activator inhibitor 1 in the progression of node-negative breast cancer. Cancer Res 2003;63(5):1101–5.

85. Tolgay Ocal I, Dolled-Filhart M, D'Aquila TG, Camp RL, Rimm DL. Tissue microarray-based studies of patients with lymph node negative breast carcinoma show that met expression is associated with worse outcome but is not correlated with epidermal growth factor family receptors. Cancer 2003;97(8):1841–8.

86. Liang TJ, Reid AE, Xavier R, Cardiff RD, Wang TC. Transgenic expression of trp-met oncogene leads to development of mammary hyperplasias and tumors. J Clin Invest 1996;97(12):2872–7.

87. Jeffers M, Fiscella M, Webb CP, Anver M, Koochekpour S, Vande Woude GF. The mutationally activated Met receptor mediates motility and metastasis. Proc Natl Acad Sci U S A 1998;95(24):14417–22.

88. Schmidt L, Duh FM, Chen F, et al. Germline and somatic mutations in the tyrosine kinase domain of the *MET* proto-oncogene in papillary renal carcinomas. Nat Genet 1997;16(1):68–73.

89. Jeffers M, Schmidt L, Nakaigawa N, et al. Activating mutations for the met tyrosine kinase receptor in human cancer. Proc Natl Acad Sci U S A 1997;94(21):11445–50.

90. Takayama H, LaRochelle WJ, Sharp R, et al. Diverse tumorigenesis associated with aberrant development in mice overexpressing hepatocyte growth factor/scatter factor. Proc Natl Acad Sci U S A 1997;94(2):701–6.

91. Gallego MI, Bierie B, Hennighausen L. Targeted expression of HGF/SF in mouse mammary epithelium leads to metastatic adenosquamous carcinomas through the activation of multiple signal transduction pathways. Oncogene 2003;22(52):8498–508.

92. Maggiora P, Marchio S, Stella MC, et al. Overexpression of the *RON* gene in human breast carcinoma. Oncogene 1998;16(22):2927–33.
93. Lee WY, Chen HH, Chow NH, Su WC, Lin PW, Guo HR. Prognostic significance of co-expression of RON and MET receptors in node-negative breast cancer patients. Clin Cancer Res 2005;11(6):2222–8.
94. Zinser GM, Leonis MA, Toney K, et al. Mammary-specific Ron receptor overexpression induces highly metastatic mammary tumors associated with β-catenin activation. Cancer Res 2006;66(24):11967–74.
95. Nusse R, Varmus HE. Many tumors induced by the mouse mammary tumor virus contain a provirus integrated in the same region of the host genome. Cell 1982;31(1):99–109.
96. Tsukamoto AS, Grossschedl R, Guzman RC, Parslow T, Varmus HE. Expression of the *int-1* gene in transgenic mice is associated with mammary gland hyperplasia and adenocarcinomas in male and female mice. Cell 1988;55(4):619–25.
97. Guy CT, Cardiff RD, Muller WJ. Induction of mammary tumors by expression of polyomavirus middle T oncogene: A transgenic mouse model for metastatic disease. Mol Cell Biol 1992;12(3):954–61.
98. Lin EY, Jones JG, Li P, et al. Progression to malignancy in the polyoma middle T oncoprotein mouse breast cancer models provides a reliable model for human diseases. Am J Pathol 2003;163(5):2113–26.
99. Webster MA, Hutchinson JN, Rauh MJ, et al. Requirement for both Shc and phosphatidylinositol 3′ kinase signaling pathways in polyomavirus middle T-mediated mammary tumorigenesis. Mol Cell Biol 1998;18(4):2344–59.
100. Xiong Y, Zhang H, Beach D. D type cyclins associate with multiple protein kinases and the DNA replication and repair factor PCNA. Cell 1992;71(3):505–14.
101. Meyerson M, Harlow E. Identification of G1 kinase activity for cdk4, a novel cyclin D partner. Mol Cell Biol 1994;14(3):2077–86.
102. Ormandy CJ, Musgrove EA, Hui R, Daly RJ, Sutherland RL. Cyclin D1, EMS1 and 11q13 amplification in breast cancer. Breast Cancer Res Treat 2003;78(3):323–35.
103. Buckley MF, Sweeney KJ, Hamilton JA, et al. Expression and amplification of cyclin genes in human breast cancer. Oncogene 1993;8(8):2127–33.
104. Keyomarsi K, Pardee AB. Redundant cyclin overexpression and gene amplification in breast cancer cells. Proc Natl Acad Sci U S A 1993;90(3):1112–6.
105. Gillett C, Fantl V, Smith R, et al. Amplification and overexpression of cyclin D1 in breast cancer detected by immunohistochemical staining. Cancer Res 1994;54(7):1812–7.
106. Alle KM, Henshall SM, Field AS, Sutherland RL. Cyclin D1 protein is overexpressed in hyperplasia and intraductal carcinoma of the breast. Clin Cancer Res 1998;4(4):847–54.
107. Wang TC, Cardiff RD, Zukerberg L, Lees E, Arnold A, Schmidt EV. Mammary hyperplasia and carcinoma in MMTV-cyclin D1 transgenic mice. Nature 1994;369(6482):669–71.
108. Bartkova J, Zemanova M, Bartek J. Abundance and subcellular localisation of cyclin D3 in human tumours. Int J Cancer 1996;65(3):323–7.
109. Wong SC, Chan JK, Lee KC, Hsiao WL. Differential expression of p16/p21/p27 and cyclin D1/D3, and their relationships to cell proliferation, apoptosis, and tumour progression in invasive ductal carcinoma of the breast. J Pathol 2001;194(1):35–42.
110. Pirkmaier A, Dow R, Ganiatsas S, et al. Alternative mammary oncogenic pathways are induced by D-type cyclins; MMTV-cyclin D3 transgenic mice develop squamous cell carcinoma. Oncogene 2003;22(28):4425–33.
111. Vennstrom B, Sheiness D, Zabielski J, Bishop JM. Isolation and characterization of c-*myc*, a cellular homolog of the oncogene (v-*myc*) of avian myelocytomatosis virus strain 29. J Virol 1982;42(3):773–9.
112. Escot C, Theillet C, Lidereau R, et al. Genetic alteration of the c-*myc* protooncogene (MYC) in human primary breast carcinomas. Proc Natl Acad Sci U S A 1986;83(13):4834–8.
113. Ried T, Just KE, Holtgreve-Grez H, et al. Comparative genomic hybridization of formalin-fixed, paraffin-embedded breast tumors reveals different patterns of chromosomal gains and losses in fibroadenomas and diploid and aneuploid carcinomas. Cancer Res 1995;55(22):5415–23.

Chapter 7 / Modeling Human Breast Cancer: The Use of Transgenic Mice 119

114. Tirkkonen M, Tanner M, Karhu R, Kallioniemi A, Isola J, Kallioniemi OP. Molecular cytogenetics of primary breast cancer by CGH. Genes Chromosomes Cancer 1998;21(3):177–84.
115. Janocko LE, Brown KA, Smith CA, et al. Distinctive patterns of Her-2/neu, c-myc, and cyclin D1 gene amplification by fluorescence in situ hybridization in primary human breast cancers. Cytometry 2001;46(3):136–49.
116. Schoenenberger CA, Andres AC, Groner B, van der Valk M, LeMeur M, Gerlinger P. Targeted c-*myc* gene expression in mammary glands of transgenic mice induces mammary tumours with constitutive milk protein gene transcription. EMBO J 1988;7(1):169–75.
117. D'Cruz CM, Gunther EJ, Boxer RB, et al. c-MYC induces mammary tumorigenesis by means of a preferred pathway involving spontaneous *Kras2*. Nat Med 2001;7(2):235–9.
118. Sinn E, Muller W, Pattengale P, Tepler I, Wallace R, Leder P. Coexpression of MMTV/v-Ha-*ras* and MMTV/c-*myc* genes in transgenic mice: Synergistic action of oncogenes *in vivo*. Cell 1987;49(4):465–75.
119. Amundadottir LT, Johnson MD, Merlino G, Smith GH, Dickson RB. Synergistic interaction of transforming growth factor α and c-*myc* in mouse mammary and salivary gland tumorigenesis. Cell Growth Differ 1995;6(6):737–48.
120. Bearss DJ, Lee RJ, Trover DA, Pestell RG, Windle JJ. Differential effects of p21$^{(WAF1/CIP1)}$ deficiency on MMTV-*ras* and MMTV-*myc* mammary tumor properties. Cancer Res 2002; 62(7):2077–84.
121. Weaver ZA, McCormack SJ, Liyanage M, et al. A recurring pattern of chromosomal aberrations in mammary gland tumors of MMTV-*cmyc* transgenic mice. Genes Chromosomes Cancer 1999;25(3):251–60.
122. Leder A, Pattengale PK, Kuo A, Stewart TA, Leder P. Consequences of widespread deregulation of the c-*myc* gene in transgenic mice: multiple neoplasms and normal development. Cell 1986;45(4):485–95.
123. Cardiff RD, Sinn E, Muller W, Leder P. Transgenic oncogene mice. Tumor phenotype predicts genotype. Am J Pathol 1991;139(3):495–501.
124. Bocchinfuso WP, Lindzey JK, Hewitt SC, et al. Induction of mammary gland development in estrogen receptor-α knockout mice. Endocrinology 2000;141(8):2982–94.
125. Frech MS, Halama ED, Tilli MT, et al. Deregulated estrogen receptor α expression in mammary epithelial cells of transgenic mice results in the development of ductal carcinoma *in situ*. Cancer Res 2005;65(3):681–5.
126. Krege JH, Hodgin JB, Couse JF, et al. Generation and reproductive phenotypes of mice lacking estrogen receptor β. Proc Natl Acad Sci U S A 1998;95(26):15677–82.
127. Forster C, Makela S, Warri A, et al. Involvement of estrogen receptor β in terminal differentiation of mammary gland epithelium. Proc Natl Acad Sci U S A 2002;99(24):15578–83.
128. Guan XY, Xu J, Anzick SL, Zhang H, Trent JM, Meltzer PS. Hybrid selection of transcribed sequences from microdissected DNA: isolation of genes with amplified region at 20q11-q13.2 in breast cancer. Cancer Res 1996;56(15):3446–50.
129. Anzick SL, Kononen J, Walker RL, et al. AIB1, a steroid receptor coactivator amplified in breast and ovarian cancer. Science 1997;277(5328):965–8.
130. Bautista S, Valles H, Walker RL, et al. In breast cancer, amplification of the steroid receptor coactivator gene *AIB1* is correlated with estrogen and progesterone receptor positivity. Clin Cancer Res 1998;4(12):2925–9.
131. Kurebayashi J, Otsuka T, Kunisue H, Tanaka K, Yamamoto S, Sonoo H. Expression levels of estrogen receptor-α, estrogen receptor-β, coactivators and corepressors in breast cancer. Clin Cancer Res 2000;6(2):512–8.
132. Murphy LC, Simon SL, Parkes A, et al. Altered expression of estrogen receptor coregulators during human breast tumorigenesis. Cancer Res 2000;60(22):6266–71.
133. Bouras T, Southey MC, Venter DJ. Overexpression of the steroid receptor coactivator AIB1 in breast cancer correlates with the absence of estrogen and progesterone receptors and positivity for p53 and HER2/neu. Cancer Res 2001;61(3):903–7.
134. List HJ, Reiter R, Singh B, Wellstein A, Riegel AT. Expression of the nuclear coactivator AIB1 in normal and malignant breast tissue. Breast Cancer Res Treat 2001;68(1):21–8.

135. Tikkanen MK, Carter DJ, Harris AM, et al. Endogenously expressed estrogen receptor and coactivator AIB1 interact in MCF-7 human breast cancer cells. Proc Natl Acad Sci U S A 2000;97(23):12536–40.
136. List HJ, Lauritsen KJ, Reiter R, Powers C, Wellstein A, Riegel AT. Ribozyme targeting demonstrates that the nuclear receptor coactivator AIB1 is the rate-limiting factor for estrogen-dependent growth of human MCF-7 cancer cells. J Biol Chem 2001;276(26):23763–8.
137. Xu J, Liao L, Ning G, Yoshida-Komiya H, Deng C, O'Malley BW. The steroid coactivator SRC-3 (p/CIP/RAC3/AIB1/ACTR/TRAM-1) is required for normal growth, puberty, female reproductive function, and mammary gland development. Proc Natl Acad Sci U S A 2000;97(12):6379–84.
138. Torres-Arzavus MI, Font de Mora J, Yuan J, et al. High tumor incidence and activation of the PI3K/ AKT pathway in transgenic mice define AIB1 as an oncogene. Cancer Cell 2004;6(3):263–74.
139. Avivar A, Garcia-Macias MC, Ascaso E, Herrera G, O'Connor JE, de Mora JF. Moderate overexpression of AIB1 triggers pre-neoplastic changes in mammary epithelium. FEBS Lett 2006;580(22):5222–6.
140. Reiter R, Wellstein A, Riegel AT. An isoform of the coactivator AIB1 that increases hormone and growth factor sensitivity is overexpressed in breast cancer. J Biol Chem 2001;276(43):39736–41.
141. Reiter R, Oh AS, Wellstein A, Riegel AT. Impact of the nuclear receptor coactivator AIB1 isoform AIB1-Δ3 on estrogenic ligands with different intrinsic activity. Oncogene 2004;23(2):403–9.
142. Tilli MT, Reiter R, Oh AS, et al. Overexpression of an N-terminally truncated isoform of the nuclear receptor coactivator amplified in breast cancer 1 leads to altered proliferation of mammary epithelial cells in transgenic mice. Mol Endocrinol 2005;19(3):644–56.
143. Gray DA, McGrath CM, Jones RF, Morris VL. A common mouse mammary tumor virus integration site in chemically induced precancerous mammary hyperplasias. Virology 1986;148(2):360–8.
144. Durgam VR, Tekmal RR. The nature and expression of int-5, a novel MMTV integration locus gene in carcinogen-induced mammary tumors. Cancer Lett 1994;87(2):179–86.
145. Santner SJ, Feil PD, Santen RJ. In situ estrogen production via the estrone sulfatase pathway in breast tumors: relative importance versus the aromatase pathway. J Clin Endocrinol Metab 1984;59(1):29–33.
146. Santen RJ, Leszyczynski D, Tilson-Mallet N, et al. Enzymatic control of estrogen production in human breast cancer: relative significance of aromatase versus sulfatase pathways. Ann N Y Acad Sci 1986;464:126–37.
147. Miller WR, Forrest AP. Oestradiol synthesis by a human breast carcinoma. Lancet 1974;2(7885):866–8.
148. Reed MJ, Owen AM, Lai LC, et al. In situ oestrogen synthesis in normal and breast tumour tissues: effect of treatment with 4-hydroxyandrostenedione. Int J Cancer 1989;44(2):233–7.
149. O'Neill JS, Elton RA, Miller WR. Aromatase activity in adipose tissue from breast quadrants: a link with tumour site. Br Med J (Clin Res Ed) 1988;296(6624):741–3.
150. Bulun SE, Sharda G, Rink J, Sharma S, Simpson ER. Distribution of aromatase P450 transcripts and adipose fibroblasts in the human breast. J Clin Endocrinol Metab 1996;81(3):1273–7.
151. Lu O, Nakamura J, Savinov A, et al. Expression of aromatase protein and messenger ribonucleic acid in tumor epithelial cells and evidence of functional significance of locally produced estrogen in human breast cancers. Endocrinology 1996;137(7):3061–8.
152. Miller WR. Aromatase activity in breast tissue. J Steroid Biochem Mol Biol 1991;39(5B):783–90.
153. Tekmal RR, Ramachandra N, Gubba S, et al. Overexpression of int-5/aromatase in mammary glands of transgenic mice results in the induction of hyperplasia and nuclear abnormalities. Cancer Res 1996;56(14):3180–5.
154. Kirma N, Gill K, Mandava U, Tekmal RR. Overexpression of aromatase leads to hyperplasia and changes in the expression of genes involved in apoptosis, cell cycle, growth, and tumor suppressor functions in the mammary glands of transgenic mice. Cancer Res 2001;61(5):1910–8.
155. Tekmal RR, Kirma N, Gill K, Fowler K. Aromatase overexpression and breast hyperplasia, an in vivo model- continued overexpression of aromatase is sufficient to maintain hyperplasia without circulating estrogens, and aromatase inhibitors abrogate these preneoplastic changes in mammary glands. Endocr Relat Cancer 1999;6(2):307–14.

Chapter 7 / Modeling Human Breast Cancer: The Use of Transgenic Mice   121

156. Mandava U, Kirma N, Tekmal RR. Aromatase overexpression transgenic mice model: cell type specific expression and use of letrozole to abrogate mammary hyperplasia without affecting normal physiology. J Steroid Biochem Mol Biol 2001;79(1-5):27–34.

157. Gusterson BA, Warburton MJ, Mitchell D, Ellison M, Neville AM, Rudland PS. Distribution of myoepithelial cells and basement membrane proteins in the normal breast and in benign and malignant breast diseases. Cancer Res 1982;42(11):4763–70.

158. Rudland PS, Leinster SJ, Winstanley J, Green B, Atkinson M, Zakhour HD. Immunocytochemical identification of cell types in benign and malignant breast diseases: variations in cell markers accompany the malignant state. J Histochem Cytochem 1993;41(4):543–53.

159. Trask DK, Band V, Zajchowski DA, Yaswen P, Suh T, Sager R. Keratins as markers that distinguish normal and tumor-derived mammary epithelial cells. Proc Natl Acad Sci U S A 1990;87(6):2319–23.

160. Moinfar F, Man YG, Arnould L, Bratthauer GL, Ratschek M, Tavassoli FA. Concurrent and independent genetic alterations in the stromal and epithelial cells of mammary carcinoma: implications for tumorigenesis. Cancer Res 2000;60(9):2562–6.

8 Gene Expression Profiling in Breast Cancer: Clinical Applications

Giuseppe Russo and Antonio Giordano

SUMMARY

Breast cancer is a complex genetic disease characterized by the accumulation of multiple molecular alterations. Today, routine clinical management of breast cancer is insufficient to reflect the whole clinical heterogeneity of this disease. Recent advances in human genome research and gene expression profiling have made it possible to start uncovering biological mechanisms underlying clinically useful signatures. Here we highlight gene expression profiling in breast cancer research and discuss its most current clinical applications.

Key Words: Breast cancer; Microarrays; Gene expression profiling; Data integration; Data analysis; Molecular classification; Diagnosis and prognosis; Response to therapy

1. INTRODUCTION

Breast cancer is the most common cancer in women *(1,2)* with most cases occurring in postmenopausal women, but a significant number of younger women are afflicted, often in families with a hereditary predisposition. It is the most common malignancy and leading cause of cancer death among American women between the ages 20 and 59 and the second cause of cancer death in women aged 60 to 79 *(3)*. Known risk factors include the length of the life-time exposure to estrogens, ionizing radiation, cigarette smoking, and a high-fat diet. Breast cancer is a genotypically, phenotypically, and clinically a heterogeneous complex disease. In fact, breast cancer is characterized by the accumulation of multiple molecular alterations.

From: *Current Clinical Oncology: Breast Cancer in the Post-Genomic Era,*
Edited by: A. Giordano and N. Normanno, DOI: 10.1007/978-1-60327-945-1_8,
© Humana Press, a part of Springer Science + Business Media, LLC 2009

Even though UK and US breast cancer mortality is declining because of the implementation of widespread screening mammography, earlier diagnosis, and advances in adjuvant treatment *(4)*, not all patients benefit from their treatment. In fact, current routine clinical management of breast cancer relies on a number of clinical and pathological prognostic and predictive factors and these seem insufficient to reflect the whole clinical heterogeneity of tumors and are less than perfectly adapted to each patient.

Although the strong overall association between the current standard clinicopathological variables used in breast cancer management and patients' prognosis and outcome *(5)*, it is clear that patients with similar clinical and pathological features may show distinct outcomes and vary in their response to therapy *(6)*. Even though algorithms based on clinicopathological data are now regularly used to define prognostically significant groups and to tailor systemic therapy for breast cancer patients, further improvements are required. In fact, several studies have shown that approximately 30% of lymph node-negative breast cancer patients who are classified as lying within a "good prognostic group" develop recurrence *(7)*, whereas a similar proportion of node-positive patients remain free from development of distant metastases *(8)*. Alternatively, a significant proportion of patients allocated to a poor prognosis group will never develop distant recurrence *(9)*. For this reason, there is an increasing need for additional prognostic factors to improve patients' risk stratification and the targeting of treatment. Today's goal in breast cancer research is aimed at tailoring treatment for the individual patient, known as "personalized medicine" *(10)*. This requires developing an accurate prognostic profile to define which patients should receive systemic therapy (hormone or chemotherapy) before and/or after surgery, and to decide which systemic treatments are most suitable for a given patient.

The final deciphering of the complete human genome, together with the improvement of high-throughput molecular technologies, has caused a fundamental transformation in breast cancer research, beginning to tackle the molecular complexity of breast cancer and contributing to the realization that the biological heterogeneity of breast cancer has implications for treatment. Gene expression profiling is any method that can analyze the expression of genes in selected samples and has been widely applied to cancer research in the past few years. These techniques consist of differential display *(11)*, serial analysis of gene expression *(12)*, various proteomics approaches *(13)*, and gene expression microarrays *(14)*. The recent development of microarray and related technologies provides an opportunity to perform more detailed and individualized breast tumor characterization. This assay is a powerful molecular technology that allows the simultaneous study of the expression of thousands of genes or their RNA products, giving an accurate picture of gene expression in the cell or the sample at the time of the study (Fig. 1). The two main types of microarrays are cDNA microarrays and oligonucleotide microarrays *(14,15)*. Both types of microarray are hybridized with cDNA or RNA samples obtained from tissues/cells of interest to assess changes in their expression levels. Technical details about microarrays are beyond the scope of this chapter, and readers are recommended to access the different excellent reviews on this subject.

Besides these global expression profiling approaches yielding candidate genes that requires validation, other "-omic" techniques have been used. Reverse transcriptase polymerase chain reaction (RT-PCR) (Fig. 2) allows simultaneous PCR amplification and detection of target DNA or cDNA sequences and provides semiquantitative estimation of the relative abundance of specific transcripts using specific primers. More, tissue microarrays (TMAs) *(16)* offer a method for high-throughput protein expression analysis of large cohorts of archival formalin-fixed paraffin-embedded tissue samples that can be readily linked to long-term follow-up and clinicopathological databases. The development and application of these high-throughput molecular techniques have contributed to the know-how for comprehensive studies of genes, gene products, and signaling pathways involved in the molecular biology of breast cancer.

Microarray expression profiling

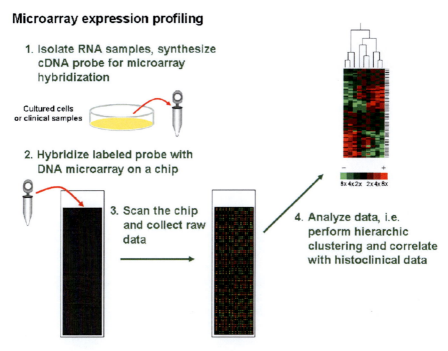

Fig. 1. Microarray expression profile. Schematic overview of an experiment of gene expression profiling by microarray.

RT - Polymerase Chain Reaction (RT-PCR)

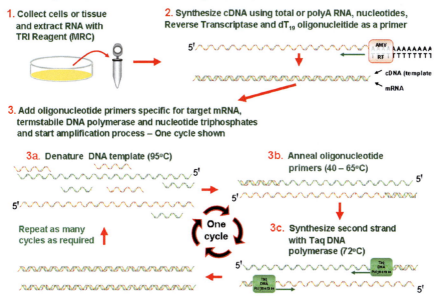

Fig. 2. RT-Polymerase Chain Reaction. Detailed overview of reverse transcriptase polymerase chain reaction.

Because of the huge dimension of the promise of microarray technology, we will focus on the contribution of microarray-based expression profiling analysis.

Microarray platform, with its ability to simultaneously analyze the expression of the entire genome of an organism, has transformed our understanding of human breast cancer. Previously, historical classification systems were based on light microscopic results and single marker-tumor features (e.g., estrogen receptor). Expression profiling and other technologies helped in discovering relevant signatures potentially related to prognosis (clinical outcome), prediction (tumor response to a specific therapy), and provide further insights into tumor biology informing both the clinician and the scientist.

Generally, molecular profiling of breast cancers by gene expression microarrays can be performed in two ways: unsupervised or supervised analysis. Unsupervised analysis is a statistical method for microarrays that does not use information derived about the data (samples or genes) to be analyzed. The outputs are simply a description of the relationships among the samples or genes based on gene expression patterns. It is an extensive set of methods, of which hierarchical clustering analysis is the most popular (17). The main objective of this approach is to determine whether discrete subsets can be defined on the basis of gene expression profiles and to identify new classes (class discovery) potentially having clinical significance in order to develop a new molecular taxonomy. In supervised analysis external information is used to group the samples (tumor grade, gender, response to therapy) or the genes (functional class, chromosomal location) and relate the grouping with gene expression data. There are two main subtypes of supervised analysis: class comparison and class prediction. The first aims to identify the transcriptomic differences between two classes of tumors, whereas the goal of the second one is the development of a "gene signature" (18,19).

2. MOLECULAR CLASSIFICATION

The identification of particular tumor subtypes is essential in order to design possible therapeutic intervention. Breast cancer heterogeneity has been confirmed at gene expression level (20). Multiple breast cancer subtypes with distinct gene expression patterns and different prognoses have been identified in primary breast cancers and their metastases. Different studies established that breast cancers can be classified into five distinct molecular subtypes based on their microarray expression (21–28). Early studies divided breast tumors in two different branches, each arising from one of the two types of breast cancer cells: basal and luminal cells. By recent inclusion of larger number of samples and meta-analysis (merging data from multiple studies) we know that luminal tumors can be subdivided into luminal A and luminal B types, and basal tumors gave rise to three major groups: normal-like, basal, and ERBB2.

Perou et al. (22) originally showed that ER status defines two groups of breast tumor samples. ER-positive tumors represent 34–66% of all breast cancers (24,29,30). Tumors in the ER-positive group have expression patterns reminiscent of the luminal epithelial cells of the breast [e.g., ER (ESR1) and luminal cytokeratins 8/18]. There are at least two subtypes of ER positive tumors (23), luminal A and luminal B (now also known as highly proliferating luminals) (31). These two tumor classes are characterized by gene expression patterns and different clinical outcomes. In general, luminal A tumors represent 19–39% of all breast cancers, have the highest expression of ER and ER-related genes, and show the best prognosis. Luminal B tumors represent 10–23% of all breast cancers, have profiles enriched for luminal genes, and show low to moderate expression of ER-related genes, relatively high expression of proliferation and cell cycle-related genes. If compared with luminal A, luminal B tumors might have a higher proliferation rate, and are associated with less favorable outcome.

Hormone receptor negative breast cancers represent 30–45% of all breast cancer, are characterized by lack of HR expression and low to absent expression of some other luminal markers. This class is further subclassified into at least three distinct subtypes sharing a common feature (e.g., HR and GATA3 negative expression), but are otherwise molecularly and biologically different: basal-like, ERBB2/HER2/neu/+, and normal breast-like. Basal-like represent 16–37% of all breast cancers *(24,30,32–34)*, express genes characteristic of basal myoepithelial cells *(a6-integrin, CK5, CK17, c-KIT, EGFR, fatty acid binding protein 7, integrin 4, laminin, metallothionein 1X, NF-kappaB, and P-cadherin) (22,27,35–37)*. Moreover, recent studies confirmed that tumors from patients carrying *BRCA1* mutations fall within the basal-like subgroup *(29,38,39)*. Basal-like tumors usually have aggressive features such as high tumor grade and *TP53* mutations *(24,31,40)* and poor outcome.

ERBB2/HER2/neu/+ tumors represent 4–10% of all breast cancers *(29,30,41,42)* and, compared with basal-like group, share comparatively poor outcomes. This subtype is characterized by overexpression of genes in a 17q11 amplicon that include *ERBB2, GRB7, GATA4,* and high levels of *NF-kappaB* activation. Like the basal-like subtype, *ERBB2*-overexpressing tumors have a high proportion of *TP53* mutations, and are significantly more likely to be grade III.

Normal breast-like subtype represents up to 10% of all breast cancer *(23,43,44)*. These tumors are sometimes called unclassified, undetermined, or null subtype *(40,45,46)*. Normal breast-like tumors have some characteristics in common with normal breast tissue, including adipose and other non-epithelial tissue components of the tumor microenvironment. These tumors share with normal breast tissue relative overexpression of basal epithelial genes and relative underexpression of luminal epithelial genes. The distinct subtypes of breast cancer have also been characterized by immunohistochemical protein markers (e.g., basal cytokeratins ER, HER1/EGFR, HER2, and PR) *(47)*. Invasive lobular breast cancers often show normal-like expression profiles *(23,29)*. These tumors have a prognosis that seems to be better than that of basal-like cancers *(23,43)* and do not appear to respond to neoadjuvant chemotherapy at the same rates as other tumors pertaining to the ER-cluster *(48)*.

A possible new subtype characterized by high expression of interferon (IFN)-regulated genes has been identified and linked to lymph node metastasis and poor prognosis *(27)*.

Different studies have reported that the best prognosis is seen in patients with luminal (ER+) tumors and, in particular, those of luminal A subtype when subclassified, and the worst prognosis in HER2 and basal-like (mainly ER⁻) tumors. Although these findings are known already, certain points of clinical importance must be underlined: (1) ER+ tumors are not a single entity and one subclass (luminal B) is reported to show a poor outcome, comparable to the ER⁻ basal-like and HER2 tumors; (2) Most basal-like and HER2 tumors have poor prognostic features as defined by routine pathology methods, which may have important implications for outcome and clinical management; (3) transcriptomic analysis has provided some leads on genes that may drive each molecular subgroup. These genes, or their protein products, could potentially suggest new therapeutic targets (e.g., epidermal growth factor receptor and c-kit in basal-like cancers). Unfortunately, today's variation in methodology and defining criteria for each class is still cause of difference in the clinical significance of the resulting molecular classification. In order for this molecular classification to be translated into a clinically useful assay, a definitive gene signature with predictive accuracy needs to be defined, and tested. To date, such set of intrinsic genes has yet to be completely defined. Further studies on larger cohorts of patients are needed. There is already the EORTC-MINDACT (Microarray In Node-negative Disease may Avoid ChemoTherapy) Trial that was launched by the Breast Cancer International Group. This trial is based on upfront patient stratification using the 70-gene predictor and aims to recruit 6,000 patients in this study.

Future analyses of these data together with meta-analyses of public data will provide more precise intrinsic gene signatures predictive of breast cancer molecular subtypes.

3. DIAGNOSIS AND PROGNOSIS

Metastases are the main cause of death in breast cancer patients. The failure of current predictive factors (factors correlating with response to, or benefit from, a given treatment according to specific patient or tumor characteristics) as well as prognostic factors (sources of information on the prognosis for different subgroups of patients, describing the natural course and outcome, unrelated to different therapeutic interventions) prompted clinicians to look for something new to try. The prevention of using aggressive adjuvant therapy for patients who in the end would not benefit is a hot field, but current pathological markers do not have the ability to classify such patients based on initial diagnosis yet. Genomic-based tests predicting the likelihood of tumor recurrence provide information about the molecular biology of metastasis and provide a measure of outcome for new cases *(9,20,21,24,49,50)*. At present, therapies based on molecular diagnosis are limited to hormonal-based chemotherapy such as tamoxifen for estrogen-responsive tumors or treatment of ERBB2/HER2/neu/+ tumors with Herceptin.

A 70-gene prognosis signature was identified by van't Veer et al. *(51)*. In this study, ER status and other clinical variables were not considered when the molecular predictor was developed. A 70-gene marker set was developed to classify tumors into good and poor prognosis groups. Genes significantly up-regulated in the poor prognosis signature included those involved angiogenesis, in cell cycle, invasion and metastasis, and signal transduction. This prognostic signature was found to be strongly predictive of a short interval to distant metastasis in lymph node-negative patients. The prognostic ability of the 70-gene signature has been supported by subsequent studies from this research team *(52,53)* even though some concern regarding the design and statistical analysis used to derive the original 70-gene signature have been raised *(54,55)*. The US Food and Drug Administration (FDA) approved the commercial version of the 70-gene signature, MammaPrint®, developed by Agendia (Amsterdam, Netherlands) as the first in vitro diagnostic multivariate index assay device. This array will be used as a test to distinguish lymph node-negative breast cancer patients who would benefit from additional therapy and those who would not (the ongoing European MINDACT clinical trial will examine the MammaPrint® test).

Another gene expression signature assay developed from microarray studies of breast cancer commercially available is the 21-gene Oncotype DX™ assay *(56)*. Genomic Health released the Oncotype DX Recurrence Score (RS) gene signature of breast cancer prognosis test in 2004. This test tracks a 21-gene expression signature using qRT-PCR and can be performed on formalin-fixed, paraffin-embedded tumors tissue. The TAILORx study sponsored by the US National Cancer Institute and led by the Eastern Cooperative Oncology Group will test the Oncotype DX™ assay. This study plans to enroll more than 10,000 women with hormone-positive (ESR1+ and/or PgR+), ERBB2 breast cancer that has not spread to the lymph nodes. The Oncotype DX™ assay will be used to determine which women will receive adjuvant chemotherapy in addition to hormone therapy. Initial studies of the 21-gene Oncotype DX™ assay signature are inconclusive but more studies are indeed required to establish the clinical usefulness of this assay.

CellSearch™ (Veridex, LLC; Warren, NJ) is a method to detect circulating tumor cells (CTCs) that are characterized by the lack of expression of CD45 cell surface antigen and by positive staining for epithelial cell adhesion molecule and cytokeratins 8, 18, and/or 19 *(57)*. These cells can be detected in the peripheral blood of some breast cancer patients. It is an

Chapter 8 / Gene Expression Profiling in Breast Cancer

opinion that these cells might be involved in the spread of metastases. Patients with metastatic breast cancer with more than five CTCs at baseline and first follow-up had a worse prognosis than patients with fewer than five CTCs *(58–60)*. The CellSearch™ assay is actually approved in the USA for risk stratification of patients with metastatic breast cancer based on the detection of CTCs in the peripheral blood. A recent study also demonstrated that changes in CTC count in response to therapy were also predictive of outcome *(58)*. A clinical trial is under way to examine the clinical utility of this test in switching treatment in patients not responding to initial treatment with a dropping CTC count.

A diagnostic test (VDX2) is also being developed by Veridex, (Veridex, LLC; Warren, NJ), using a set of 76 genes (the Rotterdam gene set) that were identified in a study of gene expression profiles of 286 lymph node-negative patients who had not received adjuvant systemic treatment *(9,61)*. This signature was able to predict distant metastatic recurrence with a sensitivity of 93% and a specificity of 48% *(9)*. This prognostic indicator performed better than standard, clinical variables in a multivariate analysis. The ongoing European MINDACT clinical trial may prospectively evaluate the 76-gene Veridex signature.

Mammostrat® (Applied Genomics, Inc.; Huntsville, AL) is a five-antibody panel. These antibodies were selected because of their ability to distinguish tumors with a high versus low risk for recurrence *(62)*. Mammostrat® panel was validated in two cohorts of patients, with the Cox model distinguishing ER-positive patients with poor outcomes from patients with good or moderate outcomes, but this model was not useful for ER patients. Different clinical trials indicated that the greatest clinical utility of Mammostrat® panel may be in postmenopausal patients.

Not only it is important having assays helping in decision making regarding whether patients should undergo adjuvant therapy, we need also molecular tests for prediction of risk of local or distant recurrence. Kreike et al. *(63)* and Nuyten et al. *(64)* were both independently unable to recover gene predictors of recurrence in their recent breast cancer studies in which they used unsupervised and supervised approach. A successful predictor of local recurrence identified is the wound-healing (or wound response indicator, WRI) signature *(65)*, which correctly predicted local recurrence in 7 out of 8 cases of the test dataset (88% sensitivity) with a specificity of 74% (53 out of 72). However, the number of local recurrences in the dataset was low (17/161), and these results should be confirmed in a larger study.

Several of the gene expression-based predictors mentioned in this chapter (e.g., MammaPrint® test, WRI, and Oncotype DX™ assay) have been compared. The comparison study used a single dataset of breast cancer samples from 295 women *(43)*. The indicators showed high rates of concordance in predicted outcome for individual patients, regardless of the minimal gene overlap among the assays. These results suggest that the concordance of the predictors is a result of common cellular phenotypes that are detected by the various predictors *(66)*. Even though there was discordance among the involved genes, these indicators all detected common sets of biological characteristics determining patient outcomes.

4. GENE EXPRESSION PROFILING FOR PREDICTION OF RESPONSE TO THERAPY

Breast cancer is one of the most sensitive to chemotherapy compared to other solid tumors. Systemic therapy for breast cancer includes chemotherapy, hormonal therapy, and novel agents. Several single agent and combination chemotherapy regimens are successful treatments for breast cancer, such as cyclophosphamide, doxorubicin, 5-fluorouracil (5-FU), and taxanes. Since in clinical practice chemotherapy is applied empirically despite the fact that not all patients benefit from those agents, there is an effective need to identify predictive biomarkers for its efficacy.

Evaluation of ER status is an essential component of the pathological breast cancer because ER status is used to determine candidacy for endocrine therapy. ER status is determined by performing immunohistochemistry (IHC) on formalin-fixed, paraffin-embedded tumor tissue, but these assays are known to have considerable variation in tissue fixation, antigen retrieval, staining techniques, and interpretation of results across laboratories. Studies suggested that benefit of estrogen therapy is proportional to the level of ER expression; therefore, further quantitative ER measurements assays are important *(67)*. Today, the expression of the ER is measured at the mRNA level using RT-PCR or microarrays, which are more quantitative than IHC *(68)*.

Taxanes are a class of antimicrotubule agents that are proven to be effective and are routinely used in multidrug therapy of breast cancer *(69–72)*. A 92-gene panel was developed as potential predictor of response to taxanes. Tumors from patients ($n = 24$) with primary breast cancer were biopsied prior to neoadjuvant treatment with docetaxel *(73)*. Gene expression patterns were then correlated with a response to docetaxel (one of the most active agents in this disease). In cross-validation experiments, the resultant 92-gene predictor detected docetaxel-sensitive and docetaxel-resistant tumors with 92% specificity and 83% sensitivity. More studies with larger sample sizes are needed to further validate this predictor.

A Japanese group studied 44 primary or locally recurrent breast cancers treated with docetaxel using a 2,453-gene high-throughput RT-PCR technique *(74)*. They developed an 85-gene classifier for partial or complete response, and it was validated in an additional 26 patients.

Topoisomerases are enzymes regulating the coiling of DNA and are essential components of the cell division machinery. It was recently demonstrated that patients with advanced breast cancer also showed that topoisomerase *TOP2A* overexpression was associated with a higher probability of response to single-agent doxorubicin but not to single-agent docetaxel *(75)*. Recently, FDA approved a *TOP2A* fluorescence in situ hybridization (FISH) assay (TOP2A FISH pharmDx™; Dako, Glostrup, Denmark) to measure amplification of this gene in breast cancer specimens.

Two years ago a group from Germany reported a 512-gene signature, enriched for genes involved in transforming growth factor beta and RAS-mediated signaling pathways, to predict pathologic complete response to primary systemic therapy with chemotherapy drugs docetaxel, epirubicin, and gemcitabine in primary breast cancers *(76)*. Although all groups reported an association between gene expression profile and treatment outcome, the predictive power was too low for current clinical use and larger validation studies are certainly needed.

Several small studies have provided "proof-of-principle" that the gene expression profile of cancers highly sensitive to chemotherapy is different from the gene expression profile of tumors that are resistant to treatment *(77)*. The largest study included 133 patients with stage I–III breast cancer who received preoperative weekly paclitaxel and 5-fluorouracil, doxorubicin, and cyclophosphamide (T-FAC) chemotherapy *(78)*. The first 82 cases were used to develop a multigene signature predictive of a pathological complete response (pCR), and the remaining 51 cases were used to test the accuracy of the predictor. The overall pCR rate was 26% in both cohorts. A 30-gene predictor correctly identified all but one of the patients who achieved a pCR (12 of 13) and all but one of those who had residual cancer (27 of 28) in the validation set. It showed a significantly higher sensitivity (92% vs. 61%) than a clinical variable-based predictor that included age, ER status, and nuclear grade.

Tamoxifen reduces recurrence rates in patients with early stage, ER-positive breast cancer, but a better identification of people who actually benefit from this drug is needed *(79)*. A comparison of ER-positive tumors obtained from tamoxifen responders and non-responders with advanced breast cancer led to the identification of 44 genes that are differentially

Chapter 8 / Gene Expression Profiling in Breast Cancer

expressed in these tissues. The predictive power of this signature was considerably superior to that of traditional predictive factors in a univariate analysis and it was associated with a longer progression-free survival time in univariate and multivariate analyses. It was also demonstrated that a two-gene ratio (*HOXB13/IL17BR*) was predictive of disease-free survival in patients with early-stage, ER-positive breast cancer who received treatment with tamoxifen *(79)*. An RT-PCR based method to assess this ratio from paraffin-embedded tissue samples is now commercially available (AviaraDx H/ITM; AviaraDx, Carlsbad, CA).

5. INTEGRATED DATA ANALYSIS OF MICROARRAY PLATFORMS

Several public repositories have been established to collect the publicly available microarray data (Table 1). A researcher can query these databases for all experiments of a given type and retrieve the respective data, which then can be combined with the researcher's own data or used for designing new experiments. These repositories represent a large data resource. With growing amounts of microarray data, improving quality, and new analysis methods being developed, these databases are a rich resource for both data mining and validation of "-omic" studies of breast cancer. Datasets can also be combined in meta-analysis. Since the cost and availability of biopsy tissues limit the number of samples analyzed, low case-to-feature ratio remains an issue. For this reason, meta-analysis is an attractive option. Meta-analysis of many gene expression datasets has been applied to define the number of well-supported molecular subtypes of breast cancer *(80)* and to obtain more robust breast cancer gene signatures *(81)*. New integrated meta-analysis methods are being developed and applied to many types of "-omic" data from ongoing large clinical trials and other studies. The analyses of these integrated datasets might yield a more complete understanding and insight than can be obtained from any single approach regarding gene expression profiling of breast cancer.

6. CONCLUSIONS

The completing of the human genome sequencing, together with the development of high-throughput technologies, such as gene expression profiling, is giving us the opportunity to describe biological features in a quantitative manner. In the past decade, high-throughput biology and gene expression profiling have matured considerably. Gene expression profiles by

Table 1
Omics data in public repositories

Repository	Experiments	Number of arrays	URL
ArrayExpress	3,720	110,731	http://www.ebi.ac.uk/arrayexpress
Oncomine	360	25,447	http://www.oncomine.org
CIBEX	30	50	http://cibex.nig.ac.jp
RAD	85	86	http://www.cbi1.upenn.edu/RAD
GENEVESTIGATOR		20 024	https://www.genevestigator.ethz.ch

CIBEX, Center for Information Biology gene Expression database; RAD, RNA Abundance Database. An array is a single-microarray hybridization; an experiment is a collection of arrays. Counts compiled June 2008 microarray analysis of breast cancer samples have allowed researchers the development of profiles that can distinguish, identify, and classify discrete subsets of disease, predict the disease outcome, or the response to therapy. Currently, most breast tumors are detected in breast examination and mammography, and when abnormalities are found, these are followed up with invasive needle or surgical biopsy. For this reason, less-invasive approaches would be a significant advance. The gene expression profiling has the incredible potential to change the prognostication and treatment options for patients with breast cancer. More, an important potential of microarray-based tests is that multiple predictions, including prognosis and sensitivity to various treatment modalities, may be generated from a single experiment. These assays would use information from different sets of genes measured from the same tissue for different predictions, substantially improving the cost-effectiveness of these promising tests.

While reports of microarray studies in breast cancer research are exciting, the use of this technology has not yet been completely implemented clinically. Different signatures are reported by different studies of the same disease, resulting in classifiers with little overlap between predictive gene lists for the same cancer, even when the same microarray platform is used *(19,43,55,82–84)*. Among the many limitations to deriving a stable molecular predictor for new cases of breast cancer is variability in technique platform, patient selection criteria, statistical methods of data analysis, noise and bias analysis, sample size, and prediction rules *(14,50,53,83,85–87)*. In most studies, the number of tumors assayed is an order of magnitude smaller than the number of genes analyzed, leading to a lack of statistical power. Moreover, when large numbers of genes are involved in the analysis, traditional approaches to multiple hypothesis correction are too conservative, finding only few of any significant genes. Many of the currently available tests are based on retrospective studies performed on archival material, and thus, they do not provide the level of evidence that can only be gained from prospective, randomized, high-powered clinical trials. Currently, the MammaPrint® test 70-gene set is being validated in the MINDACT clinical trial, and Oncotype DX™ assay is being evaluated in the TAILORx clinical trial. These trials might provide clinicians with better information regarding the clinical utility of these tests, serving as models for future efforts addressing the clinical impact of gene expression profiling in this disease.

As discussed above, several gene expression profiles that have successfully predicted survival in patients with breast cancer have been identified; however, it remains to be determined whether these gene sets will be used individually, in conjunction, or if there will be a gene signature to rule them all. Moreover, we are still uncertain about the clinical value of these assays and their potential superiority to standard clinicopathological parameters *(83,88)*.

In conclusion, expression profiling technology holds the promise to help improve clinical management. Profiling of experimental models with activation of specific oncogenic pathways might be used to find the molecular events involved in the establishment and development of breast tumors and, consequently, these models could be validated as tools for preclinical therapy. Moreover, the detailed analysis of gene expression deregulation after response to the therapies in such models might allow us to predict the response to specific drugs, and to target the therapies to patients in search for individualized management of breast cancer. Recent advances in microarray technology have demonstrated improved reproducibility, which will make its clinical application more achievable and highly possible that this technology will improve and refine, rather than replace current prognostic and predictive tools.

Acknowledgments: This study was supported by NIH grants (A.G.) and the Sbarro Health Research Organization (A.G. and G.R.)

REFERENCES

1. Kamangar F, Dores GM, Anderson WF. Patterns of cancer incidence, mortality, and prevalence across five continents: defining priorities to reduce cancer disparities in different geographic regions of the world. J Clin Oncol 2006;24(14):2137–50.
2. Parkin DM, Bray F, Ferlay J, Pisani P. Estimating the world cancer burden: Globocan 2000. Int J Cancer 2001;94(2):153–6.
3. Jemal A, Siegel R, Ward E, et al. Cancer statistics, 2006. CA Cancer J Clin 2006;56(2):106–30.
4. Peto R, Boreham J, Clarke M, Davies C, Beral V. UK and USA breast cancer deaths down 25% in year 2000 at ages 20–69 years. Lancet 2000;355(9217):1822.
5. Elston CW, Ellis IO, Pinder SE. Pathological prognostic factors in breast cancer. Crit Rev Oncol Hematol 1999;31(3):209–23.
6. Alizadeh AA, Ross DT, Perou CM, van de Rijn M. Towards a novel classification of human malignancies based on gene expression patterns. J Pathol 2001;195(1):41–52.
7. Polychemotherapy for early breast cancer: an overview of the randomised trials. Early Breast Cancer Trialists' Collaborative Group. Lancet 1998;352(9132):930–42.
8. Feng Y, Sun B, Li X, et al. Differentially expressed genes between primary cancer and paired lymph node metastases predict clinical outcome of node-positive breast cancer patients. Breast Cancer Res Treat 2007;103(3):319–29.
9. Wang Y, Klijn JG, Zhang Y, et al. Gene-expression profiles to predict distant metastasis of lymph-node-negative primary breast cancer. Lancet 2005;365(9460):671–9.
10. Stearns V, Davidson NE, Flockhart DA. Pharmacogenetics in the treatment of breast cancer. Pharmacogenomics J 2004;4(3):143–53.
11. Liang P, Pardee AB. Differential display of eukaryotic messenger RNA by means of the polymerase chain reaction. Science 1992;257(5072):967–71.
12. Velculescu VE, Zhang L, Vogelstein B, Kinzler KW. Serial analysis of gene expression. Science 1995;270(5235):484–7.
13. Geisow MJ. Proteomics: one small step for a digital computer, one giant leap for humankind. Nat Biotechnol 1998;16(2):206.
14. Russo G, Zegar C, Giordano A. Advantages and limitations of microarray technology in human cancer. Oncogene 2003;22(42):6497–507.
15. Russo G, Claudio PP, Fu Y, et al. pRB2/p130 target genes in non-small lung cancer cells identified by microarray analysis. Oncogene 2003;22(44):6959–69.
16. Kononen J, Bubendorf L, Kallioniemi A, et al. Tissue microarrays for high-throughput molecular profiling of tumor specimens. Nat Med 1998;4(7):844–7.
17. Quackenbush J. Computational analysis of microarray data. Nat Rev Genet 2001;2(6):418–27.
18. Reis-Filho JS, Westbury C, Pierga JY. The impact of expression profiling on prognostic and predictive testing in breast cancer. J Clin Pathol 2006;59(3):225–31.
19. Simon R, Radmacher MD, Dobbin K, McShane LM. Pitfalls in the use of DNA microarray data for diagnostic and prognostic classification. J Natl Cancer Inst 2003;95(1):14–8.
20. Jeffrey SS, Lonning PE, Hillner BE. Genomics-based prognosis and therapeutic prediction in breast cancer. J Natl Compr Canc Netw 2005;3(3):291–300.
21. Perou CM, Jeffrey SS, van de Rijn M, et al. Distinctive gene expression patterns in human mammary epithelial cells and breast cancers. Proc Natl Acad Sci U S A 1999;96(16):9212–7.
22. Perou CM, Sorlie T, Eisen MB, et al. Molecular portraits of human breast tumours. Nature 2000;406(6797):747–52.
23. Sorlie T, Perou CM, Tibshirani R, et al. Gene expression patterns of breast carcinomas distinguish tumor subclasses with clinical implications. Proc Natl Acad Sci U S A 2001;98(19):10869–74.
24. Sotiriou C, Neo SY, McShane LM, et al. Breast cancer classification and prognosis based on gene expression profiles from a population-based study. Proc Natl Acad Sci U S A 2003;100(18):10393–8.
25. Yu K, Lee CH, Tan PH, et al. A molecular signature of the Nottingham prognostic index in breast cancer. Cancer Res 2004;64(9):2962–8.

26. Yu K, Lee CH, Tan PH, Tan P. Conservation of breast cancer molecular subtypes and transcriptional patterns of tumor progression across distinct ethnic populations. Clin Cancer Res 2004;10(16):5508–17.
27. Hu Z, Fan C, Oh DS, et al. The molecular portraits of breast tumors are conserved across microarray platforms. BMC Genomics 2006;7:96.
28. Cheng SH, Horng CF, West M, et al. Genomic prediction of locoregional recurrence after mastectomy in breast cancer. J Clin Oncol 2006;24(28):4594–602.
29. Sorlie T, Tibshirani R, Parker J, et al. Repeated observation of breast tumor subtypes in independent gene expression data sets. Proc Natl Acad Sci U S A 2003;100(14):8418–23.
30. West M, Blanchette C, Dressman H, et al. Predicting the clinical status of human breast cancer by using gene expression profiles. Proc Natl Acad Sci U S A 2001;98(20):11462–7.
31. Langerod A, Zhao H, Borgan O, et al. TP53 mutation status and gene expression profiles are powerful prognostic markers of breast cancer. Breast Cancer Res 2007;9(3):R30.
32. Rakha EA, Reis-Filho JS, Ellis IO. Basal-like breast cancer: a critical review. J Clin Oncol 2008;26(15):2568–81.
33. Turner NC, Reis-Filho JS, Russell AM, et al. BRCA1 dysfunction in sporadic basal-like breast cancer. Oncogene 2007;26(14):2126–32.
34. Foulkes WD, Brunet JS, Stefansson IM, et al. The prognostic implication of the basal-like (cyclin E high/p27 low/p53+/glomeruloid-microvascular-proliferation+) phenotype of BRCA1-related breast cancer. Cancer Res 2004;64(3):830–5.
35. Vogelstein B, Kinzler KW. Cancer genes and the pathways they control. Nat Med 2004;10(8):789–99.
36. Savage K, Lambros MB, Robertson D, et al. Caveolin 1 is overexpressed and amplified in a subset of basal-like and metaplastic breast carcinomas: a morphologic, ultrastructural, immunohistochemical, and in situ hybridization analysis. Clin Cancer Res 2007;13(1):90–101.
37. Yehiely F, Moyano JV, Evans JR, Nielsen TO, Cryns VL. Deconstructing the molecular portrait of basal-like breast cancer. Trends Mol Med 2006;12(11):537–44.
38. Charafe-Jauffret E, Ginestier C, Monville F, et al. Gene expression profiling of breast cell lines identifies potential new basal markers. Oncogene 2006;25(15):2273–84.
39. Lakhani SR, Reis-Filho JS, Fulford L, et al. Prediction of BRCA1 status in patients with breast cancer using estrogen receptor and basal phenotype. Clin Cancer Res 2005;11(14):5175–80.
40. Carey LA, Perou CM, Livasy CA, et al. Race, breast cancer subtypes, and survival in the Carolina Breast Cancer Study. JAMA 2006;295(21):2492–502.
41. Bertucci F, Borie N, Ginestier C, et al. Identification and validation of an ERBB2 gene expression signature in breast cancers. Oncogene 2004;23(14):2564–75.
42. Biswas DK, Iglehart JD. Linkage between EGFR family receptors and nuclear factor kappaB (NF-kappaB) signaling in breast cancer. J Cell Physiol 2006;209(3):645–52.
43. Fan C, Oh DS, Wessels L, et al. Concordance among gene-expression-based predictors for breast cancer. N Engl J Med 2006;355(6):560–9.
44. Rody A, Karn T, Solbach C, et al. The erbB2 + cluster of the intrinsic gene set predicts tumor response of breast cancer patients receiving neoadjuvant chemotherapy with docetaxel, doxorubicin and cyclophosphamide within the GEPARTRIO trial. Breast 2007;16(3):235–40.
45. Kim MJ, Ro JY, Ahn SH, Kim HH, Kim SB, Gong G. Clinicopathologic significance of the basal-like subtype of breast cancer: a comparison with hormone receptor and Her2/neu-overexpressing phenotypes. Hum Pathol 2006;37(9):1217–26.
46. Diallo-Danebrock R, Ting E, Gluz O, et al. Protein expression profiling in high-risk breast cancer patients treated with high-dose or conventional dose-dense chemotherapy. Clin Cancer Res 2007;13(2 Pt 1):488–97.
47. Nielsen TO, Hsu FD, Jensen K, et al. Immunohistochemical and clinical characterization of the basal-like subtype of invasive breast carcinoma. Clin Cancer Res 2004;10(16):5367–74.
48. Rouzier R, Perou CM, Symmans WF, et al. Breast cancer molecular subtypes respond differently to preoperative chemotherapy. Clin Cancer Res 2005;11(16):5678–85.
49. Chang HY, Nuyten DS, Sneddon JB, et al. Robustness, scalability, and integration of a wound-response gene expression signature in predicting breast cancer survival. Proc Natl Acad Sci U S A 2005;102(10):3738–43.

Chapter 8 / Gene Expression Profiling in Breast Cancer

50. Mikhitarian K, Gillanders WE, Almeida JS, et al. An innovative microarray strategy identities informative molecular markers for the detection of micrometastatic breast cancer. Clin Cancer Res 2005;11(10):3697–704.

51. van't Veer LJ, Dai H, van de Vijver MJ, et al. Gene expression profiling predicts clinical outcome of breast cancer. Nature 2002;415(6871):530–6.

52. van de Vijver MJ, He YD, van't Veer LJ, et al. A gene-expression signature as a predictor of survival in breast cancer. N Engl J Med 2002;347(25):1999–2009.

53. Buyse M, Loi S, van't Veer L, et al. Validation and clinical utility of a 70-gene prognostic signature for women with node-negative breast cancer. J Natl Cancer Inst 2006;98(17):1183–92.

54. O'Brien SL, Fagan A, Fox EJ, et al. CENP-F expression is associated with poor prognosis and chromosomal instability in patients with primary breast cancer. Int J Cancer 2007;120(7):1434–43.

55. Ein-Dor L, Kela I, Getz G, Givol D, Domany E. Outcome signature genes in breast cancer: is there a unique set? Bioinformatics 2005;21(2):171–8.

56. Paik S, Shak S, Tang G, et al. A multigene assay to predict recurrence of tamoxifen-treated, node-negative breast cancer. N Engl J Med 2004;351(27):2817–26.

57. Witzig TE, Bossy B, Kimlinger T, et al. Detection of circulating cytokeratin-positive cells in the blood of breast cancer patients using immunomagnetic enrichment and digital microscopy. Clin Cancer Res 2002;8(5):1085–91.

58. Cristofanilli M, Budd GT, Ellis MJ, et al. Circulating tumor cells, disease progression, and survival in metastatic breast cancer. N Engl J Med 2004;351(8):781–91.

59. Cristofanilli M. Circulating tumor cells, disease progression, and survival in metastatic breast cancer. Semin Oncol 2006;33(3 Suppl 9):S9–14.

60. Hayes DF, Cristofanilli M, Budd GT, et al. Circulating tumor cells at each follow-up time point during therapy of metastatic breast cancer patients predict progression-free and overall survival. Clin Cancer Res 2006;12(14 Pt 1):4218–24.

61. Desmedt C, Piette F, Loi S, et al. Strong time dependence of the 76-gene prognostic signature for node-negative breast cancer patients in the TRANSBIG multicenter independent validation series. Clin Cancer Res 2007;13(11):3207–14.

62. Ring BZ, Seitz RS, Beck R, et al. Novel prognostic immunohistochemical biomarker panel for estrogen receptor-positive breast cancer. J Clin Oncol 2006;24(19):3039–47.

63. Kreike B, Halfwerk H, Kristel P, et al. Gene expression profiles of primary breast carcinomas from patients at high risk for local recurrence after breast-conserving therapy. Clin Cancer Res 2006;12(19):5705–12.

64. Nuyten DS, Kreike B, Hart AA, et al. Predicting a local recurrence after breast-conserving therapy by gene expression profiling. Breast Cancer Res 2006;8(5):R62.

65. Chang HY, Sneddon JB, Alizadeh AA, et al. Gene expression signature of fibroblast serum response predicts human cancer progression: similarities between tumors and wounds. PLoS Biol 2004;2(2):E7.

66. Desmedt C, Sotiriou C. Proliferation: the most prominent predictor of clinical outcome in breast cancer. Cell Cycle 2006;5(19):2198–202.

67. Harvey JM, Clark GM, Osborne CK, Allred DC. Estrogen receptor status by immunohistochemistry is superior to the ligand-binding assay for predicting response to adjuvant endocrine therapy in breast cancer. J Clin Oncol 1999;17(5):1474–81.

68. Gong Y, Yan K, Lin F, et al. Determination of oestrogen-receptor status and ERBB2 status of breast carcinoma: a gene-expression profiling study. Lancet Oncol 2007;8(3):203–11.

69. Fisher B, Bryant J, Wolmark N, et al. Effect of preoperative chemotherapy on the outcome of women with operable breast cancer. J Clin Oncol 1998;16(8):2672–85.

70. Rivera E, Holmes FA, Frye D, et al. Phase II study of paclitaxel in patients with metastatic breast carcinoma refractory to standard chemotherapy. Cancer 2000;89(11):2195–201.

71. Wolmark N, Wang J, Mamounas E, Bryant J, Fisher B. Preoperative chemotherapy in patients with operable breast cancer: nine-year results from National Surgical Adjuvant Breast and Bowel Project B-18. J Natl Cancer Inst Monogr 2001;(30):96–102.

72. Nowak AK, Wilcken NR, Stockler MR, Hamilton A, Ghersi D. Systematic review of taxane-containing versus non-taxane-containing regimens for adjuvant and neoadjuvant treatment of early breast cancer. Lancet Oncol 2004;5(6):372–80.

73. Chang JC, Wooten EC, Tsimelzon A, et al. Gene expression profiling for the prediction of therapeutic response to docetaxel in patients with breast cancer. Lancet 2003;362(9381):362–9.
74. Iwao-Koizumi K, Matoba R, Ueno N, et al. Prediction of docetaxel response in human breast cancer by gene expression profiling. J Clin Oncol 2005;23(3):422–31.
75. Durbecq V, Paesmans M, Cardoso F, et al. Topoisomerase-II alpha expression as a predictive marker in a population of advanced breast cancer patients randomly treated either with single-agent doxorubicin or single-agent docetaxel. Mol Cancer Ther 2004;3(10):1207–14.
76. Thuerigen O, Schneeweiss A, Toedt G, et al. Gene expression signature predicting pathologic complete response with gemcitabine, epirubicin, and docetaxel in primary breast cancer. J Clin Oncol 2006;24(12):1839–45.
77. Andre F, Mazouni C, Hortobagyi GN, Pusztai L. DNA arrays as predictors of efficacy of adjuvant/neoadjuvant chemotherapy in breast cancer patients: current data and issues on study design. Biochim Biophys Acta 2006;1766(2):197–204.
78. Hess KR, Anderson K, Symmans WF, et al. Pharmacogenomic predictor of sensitivity to preoperative chemotherapy with paclitaxel and fluorouracil, doxorubicin, and cyclophosphamide in breast cancer. J Clin Oncol 2006;24(26):4236–44.
79. Ma XJ, Wang Z, Ryan PD, et al. A two-gene expression ratio predicts clinical outcome in breast cancer patients treated with tamoxifen. Cancer Cell 2004;5(6):607–16.
80. Kapp AV, Jeffrey SS, Langerod A, et al. Discovery and validation of breast cancer subtypes. BMC Genomics 2006;7:231.
81. Calza S, Hall P, Auer G, et al. Intrinsic molecular signature of breast cancer in a population-based cohort of 412 patients. Breast Cancer Res 2006;8(4):R34.
82. Ahmed AA, Brenton JD. Microarrays and breast cancer clinical studies: forgetting what we have not yet learnt. Breast Cancer Res 2005;7(3):96–9.
83. Pusztai L. Chips to bedside: incorporation of microarray data into clinical practice. Clin Cancer Res 2006;12(24):7209–14.
84. Shi L, Tong W, Goodsaid F, et al. QA/QC: challenges and pitfalls facing the microarray community and regulatory agencies. Expert Rev Mol Diagn 2004;4(6):761–77.
85. Grann VR, Troxel AB, Zojwalla NJ, Jacobson JS, Hershman D, Neugut AI. Hormone receptor status and survival in a population-based cohort of patients with breast carcinoma. Cancer 2005;103(11):2241–51.
86. Reid JF, Lusa L, De Cecco L, et al. Limits of predictive models using microarray data for breast cancer clinical treatment outcome. J Natl Cancer Inst 2005;97(12):927–30.
87. Febbo PG, Kantoff PW. Noise and bias in microarray analysis of tumor specimens. J Clin Oncol 2006;24(23):3719–21.
88. Sotiriou C, Piccart MJ. Taking gene-expression profiling to the clinic: when will molecular signatures become relevant to patient care? Nat Rev Cancer 2007;7(7):545–53.

9

TGF-β Signaling: A Novel Target for Treatment of Breast Cancer?

Jason D. Lee and Gerard C. Blobe

SUMMARY

Targeted therapies for breast cancer rely on an understanding of cellular signaling in both normal and neoplastic tissue. The transforming growth factor-beta (TGF-β) signaling pathway is an important regulator of both normal mammary gland development and mammary carcinogenesis. The TGF-β signaling pathway regulates numerous cellular processes in breast tissue, including proliferation, apoptosis, migration, and invasion, in addition to contributing to angiogenesis and modulation of the immune system. TGF-β often has opposing effects on these cellular processes, with its effects being both cell and context specific. Moreover, TGF-β possesses a unique dichotomy of function in breast cancer progression, acting as a tumor suppressor early in breast cancer carcinogenesis and then as a tumor promoter in the later stages of breast cancer progression. Highlighting the complexities inherent in TGF-β signaling, along with our current efforts to better our understanding of it, we outline several strategies that may enable us to create focused therapies in the prevention and treatment of breast cancer.

Key Words: TGF-β: Breast cancer; Metastasis; Apoptosis; Proliferation; Invasion; Angiogenesis; Immune system; Targeted therapy

1. INTRODUCTION

Worldwide, breast cancer is one of the most significant causes of cancer morbidity and mortality with over one million new cases and 400,000 deaths every year globally *(1)*. Through advances in detection and treatment modalities, the number of women with poor outcomes after diagnosis has steadily decreased. The prevalence of breast cancer remains

From: *Current Clinical Oncology: Breast Cancer in the Post-Genomic Era,*
Edited by: A. Giordano and N. Normanno, DOI: 10.1007/978-1-60327-945-1_9,
© Humana Press, a part of Springer Science + Business Media, LLC 2009

high, however, justifying continued studies into the etiology and biology of breast cancer with the aim of further reducing morbidity and mortality.

Chemotherapeutic and targeted agents are used in adjuvant and neoadjuvant settings in combination with surgical resection and radiation therapy for the treatment of breast cancer. Until recently, chemotherapeutic drugs were blunt instruments lacking specificity for breast cancer cells. The relatively recent introduction of targeted therapies heralded a new paradigm of breast cancer treatment, promising greater specificity and thus a lower attendant potential for toxicity. The selective estrogen receptor modulator (SERM) tamoxifen and the HER-2/ neu receptor antagonist trastuzumab, targeting ER-positive and HER-2-overexpressing breast cancers, respectively, have revolutionized the treatment of breast cancer patients. The demonstrated efficacy of these targeted drugs provides proof of principle for developing rational, targeted strategies for breast cancer therapy based on studies of both normal and tumor biology. Given this backdrop, here we examine the transforming growth factor-beta (TGF-β) signaling pathway, an important regulator of normal mammary gland development and homeostasis whose disruption is a common event during mammary carcinogenesis. We pay particular attention to the current understanding of TGF-β biology at the molecular, cellular, and systemic levels in normal and tumor states and the potential for and challenges posed by targeting the TGF-β pathway in the prevention and treatment of breast cancer.

2. THE TGF-β SIGNALING PATHWAY

The canonical signaling cascade for TGF-β involves the binding of TGF-β ligand dimer to its cognate cell surface receptors. TGF-β binds either to the type III TGF-β receptor (TβRIII, or betaglycan) dimer, which in turn presents TGF-β to the dimeric type II TGF-β receptor (TβRII), or directly to TβRII. Once either of these occurs, ligand binding to TβRII favors recruitment and interaction with the type I receptor (TβRI) dimer, forming a mul-timeric ligand–receptor complex. In this complex, TβRII transphosphorylates serine residues on TβRI in the cytoplasmic domain, thereby activating TβRI serine/threonine kinase activity. Activated TβRI then recruits and phosphorylates the Smad2 or Smad3 transcription factors, members of a family of receptor Smads. Once phosphorylated, Smad2/3 binds to Smad4, a co-Smad. This complex then translocates to the nucleus and directly interacts with other transcription factors to regulate expression of TGF-β-responsive genes in a cell- and context-specific manner *(2)* (Fig. 1).

3. EFFECTS OF TGF-β ON BREAST CANCER BIOLOGY

The relative simplicity of the canonical TGF-β signaling pathway as outlined above belies the complexities of TGF-β-mediated biology. The TGF-β superfamily of growth factors influences a wide variety of biological processes in both normal and disease states. Physiologically, TGF-β plays prominent roles in development, wound healing, and modulating immune system responses. Subversion of these normal processes by TGF-β misregulation can contribute, for example, to abnormal fibrotic changes, immunosuppression, and carcino-genesis. Underlying these systemic manifestations, TGF-β signaling is involved at the cellular level in the intricate regulation of proliferation, apoptosis, differentiation, extracel-lular matrix deposition, migration, and invasion. We will briefly discuss below the role of TGF-β signaling in cellular and systemic processes relevant to breast cancer development and progression.

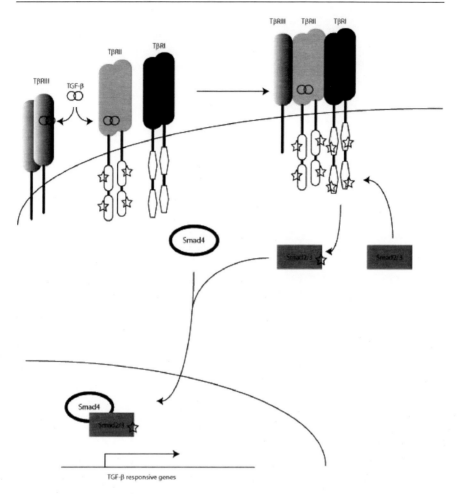

Fig. 1. The TGF-β signaling pathway. TGF-β binds to either TβRIII or TβRII which leads to complex formation with TβRI. Activated TβRI phosphorylates Smad2 or Smad3. The Smad2/3 complex with Smad4 translocates to the nucleus and regulates target gene transcription.

3.1. Regulation of Proliferation

Proliferation is perhaps the most well-characterized role for TGF-β in carcinogenesis. Normally, TGF-β acts as a potent inhibitor of proliferation. TGF-β activation leads to cell cycle arrest at the G1/S phase, primarily through the upregulation of cyclins and the cyclin-dependent kinase inhibitors p15 *(3)* and p21 *(4)* and additionally via repression of c-myc *(5)*. During cancer progression, however, cells become resistant to TGF-β-mediated inhibition of proliferation, and TGF-β signaling instead can promote malignant proliferation. In a study of TGF-β modulation of mammary tumor progression, mice transgenic for activated TβRI were crossed with transgenic mice expressing oncogenic Neu (the mouse homolog of human HER-2/neu). Mice singly transgenic for oncogenic Neu developed mammary tumors with minimal metastases to the lung (6). Overexpression of TβRI reduced the mitotic index and proliferation rate of the Neu-driven primary tumors but enhanced pulmonary metastasis (7). Thus, TGF-β signaling acts early in carcinogenesis to suppress tumor proliferation but potentiates tumorigenesis in later stages.

3.2. Regulation of Apoptosis

In contrast to proliferation, another mechanism by which cell number can be controlled is apoptosis, or programmed cell death. TGF-β mediates the induction of apoptosis in normal epithelia. TGF-β and its family members influence prototypical regulators of apoptosis, including upregulation of the pro-apoptotic factors Bax and caspases (8,9), and downregulation of the anti-apoptotic Bcl-2 family members (10). In the context of apoptosis regulation in cancer, TGF-β modulates the tumor suppressor p53 by inducing p53 activity and consequent apoptosis in a Smad-dependent manner (11). In addition, MCF-7 breast cancer cells overexpressing dominant negative TβRII or treated with a TβRI inhibitor exhibit increased apoptosis compared to normal breast epithelia (12), revealing a potential mechanism of therapy.

3.3. Regulation of Migration and Invasion

The TGF-β signaling pathway is a key regulator of cellular migration and invasion through effects on cellular adhesion, motility, and the extracellular matrix. In normal epithelia and in early tumorigenesis, TGF-β facilitates extracellular matrix deposition by increasing the biosynthesis of extracellular matrix proteins and by inhibiting the degradation of extracellular matrix proteins via upregulation of PAI-1 and TIMP-1 (13). In the later stages of carcinogenesis, however, TGF-β fosters a permissive environment for migration and invasion by upregulating matrix metalloproteases (MMPs) and other enzymes that degrade extracellular matrix (14). In an immunohistochemical analysis of breast tumors, TGF-β staining was concentrated at the tumor periphery as compared to the central tumor bulk (15), supporting a role at the invasive front. Furthermore, in a pre-neoplastic breast epithelial line, TGF-β triggered the transcriptional induction of MMP-2 (16) and MMP-9 (17). Interestingly, while TGF-β modulates p53-mediated apoptosis, p53 affects TGF-β-mediated migration. A p53 mutant was shown to downregulate TβRII and attenuate Smad2/3 phosphorylation, thereby decreasing migration in vitro (18). Taken together, current studies suggest that TGF-β inhibits migration and invasion early in carcinogenesis but promotes metastatic potential later in cancer progression.

3.4. Regulation of Angiogenesis

Tumor progression requires the recruitment of new blood vessels to support ongoing tumor growth, making angiogenesis an attractive target for pharmacotherapy. The efficacy of bevacizumab, a monoclonal antibody directed against the angiogenic activator VEGF, in treating metastatic colon and non-small cell lung cancers validates the clinical utility of anti-angiogenic agents. TGF-β induces VEGF expression in a smooth muscle cell model (19), while genetic analysis directly implicates TGF-β signaling in vascular development. Mutations of the type III TGF-β receptor endoglin and type I receptor ALK-1 in humans are linked to defective vascular formation in hereditary hemorrhagic telangiectasia type 2 (HHT-2) (20,21).

Chapter 9 / TGF-β Signaling: A Novel Target for Treatment of Breast Cancer? 141

Interestingly, we have shown that overexpressing TβRIII in a xenograft breast cancer model decreases angiogenesis in both the primary and metastatic tumor *(22)*. Finally, TGF-β upregulation of MMP-9, related to invasive and metastatic potential as discussed above, also induces angiogenesis in a breast cancer line *(23)*. Thus, TGF-β signaling generally enhances angiogenesis.

3.5. Regulation of the Immune System

Another facet that affects breast cancer progression is the systemic surveillance of cancer cells, for which the immune system is responsible. Among the many roles that TGF-β plays is its modulation of the immune system. TGF-β signaling has an overall suppressive effect on the immune system, specifically on cellular immunity mediated by T-cells and antigen presenting cells (APCs). TGF-β influences T-cell development at the level of both proliferation and differentiation. TGF-β suppresses T-cell proliferation, as seen in CD4+ cells *(24)* and CD8+ cells *(25)*, but promotes T-cell differentiation, as exemplified by the conversion of naïve CD4+ CD25 T-cells to regulatory CD4+ CD25+ T-cells *(26)* and by the conversion of naïve T-cells to helper T-cells *(27)*. Given the intimate interaction between T-cells and APCs required for cell-mediated immunity, it is not surprising that TGF-β also regulates APCs themselves. Mice with conditional dendritic cell knockout of a TGF-β-activating integrin lack regulatory T-cell activity and display an autoimmune phenotype in the colon *(28)*. TGF-β also inhibits macrophage activation *(29)* and Langerhans cell development *(30)*. The higher TGF-β levels associated with increased tumor burden, therefore, would be predicted to promote immunosuppression, thereby allowing cancer cells to more effectively evade immune system surveillance.

3.6. Evidence of TGF-β Alterations in Human Breast Cancer

The cellular and systemic activities of TGF-β take on great clinical and therapeutic significance in the face of evidence that several human cancers feature alterations in the TGF-β signaling pathway. TGF-β ligand expression is elevated in the later stages of a wide variety of cancers, including breast, colon, lung, gastric, pancreatic, and hepatic carcinomas *(31)*. All three TGF-β receptors display evidence of mutation, deletion, or reduced protein expression with corresponding implications for tumor biology and clinical prognosis. TβRI mutations are associated with advanced stages of breast cancer *(32,33)*. Reduced expression or mutation of TβRII receptor has been observed in some breast and colon cancers *(34,35)*. Loss of TβRII expression in hyperplastic breast lesions is associated with an increased risk of invasive breast cancer *(36)*, while reduced TβRII expression is associated with higher tumor grades *(37)*. TβRIII displays reduced expression in breast, prostate, and ovarian cancers *(22,38,39)*. With regards to downstream mediators, microarray analysis of human breast carcinomas reveals that decreased levels of phosphorylated Smad2 are associated with decreased survival times in patients with stage II breast cancer *(40)*.

Notably, a plethora of evidence points to TGF-β as a major player in breast cancer progression. Increasing circulating TGF-β levels are correlated with advancing stages of breast cancer *(41)*, and elevated TGF-β levels, as well as those of the family member BMP-7, are prognostic of a poorer outcome for breast cancer patients *(42,43)*. After surgical removal of cancerous breast tissue, circulating TGF-β levels decline, suggesting that reduced tumor burden leads to a decrease in TGF-β secretion *(44)*. In addition, an aggressive subpopulation of breast cancers featuring increased invasion and poorer outcome was associated with increased TβRII expression and TGF-β activation *(45)*. These findings demonstrate that increased TGF-β levels or activity are associated with later stages of breast cancer and less favorable prognoses.

Taken together with our current understanding of the biology of TGF-β signaling, these findings are seemingly paradoxical. Losses or deficiencies in TGF-β signaling are associated with increasingly malignant tumors, suggesting that decreased TGF-β signaling output is associated with advancing stages of cancer and that TGF-β acts as a tumor suppressor. Increased TGF-β levels, however, are also associated with increased tumor progression and poorer survival, suggesting that TGF-β promotes tumorigenesis. This dichotomy of TGF-β activity remains a central and fundamental focus of investigation. Delving into the intricacies of the complex interplay of tumor-suppressing and tumor-promoting activities is critical to our eventual understanding of TGF-β in cancer and, importantly, in developing sound therapeutic strategies in breast cancer treatment (Fig. 2).

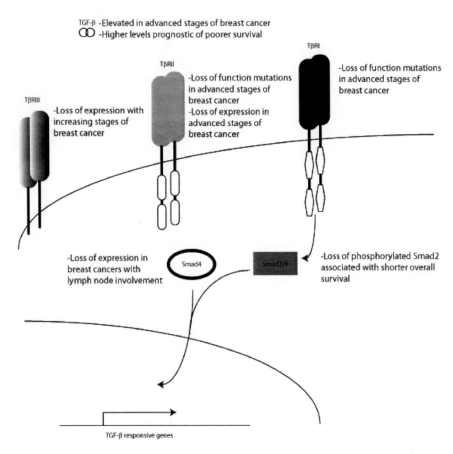

Fig. 2. Alterations in the TGF-β signaling pathway in breast cancer. The progression of human breast cancer is linked to changes at different levels of the TGF-β signaling cascade, from the levels of TGF-β ligand and its cognate receptors to the expression and activation of the downstream signaling mediator Smads.

4. DICHOTOMY OF TGF-β SIGNALING

How do we start to understand the apparent dichotomy of TGF-β signaling? A widely regarded explanation for the dichotomy of TGF-β-mediated effects is that cells develop altered responsiveness to TGF-β or insensitivity to TGF-β signaling. Indeed, unlike other TGF-β-associated cancers such as pancreatic or colon cancers, breast cancer is more likely to be associated with subtle alterations in cellular responses to TGF-β. The majority of breast cancers is not associated with overt loss of function or expression of TβRII or TβRI, though TβRIII is lost at both the mRNA and protein levels in the progression from early to later stages of breast cancer (22). Smads, including Smad2 and Smad4, are also not frequently altered or mutated in human breast cancer (40,46).

Indeed, the scaffolding of the TGF-β signaling pathway remains largely intact in human breast cancers. What ultimately determines TGF-β's role during cancer progression – tumor suppression or tumor promotion – is the milieu and time point in which cells are exposed. Generally, TGF-β tends to act in a tumor suppressor role in normal tissue and in early carcinogenesis but as a tumor promoter in the later stages of carcinogenesis. Studies in animal models support this dual, context-dependent role for TGF-β. Targeted mammary expression of dominant-negative TβRII in the context of chemically induced breast cancer enhanced the tumorigenicity of both mammary and pulmonary tumors (47). In contrast, expression of dominant-negative TβRII in a mouse model of oncogenic Neu-driven breast cancer not only decreased tumor but also decreased lung metastatic potential (7). Targeted expression of activated TβRI in the mammary glands of oncogenic Neu mice elicited yet another response: delayed initial tumor onset but increased lung metastasis (7).

The precise mechanisms underlying the switch in the functional effects of TGF-β signaling remain unclear. An attractive possibility is that early tumor epithelia become gradually more resistant to the anti-proliferative effects of TGF-β, effectively driving an anomalous feedback cycle that increases TGF-β signaling. This TGF-β signaling eventually leads to autocrine and paracrine effects, both on the adjacent epithelia and the extracellular environment. In an increasingly unregulated fashion, TGF-β signaling ramps up to a critical point at which it becomes pro-oncogenic.

In this context, it should be noted that TGF-β effects depend not only on the epithelia in situ but also on the surrounding extracellular matrix. The differential effects of TGF-β in epithelial versus mesenchymal cells is long-established, but more intense study of the interplay between the tumor and its microenvironment has been undertaken only recently (48). Stromal secretion of TGF-β contributes to the inhibition of proliferation and tumor progression in the epithelia (49). Changes in stromal TGF-β signaling can also dictate cancer progression and the balance of oncogenic potential. One study demonstrated, for example, that fibroblasts lacking TβRII are able to induce an invasive phenotype in adjacent carcinomas, featuring increased proliferation rate, greater angiogenesis, and reduced apoptosis (50). Furthermore, TβRII-null fibroblasts grafted into the mammary fat pads of wild-type mice induced epithelial changes in the new local microenvironment (50).

This interplay between the stromal and epithelial compartments lends credence to another explanation for the functional dichotomy of TGF-β in cancer progression. In this model, the carcinoma in situ derived from an epithelial cell type acquires traits of a mesenchymal cell in the process termed epithelial-mesenchymal transition (EMT). Epithelial cells are characterized by a low level of motility, enhanced cell–cell contact, and flattened morphology. In contrast, mesenchymal cells exhibit relatively higher levels of motility and invasiveness, decreased cell–cell contact, and a spindle-like morphology. A subset of cancer cells at the primary site switch to a more mesenchymal phenotype. The more invasive mesenchymal cells can then break through the immediate extracellular matrix, including the basement membrane, greatly facilitating metastasis to secondary sites *(51)*. Interestingly, differences in TGF-β signaling in epithelial cells and mesenchymal cells parallel those of early and late carcinogenesis; that is, TGF-β in epithelial cells inhibits proliferation, migration, and invasion, whereas TGF-β tends to promote these processes in mesenchymal cells. We have found that TβRIII modulates the EMT-associated migration and invasion of pancreatic carcinomas. Specifically, during EMT TβRIII expression decreases, and either membrane-bound or soluble TβRIII can inhibit this EMT-associated migration and invasion *(52)*. Evidence also implicates TGF-β and EMT in breast cancer progression. In one model, TGF-β induced EMT and consequent migration in a PI3K-dependent manner *(53)*. In another cell culture model of breast cancer, dominant negative TβRII was associated with a decrease in tumor progression with concomitant inhibition of EMT *(54)*. Thus, the EMT model presents an attractive explanation for the dichotomy of TGF-β signaling.

5. TGF-β AS A TARGET FOR BREAST CANCER THERAPY

Efforts are underway to target the TGF-β pathway for the prevention or treatment of breast cancer. Unlike other targeted therapies, however, the therapeutic strategy for TGF-β is not straightforward. The complex and sometimes diametrically opposed aspects of TGF-β signaling render the outcome of TGF-β inhibition difficult to predict. Nevertheless, the varying degrees of success in initial forays into this field of TGF-β targeted therapy have laid the groundwork for more promising approaches.

Given the observed anti-proliferative effect of TGF-β in early carcinogenesis, one potential strategy for preventing the initiation or progression of early stage breast cancer is to functionally increase local TGF-β signaling. TGF-β seems to play an inhibitory role in the early stages of hormone-dependent breast cancers in particular *(55)*. In fact, tamoxifen use in ER-positive breast cancers augments TGF-β secretion and consequent growth inhibition *(56)*. In addition, a human breast cancer line treated with a histone deacetylase inhibitor displayed increased expression of TβRII, consequent downstream TGF-β signaling, and inhibition of cancer cell proliferation *(57)*.

Despite these telling findings, to date no definitive evidence demonstrates high efficacy in directly exploiting the early anti-proliferative effects of TGF-β. The difficulties in employing a strategy of functionally increasing TGF-β signaling for prevention and treatment of early breast cancer are compounded by the contrasting role of TGF-β in later stages of cancer. Given that several models suggest that primary tumors initially inhibited by TGF-β signaling eventually give rise to more aggressive and malignant tumors, some serious considerations must be made. First, what constitutes an "early stage" of breast cancer in the spectrum of TGF-β function must be defined so as to avoid a scenario in which artificially enhanced TGF-β signaling unintentionally becomes tumor-promoting. The association of stage or grade with TGF-β functionality has not yet been rigorously established. Second, the present benefit of TGF-β-mediated delay in tumor onset must be weighed against the future risk of a more aggressive tumor phenotype. The risk–benefit ratio for each individual patient would need to account for improvements in morbidity and quality of life as well as the availability and efficacy of treatment strategies for the contingency of an increasingly aggressive tumor.

In comparison to the complications inherent to exploiting TGF-β's tumor suppressing role in early carcinogenesis, the approach of targeting increased TGF-β signaling in later stages of cancer is much more straightforward. A number of therapeutic strategies designed to inhibit TGF-β signaling locally or systemically are currently being evaluated.

Chapter 9 / TGF-β Signaling: A Novel Target for Treatment of Breast Cancer?   145

One attractive strategy for targeting breast carcinomas directly: one exploits the fact that both TβRI and TβRII are receptor kinases whose downstream effects are mediated by the phosphorylation of their target residues. High-throughput screening for specific activity against the TβRI and TβRII kinase domains has identified many promising small molecule inhibitors. A few compounds, including SB-431542, SB-505124, and SB-203580, have been shown to specifically inhibit TβRI with consequent inhibition of proliferation, angiogenesis, motility, and TGF-β-dependent transcription *(58–60)*. Another small molecule inhibitor, Ki26894, has been shown to selectively and effectively inhibit TGF-β responsiveness in a breast cancer-specific assay. In a xenograft mouse model of a highly metastatic human breast cancer cell line, application of Ki26894 significantly inhibited metastatic potential and prolonged survival time *(61)*. Continued small molecule discovery combined with testing in preclinical trials promises to expand the possibilities of carcinoma-directed TGF-β therapy.

A complementary approach for TGF-β inhibition is based on limiting the bioavailability of the TGF-β ligand itself. Increased circulating serum TGF-β levels are correlated with increasing tumor grade *(31)*, making the attenuation of TGF-β ligand another avenue of intense investigation. At the cellular level, increased availability of TGF-β for autocrine and paracrine signaling is thought to contribute to tumor-promoting activity, and TGF-β mediates important interplay between the epithelial and stromal compartments in the tumor microenvironment *(48)*. The use of neutralizing antibodies to sequester TGF-β ligand has yielded encouraging results. One such antibody has been used in a mouse xenograft model to abrogate TGF-β-mediated tumor progression and metastasis of the human breast cancer line MCF-7 *(62)*, with similar results reported using another human cancer line MDA-MB231 *(63)*. Another way to sequester TGF-β ligand is to utilize soluble forms of the cognate TGF-β receptors which, when circulated, bind to free serum TGF-β and prevent signaling to cell surface receptors. A soluble form of recombinant TβRII has been used to inhibit breast cancer progression in a mouse model, both increasing apoptosis in the primary tumor and decreasing pulmonary metastatic potential *(64)*. Similarly, introduction of a soluble recombinant TβRIII reduced metastasis and angiogenesis in a xenograft of a human breast cancer line *(65)*. Importantly, soluble TβRIII affects other important mediators of breast cancer progression, including apoptosis *(66)*, migration, and invasion *(22)*.

In addition to carcinoma-directed strategies, therapies are now increasingly geared toward modulation of TGF-β specifically in the immune system. As TGF-β signaling suppresses the immune system in general and cell-mediated immunity in particular, an approach inhibiting TGF-β signaling in the immune compartment would be predicted to bolster immune surveillance of rogue cancer cells. In experiments demonstrating proof-of-principle using a syngeneic mouse model, expression of dominant negative TβRII in T-cells led to a marked decrease in metastases of murine melanoma and lymphoma lines *(67)*. In another experiment, CD8+ T-cells were sensitized in a nude mouse xenograft model of prostate cancer, manipulated to express dominant negative TβRII, and then re-introduced into the mice. Remarkably, introduction of modified T-cells reduced metastasis compared to introduction of unmodified control T-cells *(68)*. These results illustrate the significant role of TGF-β in the interplay between tumor and cell-mediated immunity. Further, continued research into immune-targeted approaches for breast cancer therapy is justified, with simultaneous consideration for the undesired side effects of immunosuppression.

Because TGF-β's sometimes antithetical effects depend on temporal and spatial context, a straightforward approach to utilizing TGF-β-modulating chemotherapeutic or biologic agents in the treatment of breast cancer is unlikely. However, initial preclinical investigations reveal opportunities which may be exploited to enhance the mode and timing of treatment. As our understanding of TGF-β signaling in proliferation, apoptosis, migration, invasion, angiogenesis, and immune system modulation continues to advance, so will our knowledge of how these diverse biological processes are implicated in breast cancer progression. As further efforts reveal the nuances of the TGF-β pathway, a wider range of successful therapeutic strategies will be developed. TGF-β-targeted therapies that minimize serious side effects while selectively and potently targeting breast cancer cells will add alternatives to traditional therapies to the clinician's armamentarium.

REFERENCES

1. Kamangar F, Dores GM, Anderson WF. Patterns of Cancer Incidence, Mortality, and Prevalence Across Five Continents: Defining Priorities to Reduce Cancer Disparities in Different Geographic Regions of the World. J Clin Oncol 2006;24:2137–50.
2. Massague J. TGF-beta signal transduction. Annu Rev Biochem 1998;67:753–91.
3. Hannon GJ, Beach D. pl5INK4B is a potential effector of TGF-[beta]-induced cell cycle arrest. Nature 1994;371:257–61.
4. Datto MB, Li Y, Panus JF, Howe DJ, Xiong Y, Wang X. Transforming Growth Factor {beta} Induces the Cyclin-Dependent Kinase Inhibitor p21 through a p53-Independent Mechanism. Proceedings of the National Academy of Sciences 1995;92:5545–9.
5. Pietenpol JA, Stein RW, Moran E, et al. TGF-[beta]1 inhibition of c-myc transcription and growth in keratinocytes is abrogated by viral transforming proteins with pRB binding domains. Cell 1990;61:777–85.
6. Siegel PM, Ryan ED, Cardiff RD, Muller WJ. Elevated expression of activated forms of Neu/ErbB-2 and ErbB-3 are involved in the induction of mammary tumors in transgenic mice: implications for human breast cancer. EMBO J 1999;18:2149–64.
7. Siegel PM, Shu W, Cardiff RD, Muller WJ, Massague J. Transforming growth factor beta signaling impairs Neu-induced mammary tumorigenesis while promoting pulmonary metastasis. Proc Natl Acad Sci U S A 2003;100:8430–5.
8. Lagna G, Nguyen PH, Ni W, Hata A. BMP-dependent activation of caspase-9 and caspase-8 mediates apoptosis in pulmonary artery smooth muscle cells. Am J Physiol Lung Cell Mol Physiol 2006;291:L1059–67.
9. Inman GJ, Allday MJ. Apoptosis induced by TGF-beta 1 in Burkitt's lymphoma cells is caspase 8 dependent but is death receptor independent. J Immunol 2000;165:2500–10.
10. Motyl T, Grzelkowska K, Zimowska W, et al. Expression of bcl-2 and bax in TGF-beta 1-induced apoptosis of L1210 leukemic cells. Eur J Cell Biol 1998;75:367–74.
11. Zhang S, Ekman M, Thakur N, et al. TGFbeta1-induced activation of ATM and p53 mediates apoptosis in a Smad7-dependent manner. Cell Cycle 2006;5:2787–95.
12. Lei X, Yang J, Nichols RW, Sun LZ. Abrogation of TGF[beta] signaling induces apoptosis through the modulation of MAP kinase pathways in breast cancer cells. Experimental Cell Research 2007;313:1687–95.
13. Blobe GC, Schiemann WP, Lodish HF. Role of Transforming Growth Factor {beta} in Human Disease. N Engl J Med 2000;342:1350–8.
14. Desruisseau S, Ghazarossian-Ragni E, Chinot O, Martin PM. Divergent effect of TGFbeta1 on growth and proteolytic modulation of human prostatic-cancer cell lines. Int J Cancer 1996;66:796–801.
15. Dalal BI, Keown PA, Greenberg AH. Immunocytochemical localization of secreted transforming growth factor-beta 1 to the advancing edges of primary tumors and to lymph node metastases of human mammary carcinoma. Am J Pathol 1993;143:381–9.
16. Kim E-S, Sohn Y-W, Moon A. TGF-[beta]-induced transcriptional activation of MMP-2 is mediated by activating transcription factor (ATF)2 in human breast epithelial cells. Cancer Letters 2007;252:147–56.
17. Kim ES, Kim MS, Moon A. TGF-beta-induced upregulation of MMP-2 and MMP-9 depends on p38 MAPK, but not ERK signaling in MCF10A human breast epithelial cells. Int J Oncol 2004;25:1375–82.

Chapter 9 / TGF-β Signaling: A Novel Target for Treatment of Breast Cancer?   147

18. Kalo E, Buganim Y, Shapira KE, et al. Mutant p53 attenuates the SMAD-dependent TGF-{beta}1 signaling pathway by repressing the expression of TGF-{beta} receptor type II. Mol Cell Biol 2007:MCB.00374–07.
19. Yamamoto T, Kozawa O, Tanabe K, et al. Involvement of p38 MAP kinase in TGF-beta-stimulated VEGF synthesis in aortic smooth muscle cells. J Cell Biochem 2001;82:591–8.
20. McAllister KA, Grogg KM, Johnson DW, et al. Endoglin, a TGF-beta binding protein of endothelial cells, is the gene for hereditary haemorrhagic telangiectasia type 1. Nat Genet 1994;8:345–51.
21. Johnson DW, Berg JN, Baldwin MA, et al. Mutations in the activin receptor-like kinase 1 gene in hereditary haemorrhagic telangiectasia type 2. Nat Genet 1996;13:189–95.
22. Dong M, How T, Kirkbride KC, et al. The type III TGF-beta receptor suppresses breast cancer progression. J Clin Invest 2007;117:206–17.
23. Safina A, Vandette E, Bakin AV. ALK5 promotes tumor angiogenesis by upregulating matrix met-alloproteinase-9 in tumor cells. Oncogene 2006;26:2407–22.
24. Classen S, Zander T, Eggle D, et al. Human resting CD4+ T cells are constitutively inhibited by TGF beta under steady-state conditions. J Immunol 2007;178:6931–40.
25. Cheng ML, Chen HW, Tsai JP, et al. Clonal restriction of the expansion of antigen-specific CD8+ memory T cells by transforming growth factor-{beta}. J Leukoc Biol 2006;79:1033–42.
26. Chen W, Jin W, Hardegen N, et al. Conversion of Peripheral CD4+ CD25- Naive T Cells to CD4+ CD25+ Regulatory T Cells by TGF-{beta} Induction of Transcription Factor Foxp3. J Exp Med 2003;198:1875–86.
27. Mangan PR, Harrington LE, O'Quinn DB, et al. Transforming growth factor-[beta] induces development of the TH17 lineage. Nature 2006;441:231–4.
28. Travis MA, Reizis B, Melton AC, et al. Loss of integrin alpha(v)beta8 on dendritic cells causes autoimmunity and colitis in mice. Nature 2007;449:361–5.
29. Bogdan C, Paik J, Vodovotz Y, Nathan C. Contrasting mechanisms for suppression of macrophage cytokine release by transforming growth factor-beta and interleukin-10. J Biol Chem 1992;267:23301–8.
30. Borkowski TA, Letterio JJ, Mackall CL, et al. Langerhans cells in the TGF beta 1 null mouse. Adv Exp Med Biol 1997;417:307–10.
31. Bierie B, Moses H. TGF-beta and cancer. Cytokine & growth factor reviews 2006;17:29–40.
32. Chen T, Jackson CR, Link A, et al. Int7G24A variant of transforming growth factor-beta receptor type I is associated with invasive breast cancer. Clin Cancer Res 2006;12:392–7.
33. Xu Y, Pasche B. TGF-beta signaling alterations and susceptibility to colorectal cancer. Hum Mol Genet 2007;16 Spec No 1:R14–20.
34. Markowitz S, Wang J, Myeroff L, et al. Inactivation of the type II TGF-beta receptor in colon cancer cells with microsatellite instability. Science 1995;268:1336–8.
35. Lucke CD, Philpott A, Metcalfe JC, et al. Inhibiting mutations in the transforming growth factor beta type 2 receptor in recurrent human breast cancer. Cancer Res 2001;61:482–5.
36. Gobbi H, Dupont WD, Simpson JF, et al. Transforming Growth Factor-{beta} and Breast Cancer Risk in Women With Mammary Epithelial Hyperplasia. J Natl Cancer Inst 1999;91:2096–101.
37. Gobbi, Arteaga, Jensen, et al. Loss of expression of transforming growth factor beta type II receptor correlates with high tumour grade in human breast in-situ and invasive carcinomas. Histopathology 2000;36:168–77.
38. Turley RS, Finger EC, Hempel N, How T, Fields TA, Blobe GC. The type III transforming growth factor-beta receptor as a novel tumor suppressor gene in prostate cancer. Cancer Res 2007;67:1090–8.
39. Hempel N, How T, Dong M, Murphy SK, Fields TA, Blobe GC. Loss of betaglycan expression in ovarian cancer: role in motility and invasion. Cancer Res 2007;67:5231–8.
40. Xie W, Mertens JC, Reiss DJ, et al. Alterations of Smad signaling in human breast carcinoma are associated with poor outcome: a tissue microarray study. Cancer Res 2002;62:497–505.
41. Kopp A, Jonat W, Schmahl M, Knabbe C. Transforming growth factor beta 2 (TGF-beta 2) levels in plasma of patients with metastatic breast cancer treated with tamoxifen. Cancer Res 1995;55:4512–5.
42. Ghellal A, Li C, Hayes M, Byrne G, Bundred N, Kumar S. Prognostic significance of TGF beta 1 and TGF beta 3 in human breast carcinoma. Anticancer Res 2000;20:4413–8.
43. Buijs JT, Henriquez NV, van Overveld PG, et al. Bone morphogenetic protein 7 in the development and treatment of bone metastases from breast cancer. Cancer Res 2007;67:8742–51.

44. Kong FM, Anscher MS, Murase T, Abbott BD, Iglehart JD, Jirtle RL. Elevated plasma transforming growth factor-beta 1 levels in breast cancer patients decrease after surgical removal of the tumor. Ann Surg 1995;222:155–62.

45. Shipitsin M, Campbell LL, Argani P, et al. Molecular Definition of Breast Tumor Heterogeneity. Cancer Cell 2007;11:259–73.

46. Benson JR. Role of transforming growth factor beta in breast carcinogenesis. Lancet Oncol 2004;5:229–39.

47. Bottinger EP, Jakubczak JL, Haines DC, Bagnall K, Wakefield LM. Transgenic Mice Overexpressing a Dominant-negative Mutant Type II Transforming Growth Factor {beta} Receptor Show Enhanced Tumorigenesis in the Mammary Gland and Lung in Response to the Carcinogen 7,12-Dimethyl-benz-[a]-anthracene. Cancer Res 1997;57:5564–70.

48. Stover D, Bierie B, Moses H. A delicate balance: TGF-beta and the tumor microenvironment. Journal of Cellular Biochemistry 2007;101:851–61.

49. Bhowmick NA, Chytil A, Plieth D, et al. TGF-beta signaling in fibroblasts modulates the oncogenic potential of adjacent epithelia. Science 2004;303:848–51.

50. Cheng N, Bhowmick NA, Chytil A, et al. Loss of TGF-beta type II receptor in fibroblasts promotes mammary carcinoma growth and invasion through upregulation of TGF-alpha-, MSP- and HGF-mediated signaling networks. Oncogene 2005;24:5053–68.

51. Thiery JP. Epithelial-mesenchymal transitions in development and pathologies. Curr Opin Cell Biol 2003;15:740–6.

52. Gordon KJ, Dong M, Chislock EM, Fields TA, Blobe GC. Loss of Type III Transforming Growth Factor {beta} Receptor Expression Increases Motility and Invasiveness associated with Epithelial to Mesenchymal Transition during Pancreatic Cancer Progression. Carcinogenesis 2007:bgm249.

53. Bakin AV, Tomlinson AK, Bhowmick NA, Moses HL, Arteaga CL. Phosphatidylinositol 3-kinase function is required for transforming growth factor beta-mediated epithelial to mesenchymal transition and cell migration. J Biol Chem 2000;275:36803–10.

54. Oft M, Heider KH, Beug H. TGFbeta signaling is necessary for carcinoma cell invasiveness and metastasis. Curr Biol 1998;8:1243–52.

55. Butta A, MacLennan K, Flanders KC, et al. Induction of transforming growth factor beta 1 in human breast cancer in vivo following tamoxifen treatment. Cancer Res 1992;52:4261–4.

56. Buck MB, Knabbe C. TGF-beta signaling in breast cancer. Ann N Y Acad Sci 2006;1089:119–26.

57. Lee BI, Park SH, Kim JW, et al. MS-275, a histone deacetylase inhibitor, selectively induces transforming growth factor beta type II receptor expression in human breast cancer cells. Cancer Res 2001;61:931–4.

58. Matsuyama S, Iwadate M, Kondo M, et al. SB-431542 and Gleevec inhibit transforming growth factor-beta-induced proliferation of human osteosarcoma cells. Cancer Res 2003;63:7791–8.

59. Callahan JF, Burgess JL, Fornwald JA, et al. Identification of novel inhibitors of the transforming growth factor beta1 (TGF-beta1) type 1 receptor (ALK5). J Med Chem 2002;45:999–1001.

60. Yakymovych I, Engstrom U, Grimsby S, Heldin CH, Souchelnytskyi S. Inhibition of transforming growth factor-beta signaling by low molecular weight compounds interfering with ATP- or substrate-binding sites of the TGF beta type I receptor kinase. Biochemistry 2002;41:11000–7.

61. Ehata S, Hanyu A, Fujime M, et al. Ki26894, a novel transforming growth factor-beta type I receptor kinase inhibitor, inhibits in vitro invasion and in vivo bone metastasis of a human breast cancer cell line. Cancer Sci 2007;98:127–33.

62. Arteaga CL, Carty-Dugger T, Moses HL, Hurd SD, Pietenpol JA. Transforming growth factor beta 1 can induce estrogen-independent tumorigenicity of human breast cancer cells in athymic mice. Cell Growth Differ 1993;4:193–201.

63. Arteaga CL, Dugger TC, Winnier AR, Forbes JT. Evidence for a positive role of transforming growth factor-beta in human breast cancer cell tumorigenesis. J Cell Biochem Suppl 1993;17G:187–93.

64. Muraoka RS, Dumont N, Ritter CA, et al. Blockade of TGF-beta inhibits mammary tumor cell viability, migration, and metastases. J Clin Invest 2002;109:1551–9.

65. Bandyopadhyay A, Lopez-Casillas F, Malik SN, et al. Antitumor activity of a recombinant soluble betaglycan in human breast cancer xenograft. Cancer Res 2002;62:4690–5.

Chapter 9 / TGF-β Signaling: A Novel Target for Treatment of Breast Cancer? 149

66. Lei X, Bandyopadhyay A, Le T, Sun L. Autocrine TGFbeta supports growth and survival of human breast cancer MDA-MB-231 cells. Oncogene 2002;21:7514–23.
67. Gorelik L, Flavell RA. Immune-mediated eradication of tumors through the blockade of transforming growth factor-beta signaling in T cells. Nat Med 2001;7:1118–22.
68. Zhang Q, Yang X, Pins M, et al. Adoptive transfer of tumor-reactive transforming growth factor-beta-insensitive CD8+ T cells: eradication of autologous mouse prostate cancer. Cancer Res 2005;65:1761–9.

10 DNA Methylation in Breast Cancer

Moshe Szyf

SUMMARY

The progression through the multiple steps of breast cancer from epithelial hypertrophy to highly invasive breast carcinoma involves multiple coordinated changes in gene expression programming. Such coordinated changes in gene expression are bound to be controlled by global mechanisms of gene expression programming. The genome is programmed by the epigenome, which consists of chromatin structure, a pattern of modification of DNA by DNA methylation and a profile of expression of noncoding RNAs such as microRNA. This chapter will focus on DNA methylation. Three kinds of aberrations in the DNA methylation machinery were observed in breast cancer: induction of DNA methyltransferase activity, hypermethylation of tumor suppressing genes, and hypomethylation of other genes. The main focus of attention has been hypermethylation of tumor suppressor genes and demethylation inducing therapies. Recent data suggest that hypomethylation of prometastatic genes might play an important role in cancer progression and metastasis. The implications of coexistence of hypermethylation and hypomethylation in breast for epigenetic therapy will be discussed.

Key Words: DNA methylation; Epigenetics; Global hypomethylation; Tumor suppressor genes; Chromatin modification; Histone acetylation; Trichostatin A (TSA); 5-Azacytidine (5-azaC); S-adenosylmethionine (SAM); DNA methyltransferase (DNMT); Histone acetyl transferase (HAT); Histone deacetylase (HDAC); Metastasis; Prometastatic genes

1. CHROMATIN, ITS MODIFICATIONS, AND CANCER

Breast cancer progression involves multiple changes in the transcriptome as unraveled by several microarray gene expression profiling studies. The epigenome regulates gene expression programming in eukaryotes. The epigenome consists of the chromatin structure and

From: *Current Clinical Oncology: Breast Cancer in the Post-Genomic Era,*
Edited by: A. Giordano and N. Normanno, DOI: 10.1007/978-1-60327-945-1_10,
© Humana Press, a part of Springer Science + Business Media, LLC 2009

chromatin modification, a pattern of covalent modification of the DNA by enzymatic addition of methyl groups from the methyl donor S-adenosyl methionine (SAM) at the 5′ of cytosines residing mainly at the dinucleotide sequence CG and a profile of expression of noncoding RNAs such as microRNA.

DNA is wrapped around a proteinacious core consisting of an octamer of histone molecules which constitutes the basic building block of chromatin, the nucleosome. The nucleosome is composed of a H3-H4 tetramer flanked on either side with a H2A-H2B dimer *(1)*. The N-terminal tails of these histones are extensively modified by methylation *(2)*, phosphorylation, acetylation *(3)*, sumoylation *(4)*, and ubiquitination *(5)*. The state of modification of these tails plays an important role in defining the accessibility of the DNA to the transcription machinery. Different histone variants, which replace the standard isoforms, also play a regulatory role and serve to mark active genes in some instances *(6)*. All histone modifications are a balance of modifying and demodifying enzymes. Thus, the state of chromatin could be tilted in both directions by blocking the different modification enzymes with specific antagonists. The state of modification at specific loci is defined through recruitment of chromatin-modifying and -demodifying enzymes by sequence-specific factors. The targeting factors are responsive to cellular signaling pathways, thus creating a conduit between cellular and extracellular signals and the epigenetic state *(7)*.

The most investigated histone modification is histone acetylation. H3 and H4 histones are acetylated at different positions especially in the N terminus tail; H3 at K9 residue as well as other residues *(4,14,18,23,27)* and H4 tails at a number of residues (K-5, 8, 12, 16, 20) *(8,9)*. The balance between HATs and HDACs defines the state of acetylation of given loci they associate with. Histone acetylation is believed to be a predominant signal for an active chromatin configuration *(10,11)*. Recent whole-genome ChIP on chip analyses revealed that histone acetylation is a hallmark of regulatory regions of active genes and could be utilized to identify transcriptional regulatory positions in the genome *(12–14)*.

Histone acetylation is catalyzed by histone acetyltransferases HAT which transfer an acetyl group from the cofactor acetyl CoA onto the ε position on lysine and is reversed by histone deacetylases HDACs (HDAC) *(8)*.

Histone acetylation plays a critical role in breast cancer. For example, the silencing of *E CADHERIN* a critical step in the epithelial-mesenchymal transition involves the transcriptional repressor SNAIL which recruits HDAC to the promoter of the gene resulting in deacetylation of histones associated with the promoter and silencing of gene expression *(15)*. HDAC inhibitors (HDACi) were shown to be effective in inducing tumor suppressor genes suppressed by hypoacetylation in breast cancer cells, blocking breast cancer cell growth and inducing apoptosis *(16–20)*. Histone acetylation is also important because of its bilateral relationship with DNA methylation *(21)* which will be discussed below.

HDAC inhibitors HDACi are in advanced clinical trials for blood cancers and several classes of HDAC inhibitors were developed. Vorinostsat (SAHA) was recently approved for clinical use in cutaneous T-cell lymphoma *(22)*. Although, HDACi are effective against breast cancer cells in culture it is still unclear whether HDACi will be active against breast cancer in humans. In a proof of principle study the HDAC inhibitor magnesium valproate and hydralazine an inhibitor of DNA methylation were added to neoadjuvant doxorubicin and cyclophosphamide in locally advanced breast cancer and indicated some efficacy of epigenetic treatment *(19)*.

Methylation of histones is a different class of histone modifications, which are especially important in the cross talk between DNA methylation and chromatin structure as will be discussed below. Histone methylation at lysine residues H3-K9Me, H3-K27Me, and H4-K20Me associated with promoters of genes are repressive of gene expression. In general,

Chapter 10 / DNA Methylation in Breast Cancer

these modifications are hallmarks of gene silencing as validated by genome-wide ChIP on chip analyses *(23)*. However, recent studies suggest that H3K9Me3 downstream to transcriptional start sites is associated with active genes rather than being a ubiquitous repressive marking as previously thought *(24)*. H3-K4Me, H3-K36Me, and H3-K79Me are associated on the other hand with gene activity and transcription elongation *(25)* and this is confirmed by genome-wide analyses *(23)*. There is a cross talk between histone acetylation and histone methylation. H3-K4Me3, H3-K36Me2, and H3-K79Me2 are associated with hyperacetylation and active genes, whereas H3-K9Me2, H3-K9Me3, H3-K27Me2, and H4-K20Me2 are associated with hypoacetylation *(23)*. A member of the PcG group of proteins is EZH2, which was shown to contain a SET domain and to function as histone methyltransferase (HMETase) targeting K27 and K9 in the H3 histone tail *(26,27)*. EZH2 plays an important role in silencing several tumor suppressor genes and might serve as the targeting factor for DNA methyltransferase, thus marking sequences for de novo methylation in response to an increase in DNMT levels *(28,29)*. Interestingly, however, EZH2 acts as a transcriptional activator in breast cancer cells integrating Wnt and estrogen signaling *(30)*. Thus, although histone modification and their enzymes are recognized for either their repressive or their activating function, they might in certain instances play an opposite role. Enhanced expression of EZH2 has been seen in highly metastatic and aggressive breast and prostate cancers *(31,32)*.

Activation and inactivation of chromatin necessitates movement of nucleosomes. Such a process requires energy, which is derived from ATP *(33,34)*. SWI/SNF, RSC, NURF, CHRAC, ACF, RSF, and NuRD are highly conserved chromatin remodeling complexes that utilize energy derived from ATP hydrolysis to remodel chromatin *(35)*. Interestingly, several breast cancer metastasis genes were shown to be members of the NurD complex. For example, the metastasis associated proteins (MTA) is found in the NurD complex *(36)*. The MTA family of proteins can act as either co-activators or co-repressors of nuclear receptors including estrogen receptor signaling which has an important involvement in breast cancer [for a review see *(37)*]. Another component of the NurD complex MTA3 was shown to be required for suppressing the expression of *SNAIL*. Inhibition of MTA3 leads to activation of SNAIL which in turn suppresses the expression of *E CADHERIN* leading to breast cancer invasion *(15)*.

In summary, the chromatin modification and remodeling machineries are involved in the changes in gene expression leading to breast cancer.

2. THE DNA METHYLATION PATTERN

The primary methylated sequence in vertebrates is composed of only two bases, the di-nucleotide sequence CG *(38)*. Another feature that distinguishes vertebrate methylation is the fact that only a fraction (<80%) of the methylatable CG population is methylated. Different CG sites are methylated in different tissues, creating a pattern of methylation, which is gene and tissue specific *(38)*. The pattern of methylation creates a layer of information, which confers upon a genome its specific cell-type identity. Although genomes are identical in all cells of the body, the DNA methylation pattern is different in distinct cell types. In some cases, such as parentally imprinted genes *(39)* or genes residing on the inactive X chromosome, the two alleles of the same gene are differentially methylated in the same cell *(40)*. DNA methylation is the only component of the covalent DNA structure that shows cell, parent of origin, and allele-specific identity. An identical sequence could be either methylated or nonmethylated in different cell types or in different alleles in the same cell type. The DNA methylation pattern is not copied by the DNA replication machinery, but by independent enzymatic machinery *(41)* the DNA methyltransferase(s) (DNMT). DNA methylation patterns in vertebrates are distinguished by their tight correlation with chromatin structure. Active regions of the chromatin, which enable gene expression, are associated with hypomethylated DNA whereas hypermethylated DNA is packaged in inactive chromatin *(41)*.

3. MECHANISMS OF SILENCING OF GENE EXPRESSION BY DNA METHYLATION

DNA methylation is a highly effective mechanism of silencing of gene expression in vertebrates and plants. DNA methylation silences gene expression by two principal mechanisms. The first mechanism involves direct interference of a methyl residue with the binding of a transcription factor to its recognition element in DNA resulting in silencing of gene expression *(42,43)*. A second mechanism is indirect. A certain density of DNA methylation moieties in the region of the gene attracts the binding of methylated-DNA binding proteins such as MeCP2 *(44)*. MeCP2 recruits other proteins such as SIN3A- and histone-modifying enzymes, which lead to formation of a "closed" chromatin configuration and silencing of gene expression *(44)*. Several methylated-DNA binding proteins such as MBD1, MBD2, and MBD3 suppress gene expression by a similar mechanism *(45–47)*. MBD3 does not bind directly methylated DNA but associates with the NurD complex which contains MBD2 as the methylated-DNA binding factor *(48)*.

The role of DNA methylation in expression is more complex than the well-accepted and attractively simple model presented above. This is important for interpretation of aberrant DNA methylation patterns in breast cancer. Methylation in body of genes was found to be associated with transcriptional activity in plants *(49)* and body of genes was found to be methylated in several active genes in mammals as well. Recent data suggest that the presence of epigenetic modification in the body of active genes, which are considered repressive in promoters, is not unique to DNA methylation. Hypoacetylation and repressive methylation marks were found to be associated with transcription elongation in yeast *(50)* and repressive HP-1 protein which recognizes H3-K9me and is involved in heterochromatin was also found to be associated with transcription elongation *(51)*. Perhaps one explanation for this contradiction of finding repressive marks in active genes is that repressive marks in bodies of genes act to prevent spurious firing of cryptic promoters outside the legitimate transcription start site *(50)*. It remains to be seen whether these repressive epigenetic marks are limited to body of genes or whether other regions upstream to promoters might be marked similarly. Future interpretation of epigenomic mapping must take this into consideration.

In addition to chromatin and DNA methylation, gene expression is also regulated by noncoding RNAs, antisense RNA as well as microRNA, which negatively regulate gene expression. Methylation of a promoter of a microRNA or an antisense RNA would result in suppression of the noncoding RNA release of repression and activation of the target genes. Thus, a simplistic interpretation of methylation marks as far as gene expression is concerned might be misleading. Perhaps some of the contradictions to the rule of the inverse correlation between gene expression and DNA methylation revealed in recent genomic screens might be explained by these confounding factors.

It is important to note here as well that methylated DNA binding proteins (MBDs) which were originally characterized as the repressive agents translating the DNA methylation signal could be involved in gene activation as well as gene silencing. MBD2 was shown to activate several promoters by methylation-dependent and independent pathways *(52–55)*, MBD3 was shown to be required for demethylation and expression of rRNA *(56,57)* and MeCP2 was shown to associate with many active promoters; a genome-wide analysis

Chapter 10 / DNA Methylation in Breast Cancer

revealed that 63% of MeCP2-bound promoters were actively expressed and only 6% were highly methylated *(58)*. Certain MBDs have other enzymatic activities. MBD4 is a thymidine glycosylase *(59)* and MBD2 was suggested to bear demethylase activity *(60–64)* although this activity was highly contested. This dual and opposite action of MBDs has obviously important implications and has to be considered in analysis of chromatin immunoprecipitation data and the future development of drugs targeting this important set of proteins for therapeutic interventions in breast cancer.

4. DNA METHYLATION AND DEMETHYLATION ENZYMES

The DNA methylation reaction is catalyzed by enzymes which transfer a methyl moiety from the methyl donor S-adenosylmethionine to the $5'$ position in the cytosine ring which is found in mammalian DNA in the context of the di-nucleotide CG. We differentiate between a de novo methylation event that introduces a new methylated site in the genome and maintenance methylation which copies the pattern of methylation of the template parental DNA strand accurately during cell division without adding or removing methylation sites in the genome. Three distinct phylogenic DNA methyltransferases were identified in mammals. DNMT1 shows preference for hemimethylated DNA in vitro, which is consistent with its role as a maintenance DNMT, whereas DNMT3a and DNMT3b methylate unmethylated and methylated DNA at an equal rate which is consistent with a de novo DNMT role *(65)*. Two additional DNMT homologs were found; DNMT2 whose substrate and DNA methylation activity is unclear *(66)* but was shown to methylate tRNA *(67,68)* and DNMT3L which is essential for the establishment of maternal genomic imprints but lacks key methyltransferase motifs, and is possibly a regulator of methylation rather than an enzyme that methylates DNA *(69)*. Knock-out mouse data indicate that DNMT1 is responsible for a majority of DNA methylation marks in the mouse genome *(70)* as well as the human genome *(71)*, whereas DNMT3a and DNMT3b are responsible for some but not all de novo methylation during development *(72)*.

Razin and Riggs proposed that the DNA methylation pattern is accurately inherited during replication since maintenance DNMT could only methylate hemimethylated sites. Hemimethylated sites are generated on the nascent DNA strand during DNA replication when a methylated CG dinucleotide in the template strand is replicated. DNA methylation was therefore proposed to be truly heritable by a semi-conservative mechanism similar to DNA replication *(38)*.

However, although this model of maintenance methylation might apply to a significant portion of the methylated CGs in the genome, it appears that the DNA methylation events, which are prevalent in breast as well as other cancers, require targeting and are not an automatic copying of methylated cytosines from the parental to nascent strand. Targeting is required not only for the initial triggering of a new (de novo) methylation event but also for maintaining the methylated pattern *(28,73)*. Thus, specific methylation event including those prevalent in cancer require active presence of the pathway that led to the methylation event in the first place and is not a hit and run phenomenon which is just selected by the growth advantage conferred by the aberrant methylation. If indeed DNA methylation in breast cancer is a targeted event launched by cancer-specific signaling pathways then it should be possible to reverse this change in methylation by targeting the signaling cascade rather than the global DNA methylation machinery.

Several proteins were shown to recruit DNMTs to target sequences and cause de novo methylation of target genes. It has recently been demonstrated that an additional factor is required for targeting DNMT1 to newly replicating hemimethylated DNA, the protein

UHRF1 (ubiquitin-like, containing PHD and RING finger domains 1), also known as NP95 in mouse and ICBP90 in human (74). Several lines of evidence indicate that DNMTs are targeted to specific sequences by sequence-specific factors, which recognize specific sequences of DNA. For example, the histone methyltransferase EZH2 or the oncoprotein PML-RAR target DNMTs to specific sequences in DNA (28,73). Targeting is emerging as a main principle guiding the way methylation patterns are generated, maintained during cell division, and altered by pathological processes (Fig. 1).

Another important issue for analyzing and treating aberrant DNA methylation in breast cancer is determining the differential role of the DNMT isoforms in the aberrant DNA methylation patterns observed in cancer. The original concept that only DNMT1 is responsible for copying the DNA methylation pattern in dividing cells including cancer cells is only partially true. Other DNMTs are involved and they might have different sequence selectivity. Since it is clear that breast cancer progression and metastasis involves both hypermethylation and silencing of certain genes as well as hypomethylation and activation of others (75) as

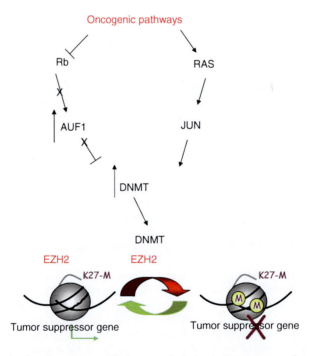

Fig. 1. A mechanism for gene-specific hypermethylation in breast cancer. Oncogenic pathways lead to activation of RAS-MAP kinase signaling pathway which in turn results in transcriptional activation of DNMT1. DNMT1 could also be activated by downregulation of Rb, which commonly occurs in cancer. Under normal conditions, RB upregulates AUF1. AUF1 normally binds the 3' of DNMT1 mRNA and destabilizes it. Downregulation of Rb leads to downregulation of AUF1 and blocks the destabilizing effects on DNMT1 resulting in increased DNMT1. The increased DNMT1 is recruited to EZH2 sites in the genome which are also histone H3K27 methylated triggering gene-specific methylation of tumor suppressor genes such as p16. This results in silencing of tumor suppressor genes and loss of cell cycle control.

will be discussed below, it is important to target the specific isoforms of DNMT responsible for methylation of tumor suppressor genes while avoiding DNMTs which are responsible for methylating and silencing of tumor promoting and prometastatic genes (Fig. 2).

It has been a prevalent dogma in the field that DNA methylation is an irreversible reaction and that demethylation occurs only during gestation but is not a major factor once the DNA methylation pattern of differentiated mature cells is established. It was proposed that if a loss of methylation occurs in somatic cells it happens through a "passive" mechanism whereby new DNA synthesized in the absence of DNMT activity avoids methylation. An active demethylation would not require new DNA synthesis. The possibility that a demethylating activity is present in breast cancer has implications on our understanding of the aberrations in DNA methylation patterns in breast cancer as well as on the design of therapeutic interventions to reverse these aberrations. Most of the literature analyzes the data from the point of view that only DNMTs are involved in defining the DNA methylation pattern in cancer and therefore the main focus of therapy is targeted toward DNMT inhibition. However, if the DNA methylation patterns are an equilibrium of methylation and demethylation as are most

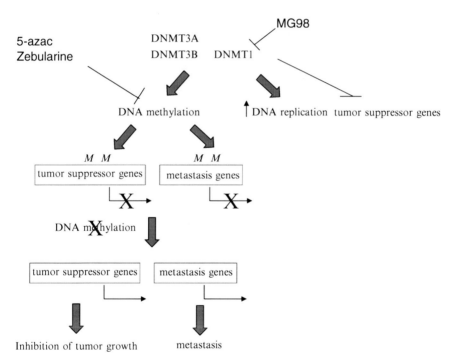

Fig. 2. Multiple effects of DNMT and DNA methylation in breast cancer. DNMTs impact cellular transformation by different mechanisms. DNMTs can lead to gene-specific methylation of both tumor suppressor genes and prometastatic genes. Different isotypes might have different gene selectivity. DNMT1 stimulates DNA replication and inhibits tumor suppressor gene expression by a DNA methylation-independent mechanism. Catalytic inhibitors of DNA methylation would block all DNMTs and cause demethylation of both tumor suppressor genes and metastasis genes. Knock down of DNMT1 will block DNA replication and thus limit passive DNA demethylation but certain tumor suppressor genes will be induced by a methylation-independent mechanism.

biological reactions as proposed here, then looking at only one side of the reaction equilibrium might be misleading and misguiding our conclusions.

The question of whether DNA methylation is a reversible reaction is the most controversial issue in the DNA methylation field. There is a long list of data from both cell culture and early mouse development supporting the hypothesis that active demethylation occurs in embryonal as well as somatic cells. There are now convincing examples of active, replication-independent DNA demethylation during development as well as in somatic differentiated tissues. Active replication-independent demethylation was demonstrated in EBV virus upon stimulation with sodium butyrate *(76)* in the myosin gene in differentiating myoblast cells *(77)*, the *INTERLEUKIN 2* gene upon T cell activation *(78)*, the *INTERFERON* gene upon exposure of memory CD8 T cells to antigens *(79)*, and in the glucocorticoid receptor gene promoter in adult rat brains upon treatment with the HDAC inhibitor TSA *(80)*. More interestingly, recent data suggest that a dynamic DNA methylation pattern is involved in memory in the brain in response to contextual fear conditioning *(81)*. The rapid demethylation–remethylation observed in post-mitotic neurons is perhaps the best evidence for a life-long dynamic and physiologically relevant DNA methylation equilibrium. A recent paper revealed dynamic cyclical DNA methylation–demethylation and transcription of an estrogen responsive promoter of the pS2/TFF gene in human breast cancer cell lines *(82)*.

Since it is becoming clear that the DNA methylation equilibrium in somatic tissues involves both methylation and demethylation, it is critical to identify the enzymatic machinery responsible for demethylation. It is impossible to understand the role of DNA methylation in normal physiology as well as its aberration in pathology by just studying one side of the DNA methylation equilibrium (Fig. 3). Moreover, designing therapeutic strategies to

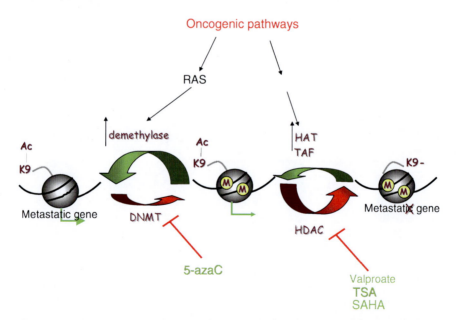

Fig. 3. Induction of demethylase activity and expression of prometastatic genes in breast cancer. Demethylation of prometastatic genes could be induced by either oncogenic signaling pathways or epigenetic drugs such as HDAC inhibitors or DNA methylation inhibitors. HDAC inhibition and increased histone acetylation will also facilitate active demethylation.

Chapter 10 / DNA Methylation in Breast Cancer

manipulate the DNA methylation pattern must take into account both sides of this equilibrium. However, the identity of the enzymes required for DNA demethylation has been extremely controversial and there was a reluctance in the field to accept the notion of enzymatic demethylation. Several candidates were proposed in the last decade but all proposed candidates were hotly contested immediately after publication. Part of the problem is the difficulty encountered in purification of active demethylation activities and the difficulty in developing a consistent cell-free assay of DNA demethylation. Nevertheless, several cell-free assays were published. In 1982, Gjerset and Martin used a cell-free radioactive assay that measured release of radioactive methyl groups from DNA to demonstrate 5-methylcytosine demethylase activity in erythrocytes extracts *(83)*, demethylase activity was shown in nuclear extract from RAS transfected p19 cells using a radioactively labeled methylated CG oligonucleotide *(84)*, A549 human lung cancer cell line *(85)*, prostate cancer cells *(86)*, and normal white matter from brain using the radioactively labeled methylated CG as a substrate *(87)*. Several enzymatic activities were proposed to bring about DNA demethylation. One proposal has been that a G/T mismatch repair glycosylase also functions as a 5-methylcytosine DNA glycosylase, recognizes methyl cytosines, and cleaves the bond between the sugar and the base. The abasic site is then repaired and replaced with a non-methylated cytosine resulting in demethylation *(88)*. An additional protein with a similar activity was recently identified, the methylated DNA binding protein 4 (MBD4) *(89)*.

A different report has proposed that methylated binding protein 2 MBD2 has demethylase activity. MBD2b (a shorter isoform of MBD2) was shown to directly remove the methyl group from methylated cytosine in methylated CpGs *(90)*. This enzyme was therefore proposed to reverse the DNA methylation reaction. However, other groups disputed this finding *(46)*. The MBD2 knock-out mouse was not found to show differences in DNA methylation; however, the assay used looked at the global state of methylation at MboI and HpaII sites in spleen and liver *(91)*. This assay does not measure the details of the DNA methylation pattern at single site resolution. Thus, it is possible that numerous changes in DNA methylation patterns would go undetected, using this assay. A more comprehensive analysis of methylation has not been performed and needs to be done to assess the effects of MBD2 depletion on DNA methylation patterns. However, although global changes in methylation were not altered in MBD2–/–, hypermethylation of several tumor suppressor genes was observed in adenomas that arose in APC Min–/+ Mbd2–/– mice *(92)*. Several follow-up studies have continued to show that MBD2 could trigger DNA demethylation in vitro *(55,60,62)* and in cells *(93)*. Knock down of MBD2 in colorectal, lung, breast, and prostate cancer cells led to inhibition of tumor growth *(94,95)*, tumor invasion, and metastasis as well as silencing and hypermethylation of hypomethylated prometastatic genes *(96,97)* supporting involvement of MBD2 in demethylation, cancer growth, and metastasis.

More recently a protein involved in DNA damage response GADD45A was proposed to trigger active DNA demethylation through a repair-mediated process *(98)*. However, this was contested by a later study *(99)*. Recently the provocative idea that the DNA methyltransferase DNMT3A acts as a demethylase possibly through a mechanism that involves deamination and excision repair of the deaminated base was proposed *(100)*. The main problem with this mechanism is that it introduces a highly mutagenic event such as deamination into the physiological process of DNA demethylation. If indeed a deamination mechanism played a physiological role in maintaining the DNA methylation equilibrium, this would constitute an almost insurmountable challenge to the maintenance of the integrity of the genome.

Understanding the mechanisms responsible for demethylation is one of the most important questions in the field and putative demethylases are candidate drug targets in combating breast cancer as will be discussed below.

5. BILATERAL RELATIONSHIP BETWEEN CHROMATIN AND DNA METHYLATION

The two main components of the epigenome chromatin and DNA methylation are tightly linked. Silencing chromatin modification such as histone hypoacetylation and histone methylation plays an important role in inhibition of expression of critical genes in breast cancer. For example, SNAIL silences *E CADHERIN*, a hallmark of epithelial to mesenchymal transition (EMT), through recruitment of HDACs resulting in histone hypoacetylation *(101)*. The HDAC inhibitor TSA activates *E CADHERIN* as expected from the mechanism of its silencing through hypoacetylation.

Certain genes are silenced by chromatin modification events exclusively but others are silenced by a combination of histone modification and DNA methylation. It was originally believed that DNA hypermethylation precedes and dictates histone modification through recruitment of histone deacetylases and histone methyltransferases by methylated DNA binding proteins *(44)*. It was thus assumed that chromatin-modifying drugs such as HDAC inhibitors would affect only histone acetylation but not the DNA methylation pattern. It was therefore believed that a combination of HDACi TSA and the DNA methylation inhibitor 5-azacytidine (5-azaC) would act synergistically to activate gene expression through 5-azaC inhibition of DNA methylation and TSA inhibition of HDAC activity *(102)*. Indeed clinical trials in several cancers were launched testing a combination of HDAC and DNA methylation inhibitors *(103)*.

However, it emerges that there is a bilateral relationship between chromatin modification and DNA methylation (Fig. 3). Not only does DNA methylation drive chromatin inactivation, chromatin modification defines DNA methylation. For example, genetic defects in chromatin remodeling proteins such as BRG1 in cancer results in aberrations in DNA methylation *(104)*, and mutation in the SWI/SNF protein ATRX results in widespread changes in DNA methylation *(105)*. The histone methyltransferase EZH2 targets tumor suppressor genes for DNA hypermethylation *(29)* and a physical association was shown to exist between HDACs and DNMTs *(106,107)*. More interestingly, HDAC inhibitors were shown to trigger active demethylation *(63,108)* and activation by demethylation of *E CADHERIN* by both histone acetylation and DNA demethylation *(109)*. Similarly, the mood stabilizer and antiepileptic drug valproic acid which was also shown to act as a HDAC inhibitor triggers active DNA demethylation and activation of genes silenced by DNA demethylation *(62,110)*. Most studies to date using HDAC inhibitors either clinically or pre-clinically have not examined the possibility that chromatin-modifying drugs could also trigger DNA methylation changes. This need to be corrected and the possibility that a classic HDAC inhibitor could also cause DNA demethylation should be examined in any clinical or pre-clinical study.

This bilateral relationship between chromatin modification and DNA methylation *(21)* has several important implications for breast cancer therapy. First, activation of signaling pathways that lead to chromatin modification could serve as a conduit for triggering gene-specific changes in DNA methylation. A good example is the role that EZH2 might be playing in targeting tumor suppressor-specific gene methylation *(28)*. Second, the long-term and broad effects that HDAC inhibitors and other chromatin-modifying agents might have on DNA methylation must be considered when assessing possible adverse effects of chromatin-based therapeutics. Third, since HDAC inhibitors trigger active replication-independent DNA demethylation, they might be used to trigger DNA demethylation in slow growing tumors in an S phase independent manner as well as in non-dividing somatic tissues.

6. ABERRATIONS IN DNA METHYLATION IN BREAST CANCER

Aberrations in DNA methylation patterns were documented in cancer in general and breast cancer in particular. These changes are postulated to be responsible in part for the broad changes in gene expression that drive cellular transformation and cancer metastasis. First, there is deregulation of normal cell cycle controlled expression of DNMT1 *(111)*. DNMT1 expression is tightly correlated with the cell cycle such that DNMT1 is expressed only during S phase of the cell cycle *(112–114)*. It was proposed that this regulation protects the genome from aberrant DNA methylation. The regulation of DNMT1 occurs at both transcriptional and post-transcriptional levels. The mitogenic RAS-JUN signaling pathway induces DNMT1 expression through AP1 sites in DNMT1 regulatory regions *(115–117)*. The tumor suppressor Rb represses DNMT1 expression through post-transcriptional mechanisms that affect RNA stability *(118)*. The RNA binding protein AUF1 degrades DNMT1 mRNA through interaction with AUF1 recognition element in the conserved 3′UTR during G0/G1 phase of the cell cycle *(119)*. Deregulated expression of DNMT1 in the wrong phase of the cell cycle results in cellular transformation *(112)*.

Overexpression of DNMT1 is postulated to trigger cellular transformation by both methylation-dependent and -independent mechanisms. DNMT1 is a multifunctional protein that has both catalytic DNMT activity and other functional domains responsible for recruitment of HDACs *(106)* associating with PCNA and the replication fork *(120)*. DNMT1 inhibition results in blocking DNA replication and launching of a DNA damage response by a mechanism independent of DNA methylation *(121–124)*. Thus, an important component of DNMT transforming action does not involve DNA methylation (Fig. 2 for a summary of DNMT and DNA methylation aberrations in breast cancer).

An expected consequence of deregulated DNMT is hypermethylation of a specific set of genes. Our recent data indicate that unscheduled expression of DNMT1 results in aberrant methylation of tumor suppressor genes. Recent data have shown that gain of function of DNMT3B promotes transformation through methylation and silencing of specific genes *(125)*. It is also important to note that although DNMT deregulation can lead to DNA methylation, it does so in a sequence-specific manner. Not all genes are equally methylated. DNMTs are targeted by specific proteins and thus the repertoire of these proteins in a given cell will define the specific targets of deregulated DNMT in the genome. Understanding the precise links between DNMTs and their targets and their relevance to breast cancer progression and metastasis is required for developing tumor-specific DNA methylation inhibitors.

In addition to deregulated expression of methylation enzymes two contradictory aberrations in the DNA methylation pattern are seen in breast cancer cells: hypermethylation of tumor suppressor genes *(126,127)* and hypomethylation of prometastatic genes *(128,129)* as well as global hypomethylation *(130)*. Indeed it is well established that two kinds of changes in the DNA methylation occur in cancer, regional hypermethylation of certain genes *(131)* and global hypomethylation *(130,132)*. This coexistence of both hypermethylation and hypomethylation in the same cancer cell has been confusing especially if one hypothesizes, as has been commonly accepted, that only one enzymatic activity maintenance DNMT is involved. However, if different enzymatic processes are involved in methylation and demethylation and they are guided to different sequences by separate signaling and targeting pathways, then this coexistence could be explained. Understanding the relationship between these two processes methylation and demethylation and the mechanisms involved is critical for both therapy of breast cancer and diagnostics and staging of breast cancer.

7. HYPERMETHYLATION OF GENES IN BREAST CANCER, ROLE IN SILENCING TUMOR SUPPRESSOR GENES

Although it has been known for some time that cancer cell are globally hypomethylated, the phenomenon of regional DNA hypermethylation and silencing of tumor suppressor genes in cancer has been the focus of attention in the last decade. A significant amount of data has established a list of genes hypermethylated in cancer and whole genome approaches have identified methylation signatures of breast cancer cells *(120,133,134)*. These methylation signatures, which are the unique combination of methylated CpG islands in a cancer cell, were correlated with breast cancer stage and have been proposed to be a diagnostic marker of breast cancer cells. In addition to their diagnostic value in breast cancer it is clear from the repertoire of methylated genes that silencing of these genes by DNA methylation plays a role in the transformation process. Among the methylated genes are tumor suppressor genes such as *p16* whose methylation is proposed to silence it, thus overriding normal cell growth regulatory signals controlled by *p16 (135,136)*. *p16* methylation in DNA prepared from plasma of breast cancer patients was associated with nodal metastasis *(137)*. Another group of methylated genes in breast cancer is composed of damage response genes such as BRCA1 *(138,139)*, which is also mutated in familial breast cancer, and mismatch repair genes hMLH1 and HMSH2 *(140)*. Disruption of repair genes might increase sporadic mutations frequency, a hallmark of cancer cells. Steroid receptor genes family members such as the *ESTROGEN RECEPTOR (126)* and *RETINOIC ACID BETA 2 (RARβ2)* receptor are methylated and silenced in a fraction of breast cancers *(16,141)*. Interaction of *RARβ2* receptor with retinoic acid might have an antiproliferative effect and its silencing confers a selective advantage on advanced breast cancer cells. Cell adhesion and cell surface molecules such as *E-CADHERIN (142)* and inhibitors of proteases such as *TIMP-3 (143)* whose silencing might promote metastasis are also found to be methylated in breast cancer. *E CADHERIN* plays an important role in EMT transition, which defines the point at which non-invasive breast cancer cells become invasive and metastatic. A new and interesting group of sequences which emerge to be hypermethylated in breast cancer are microRNA promoters *(144)*, this hypermethylation is an example of a methylation event which might result in gene activation downstream.

A recent study unraveled a hypermethylator, phenotype in a subset of breast cancer cell lines which was characterized by concurrent methylation of several genes *(CDH1, CEACAM6, CST6, ESR1, LCN2, SCNN1A) (145)*. This hypermethylator phenotype was associated with overexpression of DNMT3b. A cluster of primary breast tumors that express the hypermethylation signature, which represents 20% of breast cancers, was identified by mining microarray data. This supports the hypothesis that overexpression of DNMT results in hypermethylation of specific clusters of genes in breast cancer and illustrates the role of specific DNMT isoforms in this process. This has obvious implications on the possible therapeutic potential of isoform-specific DNMT inhibitors as will be discussed below. The involvement of a specific DNMT isotypes also begs the question of the mechanism involved in their activation in breast cancer. Several oncogenic signaling pathways were shown to upregulate DNMT expression through transcriptional activation by RAS *(115,117)* or through post-transcriptional effects resulting from *RB* knockdown *(118,119)*. Identifying breast cancers with specific hypermethylator phenotypes and deciphering the pathways linking the methylation profile with the specific DNNMT isoform responsible will facilitate targeted DNA methylation therapy as well as provide diagnostic markers for more accurate staging of breast cancer.

DNA methyltransferase inhibitors, such as the nucleoside analog 5-aza-deoxy-cytidine (5-aza-CdR) as well as antisense oligonucleotides targeting *DNMT1*, activated methylated genes in cancer supporting the hypothesis that DNA methylation plays a causal role in silencing of these genes in other cancers as well as breast cancer cells. For example, *ESTROGEN RECEPTOR (ER)* in receptor negative breast cancer cells MDA-MB-231 was demethylated and activated by either 5-aza-CdR or 5-aza-cytidine treatment *(146)*, and 5-aza-CdR demethylated and activated the *RARβ2* in receptor-negative breast cancer cells *(147)*. A *DNMT1* antisense oligonucleotide activated *ER* in ER− breast cancer cells although this activation did not involve a change in DNA methylation *(148)*. 5-aza-CdR also induced cell arrest in breast cancer cell lines and it was proposed that this was brought about by demethylation and activation of genes, which suppress tumor growth such as *RARβ2 (149)*.

However, two critical questions remain unresolved. First, although it is clear that a number of tumor suppressor genes are methylated and silenced in cancer, it is still possible that DNA methylation is not the primary event that triggered the silencing of these genes. 5-aza-CdR might be activating the genes by a different mechanism and demethylation might be a consequence rather than the cause of gene activation. Similarly, even if DNA methylation inhibitors such as 5-aza-CdR simultaneously inhibit DNA methylation, DNMT1 activity and also cause cell arrest it is still possible that DNMT1 is involved in cell growth by methylation-independent mechanisms. Understanding the precise function of DNMT1 that is the primary driver of cellular transformation is important for future development of DNMT inhibitors in breast cancer *(150)*. The main issue is that global blockage of DNMT activity as is done today in recent clinical trials in hematological cancers could result in hypomethylation and activation of genes that promote the cancer state. Thus, it is important to target DNMT functions that will not result in global demethylation.

8. THERAPEUTIC IMPLICATION OF HYPERMETHYLATION OF GENES IN BREAST CANCER

Since it is well established that inhibitors of DNA methylation can induce tumor suppressor gene expression, it was proposed that DNA methylation inhibitors might serve as anticancer agents. The induction of *ER (146)* and *RARβ2 (149)* in ER and RARβ2 negative cells by a demethylating agent also raises the prospect of combination therapy of a demethylating agent with either an estrogen antagonists or a retinoid in receptor negative tumors.

Two classes of DNA methyltransferase inhibitors are now in clinical trials. First, the nucleoside analog 5-aza-CdR, which is incorporated into DNA during replication following its phosphorylation to the trinucleotide form and traps the DNA methyltransferase as it moves along with the replication fork. As the replication fork is progressing, nascent DNA is synthesized in the absence of DNA methylation *(151)*. A second inhibitor is an antisense oligonucleotide inhibitor of DNMT1, which knocks down DNMT1 protein levels *(152)*. The two agents have somewhat different effects on DNA replication and DNA methylation reflecting their different mechanisms of action. Knock down of DNMT1 induces some tumor suppressor genes and inhibits DNA replication by a methylation-independent mechanism *(121,123,153)*. This effect on tumor suppressor expression is probably mediated by the protein–protein interactions of DNMT1. Similarly, it has recently been shown that antisense DNMT1 knockdown in ER− breast cancer cells induces ER expression without causing a change in DNA methylation supporting the hypothesis that DNMT1 regulates genes required for the transformed state by methylation-independent mechanisms *(148)*. The inhibition of replication caused by DNMT1 knockdown limits the extent of DNA methylation inhibition since nascent unmethylated DNA is not synthesized in the absence of DNMT1 *(123)*. These data point out to the possibility of targeting DNMT and its cell growth and gene regulatory functions without causing global demethylation *(150)* using a knock-down approach with either siRNA or antisense.

Several clinical trial have been launched with a nucleoside-analog pan DNMT inhibitor 5-azacytidine 5-azaC (DAC) and its deoxy analog 5-deoxycytidine in hematological cancers. Responses with tolerable adverse effects were reported in clinical trials in hematological malignancies especially in myelodysplastic syndrome (MDS) *(154)*. However, originally there was no significant success reported in solid tumors *(155)*. The weak response of solid tumors might result from pharmacokinetic issues such as delivery problems as well as dosing and scheduling. Different strategies for combining of 5-azaC and other chemotherapeutic agents or chromatin modifiers such as histone deacetylase inhibitors (HDACi) are now being tested and might be effective in solid tumors *(156)*. A recent proof of principle study in breast cancer that used a different DNMT inhibitor hydralazine in combination with the HDAC inhibitor valproic acid was somewhat promising *(19)*. It remains to be seen however whether the use of pan catalytic inhibitors of DNMT might be of utility in breast cancer or whether the lack of clinical effect observed in other solid tumors in the past reflects the adverse effects of global inhibition of DNA methylation and therefore more selective drugs need to be tested.

The main challenge here is to identify the specific isoform of DNMT responsible for silencing by hypermethylation of breast cancer targets but is not involved in methylation of prometastatic genes (Fig. 2). Alternatively, we might limit the global demethylation events and induction of prometastatic genes by knocking down DNMT1 rather than inhibiting its catalytic activity. We have recently shown that it might be possible to suppress cellular transformation by complete knock down of DNMT rather than inhibiting its catalytic activity.

9. HYPOMETHYLATION IN BREAST CANCER AND ITS THERAPEUTIC IMPLICATIONS

Although it was known for decades that the DNA of cancer cells is hypomethylated in comparison with normal DNA, the significance of this observation was not appreciated up to recent years. Several studies have now indicated that hypomethylation is widespread in cancers. Several genes heavily involved in metastasis were shown to be hypomethylated in breast cancer *(128,165–167)* although the full implication of hypomethylation on diagnosis and staging of breast cancer is not fully appreciated. Mapping the hypomethylation profile of breast tumors might reveal patterns, which could aid in staging of breast cancers and provide diagnostic tools as well as guide us to the possible mechanisms leading to hypomethylation and from hypomethylation to aggressive cancers.

It is well documented that DNA from breast cancer as well as other cancers is globally hypomethylated *(157,158)*. The extent of global hypomethylation was found in one study, which measured in vitro methylation of genomic DNA by a CG methylase as an indicator of genomic hypomethylation, to be correlated with the histological grade and malignancy *(157)*. An earlier study using methylation-sensitive restriction enzymes found global hypomethylation to characterize breast cancers but no clear correlation was found with clinical stage *(158)*. This difference might reflect the difference in sensitivity of the two assays. Repetitive sequences *(159)* and satellite DNA sequences *(130)* are hypomethylated in breast cancer. Different members of the melanoma associated cancer/testis antigens *MAGE*, which were shown to be methylated and silenced in adult tissues and hypomethylated in multiple tumors were also expressed in breast cancer cells *(160–163)*. Their expression was shown to be associated with a poorly differentiated stage in invasive ductal breast cancers *(164)*.

Chapter 10 / DNA Methylation in Breast Cancer

Unique genes such as *uPA (128,165)* and *Breast Cancer Specific Gene 1-SYNUCLEIN* γ *(166,167)* were also shown to be hypomethylated in breast cancer.

This data point out to the possibility that there is a general defect in the DNA methylation machinery in cancer cells that results in global hypomethylation. There is no reduction of DNA methyltransferase activity in cancer cells *(168)*, on the contrary upregulation of expression of DNA methyltransferase in cancers during G1 phase of the cell cycle was reported in ER− breast cancer cells *(111)*. We therefore proposed that global demethylation in cancer might be caused by an excess of demethylation activity *(150)*. We have recently shown that MBD2, that we had earlier proposed to be involved in demethylation, triggers demethylation of uPA in breast cancer cells and *uPA* and *MMP2* in prostate cancer cells *(97,129)*.

We proposed that the hypomethylation and hypermethylation observed in the same cancer cell target different components of the cancer progression program. Whereas silencing of tumor suppressor genes by hypermethylation is mainly involved in tumor growth, activation of other genes by hypomethylation seems to be targeting cancer invasiveness and metastatic potential. Indeed these two critical processes in cancer growth and invasiveness could be dissociated. Highly invasive human breast cancer cells MDA-MB-231 cells expressing ectopic RAS exhibit increased growth rate but reduced metastatic potential *(169)*.

This obviously leaves open the question of how could tumor suppressors be hypermethylated in cancer cells in an environment that is markedly hypomethylated. Recent data suggest that inactivation of the chromatin structure at the tumor suppressor *p16* gene comes about even in a colorectal cancer cell line bearing a homozygous knock out of three DNMTs DNMT 1, 3A and 3B *(170)*, suggesting that inactivation of chromatin is the primary event in silencing of *p16*. The inactivated p16 is slowly hypermethylated after chromatin structure inactivation *(170)* by residual DNMT activity suggesting that regional hypermethylation is a consequence of chromatin inactivation. Although it is yet unknown which factor recruits repressor complexes to *p16* promoter and how this leads to DNA methylation, an oncogenic transcriptional repressor such as the leukemia-promoting PML–RAR fusion protein was shown to recruit histone deacetylases HDACs and DNA methyltransferases to target promoters *(73)*. Recent data suggest that an important mechanism targeting DNMT to tumor suppressor genes is occupancy with the polycomb protein the histone methyltransferase EZH2 and H3K27me *(28)*. It is also possible that localized chromatin inactivation blocks access to demethylases and that regional chromatin structure inactivation is responsible for maintenance of regional hypermethylation even when high levels of demethylase are present in the cell. In accordance with this hypothesis, it has been shown that the InHAT complex which inhibits histone acetyltransferases can block active demethylation of ectopically methylated DNA *(108)*, thus any local change in chromatin structure such as histone deacetylation could result in local inhibition of demethylase activity. Thus, regional hypermethylation is directed by a different enzymatic process than global demethylation and could therefore coexist with global hypomethylation. An important challenge in the field is to fully understand the coordination of methylation and demethylation events during breast cancer progression, the enzymes and targeting molecules involved, the signaling pathways that regulate them, and their differential role in the different stages of breast cancer.

What are the therapeutic implications of the hypomethylation in breast cancer? The first implication is that globally inhibiting DNA methylation, although effective in activating tumor suppressor genes, could result in unleashing of genes that could drive cancer metastasis the most fatal and morbid facet of breast cancer. Thus, extreme caution should be applied before using pan inhibitors of DNA methylation such as 5-azaC in cancer therapy. Indeed we have recently shown that 5-aza C treatment of the non-invasive human breast cancer cell line MCF7 resulted in demethylation and activation of a series of prometastatic genes *(171)*.

Although the treatment inhibited growth significantly it also induced metastatic potential at the same time. Thus, it is possible to accomplish inhibition of tumor growth, which as anticipated by the classic mechanism of action of 5-azaC and at the same time plant the seeds for cancer metastasis. This should raise a red flag in evaluating current clinical trials, the immediate effects of inhibition of tumor growth might be misleading.

It is therefore imperative upon us to follow with extreme caution any therapy that involves inhibition of DNA methylation. An additional implication is that we need to develop specific DNMT inhibitors, which eliminate the growth promoting functions of DNMT without causing global demethylation and without unleashing prometastatic genes. One approach is to accurately map the hypermethylated genes at different stages of breast cancer and identify the specific DNMT isotypes responsible for their methylation. By developing isotypic-specific DNMT inhibitors and identifying isotypes that target tumor suppressor genes but not prometastatic genes it might be possible to eliminate or at least reduce the adverse demethylation events. An alternative approach would be to target the proteins that recruit DNMTs to specific tumor suppressor genes. It remains to be seen however whether it would be possible to dissociate the events leading to methylation of prometastatic genes and tumor suppressor genes. Another interesting possibility as discussed above is to target the DNA methylation-independent functions of DNMT1 and to limit global hypomethylation by knocking down the entire protein using either antisense or siRNA approaches. We have developed antisense inhibitors of *DNMT1* and showed that they cause immediate growth suppression events without causing DNA demethylation and aberrant gene activation *(121,123,124)*. MG98 a first generation DNMT1 antisense oligonucleotide was tested in phase II clinical trials *(172,173)*. Although the trials were stopped owing to lack of response in the group of patients, this approach deserves further study with altered dosing and scheduling. Although clinical use of siRNA has not been yet reported, this might be a reality in the future. Developing small molecules that target the interactions of DNMT1 with the replication fork or with PCNA rather than targeting its methylation activity might serve as an alternative approach to the current attempt to identify catalytic inhibitors of DNMT1.

The apparent role of hypomethylation in metastasis of breast and other cancers points toward a new and different DNA methylation target in breast cancer, inhibition of demethylation (Fig. 4). We have tested two approaches to inhibit DNA demethylation and to silence prometastatic genes in human breast cancer cell lines. First, as discussed above, MBD2 was found to be required for the activation of several prometastatic genes in breast cancer *(129)*. We therefore developed antisense inhibitors of MBD2 and showed that they were effective in blocking the growth of human colorectal and non-small lung cancer cells tumor cell lines implanted as xenograft growth in mice in vivo *(94,174)* as well as in blocking cell invasion and metastasis in vitro and in vivo *(129)*. Interestingly, this treatment did not result in silencing of any of the known tumor suppressor genes. Indeed, it was previously shown that MBD2 suppresses the expression of *p16* and *GSTP1* through its alternative function, recruitment of HDACs to methylated genes. Therefore, it is possible that by hitting MBD2 we will eliminate the two classes of gene expression aberrations in breast cancer, silencing of tumor suppressor genes, and activation of prometastatic genes. MBD2 is therefore an ideal candidate for intervention in breast cancer (Fig. 4).

An alternative option for inhibiting DNA demethylation in metastatic breast cancer is to treat with either SAM or an analog of SAM. SAM is the methyl donor of the DNA methylation reaction. We have previously shown that SAM inhibits active demethylation of uPA *(129)* and MMP2 *(97)* and reverses the metastatic state of breast cancer cells *(129)*. It is unclear whether SAM would be stable enough as an effective therapeutic in vivo. Analogs of SAM that inhibit demethylation might be needed to reach a therapeutic effect. Another

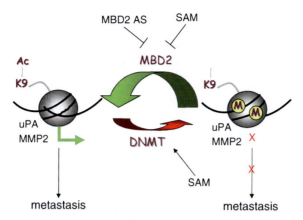

Fig. 4. Inhibition of demethylation as a potential therapy for breast cancer. In metastatic breast cancer multiple prometastatic genes (such as MMP2 and uPA) are demethylated and active. By inhibiting demethylase activity it might be possible to block demethylation and reverse the demethylated state. MBD2 AS, an antisense oligonucleotide inhibitor targeting MBD2; SAM, the methyl donor SAM.

important consideration is the possibility that diet enriched with folates or/and vitamin B12, which enhance methyl content, might protect from cancer metastasis and that SAM or its active analog might be used as a prophylactic in breast cancer (Fig. 4).

10. CONCLUSIONS AND PROSPECTIVE

Changes in DNA methylation are well established in breast cancer as well as their role in cancer growth progression and metastasis. However, it is becoming clear that the simplistic but nevertheless dominant idea that methylation in breast cancer is mainly a hypermethylation event which could be reversed using catalytic DNA methylation inhibitors needs to be revisited.

We now start understanding the multifaceted involvement of the DNA methylation machinery in breast cancer. Not only are DNMT involved but also demethylases- and chromatin-modifying enzymes and there is a strong interrelationship between these different components. We understand that loss of methylation is a critical process leading to activation of prometastatic genes and that it might be a target for therapy as much as or even more so than hypermethylation. The seemingly contradictory appearance of both hypermethylation and hypomethylation prove to be less paradoxical once the complex machinery involved in defining DNA methylation patterns and the concept of gene-specific targeting are taken into account. Just the global levels of methylating and demethylating enzymes do not define the DNA methylation pattern but these enzymes need to be targeted to specific positions in the genome by complexes which contain sequence recognition factors. Thus, by differential targeting of these enzymes both methylation and demethylation events could concurrently occur. It is also important to note that DNMTs and perhaps demethylases could have multiple actions in promoting tumorigenesis and that they might act through selective protein–protein interactions by a mechanism independent of DNA methylation. All these factors have to be taken into account in devising therapeutic strategies that involve the DNA methylation machinery (Fig. 2).

Further studies need to accurately delineate the specific involvement of the different components of the DNA methylation machinery in breast cancer and at different stages of the disease. It is important to correlate these changes in methylation machinery with specific alterations in DNA methylation profiles. This would enable to use isoform-specific inhibitors to target stage-specific methylation aberrations. Delineating the specific methylation profiles and gene expression patterns associated with them and correlating them with specific physiological and pathological outcomes will enhance our understanding of the molecular pathophysiology of breast cancer, provide important predictive markers, and guide the targeting of stage-specific epigenetic therapies.

Acknowledgments: The studies from MS laboratory discussed here were funded by a grant from the Canadian Institute of Health Research and the National Cancer Institute of Canada.

REFERENCES

1. Finch JT, Lutter LC, Rhodes D, Brown RS, Rushton B, et al. 1977. Structure of nucleosome core particles of chromatin. *Nature* 269: 29–36
2. Jenuwein T. 2001. Re-SET-ting heterochromatin by histone methyltransferases. *Trends Cell Biol* 11: 266–73.
3. Wade PA, Pruss D, Wolffe AP. 1997. Histone acetylation: chromatin in action. *Trends Biochem Sci* 22: 128–32.
4. Shiio Y, Eisenman RN. 2003. Histone sumoylation is associated with transcriptional repression. *Proc Natl Acad Sci U S A* 100: 13225–30
5. Shilatifard A. 2006. Chromatin Modifications by Methylation and Ubiquitination: Implications in the Regulation of Gene Expression. Annu Rev Biochem
6. Henikoff S, McKittrick E, Ahmad K. 2004. Epigenetics, histone H3 variants, and the inheritance of chromatin states. *Cold Spring Harb Symp Quant Biol* 69: 235–43
7. Szyf M, Weaver IC, Champagne FA, Diorio J, Meaney MJ. 2005. Maternal programming of steroid receptor expression and phenotype through DNA methylation in the rat. *Front Neuroendocrinol* 26: 139–62
8. Kuo MH, Allis CD. 1998. Roles of histone acetyltransferases and deacetylases in gene regulation. *Bioessays* 20: 615–26.
9. Lund AH, van Lohuizen M. 2004. Epigenetics and cancer. *Genes Dev* 18: 2315–35
10. Perry M, Chalkley R. 1982. Histone acetylation increases the solubility of chromatin and occurs sequentially over most of the chromatin. A novel model for the biological role of histone acetylation. *J Biol Chem* 257: 7336–47.
11. Lee DY, Hayes JJ, Pruss D, Wolffe AP. 1993. A positive role for histone acetylation in transcription factor access to nucleosomal DNA. *Cell* 72: 73–84
12. Sinha I, Wiren M, Ekwall K. 2006. Genome-wide patterns of histone modifications in fission yeast. *Chromosome Res* 14: 95–105
13. Roh TY, Wei G, Farrell CM, Zhao K. 2007. Genome-wide prediction of conserved and nonconserved enhancers by histone acetylation patterns. *Genome Res* 17: 74–81
14. Roh TY, Zhao K. 2008. High-resolution, genome-wide mapping of chromatin modifications by GMAT. *Methods Mol Biol* 387: 95–108
15. Fujita N, Jaye DL, Kajita M, Geigerman C, Moreno CS, Wade PA. 2003. MTA3, a Mi-2/NuRD complex subunit, regulates an invasive growth pathway in breast cancer. *Cell* 113: 207–19
16. Sirchia SM, Ferguson AT, Sironi E, Subramanyan S, Orlandi R, et al. 2000. Evidence of epigenetic changes affecting the chromatin state of the retinoic acid receptor beta2 promoter in breast cancer cells. *Oncogene* 19: 1556–63

Chapter 10 / DNA Methylation in Breast Cancer

17. Zhou Q, Atadja P, Davidson NE. 2007. Histone deacetylase inhibitor LBH589 reactivates silenced estrogen receptor alpha (ER) gene expression without loss of DNA hypermethylation. *Cancer Biol Ther* 6: 64–9

18. Zhou Q, Agoston AT, Atadja P, Nelson WG, Davidson NE. 2008. Inhibition of histone deacetylases promotes ubiquitin-dependent proteasomal degradation of DNA methyltransferase 1 in human breast cancer cells. *Mol Cancer Res* 6: 873–83

19. Arce C, Perez-Plasencia C, Gonzalez-Fierro A, de la Cruz-Hernandez E, Revilla-Vazquez A, et al. 2006. A proof-of-principle study of epigenetic therapy added to neoadjuvant doxorubicin cyclophosphamide for locally advanced breast cancer. *PLoS ONE* 1: e98

20. Yang X, Phillips DL, Ferguson AT, Nelson WG, Herman JG, Davidson NE. 2001. Synergistic activation of functional estrogen receptor (ER)-alpha by DNA methyltransferase and histone deacetylase inhibition in human ER- alpha-negative breast cancer cells. *Cancer Res* 61: 7025–9.

21. D'Alessio AC, Szyf M. 2006. Epigenetic tête-à-tête: the bilateral relationship between chromatin modifications and DNA methylation. *Biochem Cell Biol* 84: 463–76

22. Duvic M, Vu J. 2007. Vorinostat in cutaneous T-cell lymphoma. *Drugs Today (Barc)* 43: 585–99

23. Miao F, Natarajan R. 2005. Mapping global histone methylation patterns in the coding regions of human genes. *Mol Cell Biol* 25: 4650–61

24. Wiencke JK, Zheng S, Morrison Z, Yeh RF. 2008. Differentially expressed genes are marked by histone 3 lysine 9 trimethylation in human cancer cells. *Oncogene* 27: 2412–21

25. Santos-Rosa H, Schneider R, Bannister AJ, Sherriff J, Bernstein BE, et al. 2002. Active genes are tri-methylated at K4 of histone H3. *Nature* 419: 407–11

26. Cao R, Wang L, Wang H, Xia L, Erdjument-Bromage H, et al. 2002. Role of histone H3 lysine 27 methylation in Polycomb-group silencing. *Science* 298: 1039–43

27. Cao R, Zhang Y. 2004. SUZ12 is required for both the histone methyltransferase activity and the silencing function of the EED-EZH2 complex. *Mol Cell* 15: 57–67

28. Vire E, Brenner C, Deplus R, Blanchon L, Fraga M, et al. 2006. The Polycomb group protein EZH2 directly controls DNA methylation. *Nature* 439: 871–4

29. Schlesinger Y, Straussman R, Keshet I, Farkash S, Hecht M, et al. 2007. Polycomb-mediated methylation on Lys27 of histone H3 pre-marks genes for de novo methylation in cancer. *Nat Genet* 39: 232–6

30. Shi B, Liang J, Yang X, Wang Y, Zhao Y, et al. 2007. Integration of estrogen and Wnt signaling circuits by the polycomb group protein EZH2 in breast cancer cells. *Mol Cell Biol* 27: 5105–19

31. Raaphorst FM, Meijer CJ, Fieret E, Blokzijl T, Mommers E, et al. 2003. Poorly differentiated breast carcinoma is associated with increased expression of the human polycomb group EZH2 gene. *Neoplasia* 5: 481–8

32. Kleer CG, Cao Q, Varambally S, Shen R, Ota I, et al. 2003. EZH2 is a marker of aggressive breast cancer and promotes neoplastic transformation of breast epithelial cells. *Proc Natl Acad Sci U S A* 100: 11606–11

33. Spangenberg C, Eisfeld K, Stunkel W, Luger K, Flaus A, et al. 1998. The mouse mammary tumour virus promoter positioned on a tetramer of histones H3 and H4 binds nuclear factor 1 and OTF1. *J Mol Biol* 278: 725–39

34. Pazin MJ, Bhargava P, Geiduschek EP, Kadonaga JT. 1997. Nucleosome mobility and the maintenance of nucleosome positioning. *Science* 276: 809–12

35. Muchardt C, Yaniv M. 1999. ATP-dependent chromatin remodelling: SWI/SNF and Co. are on the job. *J Mol Biol* 293: 187–98

36. Xue Y, Wong J, Moreno GT, Young MK, Cote J, Wang W. 1998. NURD, a novel complex with both ATP-dependent chromatin-remodeling and histone deacetylase activities. *Mol Cell* 2: 851–61

37. Manavathi B, Singh K, Kumar R. 2007. MTA family of coregulators in nuclear receptor biology and pathology. *Nucl Recept Signal* 5: e010

38. Razin A, Riggs AD. 1980. DNA methylation and gene function. *Science* 210: 604–10

39. Swain JL, Stewart TA, Leder P. 1987. Parental legacy determines methylation and expression of an autosomal transgene: a molecular mechanism for parental imprinting. *Cell* 50: 719–27

40. Mohandas T, Sparkes RS, Shapiro LJ. 1981. Reactivation of an inactive human X chromosome: evidence for X inactivation by DNA methylation. *Science* 211: 393–6

41. Razin A, Cedar H. 1977. Distribution of 5-methylcytosine in chromatin. *Proc Natl Acad Sci U S A* 74: 2725–8

42. Comb M, Goodman HM. 1990. CpG methylation inhibits proenkephalin gene expression and binding of the transcription factor AP-2. *Nucleic Acids Res* 18: 3975–82

43. Inamdar NM, Ehrlich KC, Ehrlich M. 1991. CpG methylation inhibits binding of several sequence-specific DNA- binding proteins from pea, wheat, soybean and cauliflower. *Plant Mol Biol* 17: 111–23

44. Nan X, Campoy FJ, Bird A. 1997. MeCP2 is a transcriptional repressor with abundant binding sites in genomic chromatin. *Cell* 88: 471–81

45. Hendrich B, Bird A. 1998. Identification and characterization of a family of mammalian methyl-CpG binding proteins. *Mol Cell Biol* 18: 6538–47

46. Ng HH, Zhang Y, Hendrich B, Johnson CA, Turner BM, et al. 1999. MBD2 is a transcriptional repressor belonging to the MeCP1 histone deacetylase complex [see comments]. *Nat Genet* 23: 58–61

47. Fujita N, Takebayashi S, Okumura K, Kudo S, Chiba T, et al. 1999. Methylation-mediated transcriptional silencing in euchromatin by methyl- CpG binding protein MBD1 isoforms. *Mol Cell Biol* 19: 6415–26

48. Zhang Y, Ng HH, Erdjument-Bromage H, Tempst P, Bird A, Reinberg D. 1999. Analysis of the NuRD subunits reveals a histone deacetylase core complex and a connection with DNA methylation. *Genes Dev* 13: 1924–35

49. Zilberman D, Gehring M, Tran RK, Ballinger T, Henikoff S. 2007. Genome-wide analysis of Arabidopsis thaliana DNA methylation uncovers an interdependence between methylation and transcription. *Nat Genet* 39: 61–9

50. Li B, Gogol M, Carey M, Pattenden SG, Seidel C, Workman JL. 2007. Infrequently transcribed long genes depend on the Set2/Rpd3S pathway for accurate transcription. *Genes Dev* 21: 1422–30

51. Vakoc CR, Mandat SA, Olenchock BA, Blobel GA. 2005. Histone H3 lysine 9 methylation and HP1gamma are associated with transcription elongation through mammalian chromatin. *Mol Cell* 19: 381–91

52. Ego T, Tanaka Y, Shimotohno K. 2005. Interaction of HTLV-1 Tax and methyl-CpG-binding domain 2 positively regulates the gene expression from the hypermethylated LTR. *Oncogene* 24: 1914–23

53. Lembo F, Pero R, Angrisano T, Vitiello C, Iuliano R, et al. 2003. MBDin, a novel MBD2-interacting protein, relieves MBD2 repression potential and reactivates transcription from methylated promoters. *Mol Cell Biol* 23: 1656–65

54. Fujita H, Fujii R, Aratani S, Amano T, Fukamizu A, Nakajima T. 2003. Antithetic effects of MBD2a on gene regulation. *Mol Cell Biol* 23: 2645–57

55. Detich N, Theberge J, Szyf M. 2002. Promoter-specific activation and demethylation by MBD2/demethylase. *J Biol Chem* 277: 35791–4

56. Brown SE, Szyf M. 2008. Dynamic epigenetic states of ribosomal RNA promoters during the cell cycle. *Cell Cycle* 7: 382–90

57. Brown SE, Szyf M. 2007. Epigenetic programming of the rRNA promoter by MBD3. *Mol Cell Biol* 27: 4938–52

58. Yasui DH, Peddada S, Bieda MC, Vallero RO, Hogart A, et al. 2007. Integrated epigenomic analyses of neuronal MeCP2 reveal a role for long-range interaction with active genes. *Proc Natl Acad Sci U S A* 104: 19416–21

59. Hendrich B, Hardeland U, Ng HH, Jiricny J, Bird A. 1999. The thymine glycosylase MBD4 can bind to the product of deamination at methylated CpG sites. *Nature* 401: 301–4.

60. Hamm S, Just G, Lacoste N, Moitessier N, Szyf M, Mamer O. 2008. On the mechanism of demethylation of 5-methylcytosine in DNA. *Bioorg Med Chem Lett* 18: 1046–9

61. Detich N, Hamm S, Just G, Knox JD, Szyf M. 2003. The Methyl Donor S-Adenosylmethionine Inhibits Active Demethylation of DNA: A CANDIDATE NOVEL MECHANISM FOR THE PHARMACOLOGICAL EFFECTS OF S-ADENOSYLMETHIONINE. *J Biol Chem* 278: 20812–20

Chapter 10 / DNA Methylation in Breast Cancer

62. Detich N, Bovenzi V, Szyf M. 2003. Valproate induces replication-independent active DNA demethylation. *J Biol Chem* 278: 27586–92
63. Cervoni N, Szyf M. 2001. Demethylase activity is directed by histone acetylation. *J Biol Chem* 276: 40778–87.
64. Bhattacharya SK, Ramchandani S, Cervoni N, Szyf M. 1999. A mammalian protein with specific demethylase activity for mCpG DNA. *Nature* 397: 579–83
65. Okano M, Xie S, Li E. 1998. Cloning and characterization of a family of novel mammalian DNA (cytosine-5) methyltransferases [letter]. *Nat Genet* 19: 219–20
66. Vilain A, Apiou F, Dutrillaux B, Malfoy B. 1998. Assignment of candidate DNA methyltransferase gene (DNMT2) to human chromosome band 10p15.1 by in situ hybridization. *Cytogenet Cell Genet* 82: 120
67. Rai K, Chidester S, Zavala CV, Manos EJ, James SR, et al. 2007. Dnmt2 functions in the cytoplasm to promote liver, brain, and retina development in zebrafish. *Genes Dev* 21: 261–6
68. Goll MG, Kirpekar F, Maggert KA, Yoder JA, Hsieh CL, et al. 2006. Methylation of tRNAAsp by the DNA methyltransferase homolog Dnmt2. *Science* 311: 395–8
69. Bourc'his D, Xu GL, Lin CS, Bollman B, Bestor TH. 2001. Dnmt3L and the establishment of maternal genomic imprints. *Science* 294: 2536–9
70. Li E, Bestor TH, Jaenisch R. 1992. Targeted mutation of the DNA methyltransferase gene results in embryonic lethality. *Cell* 69: 915–26
71. Chen T, Hevi S, Gay F, Tsujimoto N, He T, et al. 2007. Complete inactivation of DNMT1 leads to mitotic catastrophe in human cancer cells. Nat Genet
72. Okano M, Bell DW, Haber DA, Li E. 1999. DNA methyltransferases Dnmt3a and Dnmt3b are essential for de novo methylation and mammalian development. *Cell* 99: 247–57
73. Di Croce L, Raker VA, Corsaro M, Fazi F, Fanelli M, et al. 2002. Methyltransferase recruitment and DNA hypermethylation of target promoters by an oncogenic transcription factor. *Science* 295: 1079–82.
74. Bostick M, Kim JK, Esteve PO, Clark A, Pradhan S, Jacobsen SE. 2007. UHRF1 Plays a Role in Maintaining DNA Methylation in Mammalian Cells. *Science* 317: 1760–4
75. Szyf M, Pakneshan P, Rabbani SA. 2004. DNA demethylation and cancer: therapeutic implications. *Cancer Lett* 211: 133–43
76. Szyf M, Eliasson L, Mann V, Klein G, Razin A. 1985. Cellular and viral DNA hypomethylation associated with induction of Epstein-Barr virus lytic cycle. *Proc Natl Acad Sci U S A* 82: 8090–4
77. Lucarelli M, Fuso A, Strom R, Scarpa S. 2001. The dynamics of myogenin site-specific demethylation is strongly correlated with its expression and with muscle differentiation. *J Biol Chem* 276: 7500–6.
78. Bruniquel D, Schwartz RH. 2003. Selective, stable demethylation of the interleukin-2 gene enhances transcription by an active process. *Nat Immunol* 4: 235–40
79. Kersh EN, Fitzpatrick DR, Murali-Krishna K, Shires J, Speck SH, et al. 2006. Rapid Demethylation of the IFN-{gamma} Gene Occurs in Memory but Not Naive CD8 T Cells. *J Immunol* 176: 4083–93
80. Weaver IC, Cervoni N, Champagne FA, D'Alessio AC, Sharma S, et al. 2004. Epigenetic programming by maternal behavior. *Nat Neurosci* 7: 847–54
81. Miller CA, Sweatt JD. 2007. Covalent modification of DNA regulates memory formation. *Neuron* 53: 857–69
82. Metivier R, Gallais R, Tiffoche C, Le Peron C, Jurkowska RZ, et al. 2008. Cyclical DNA methylation of a transcriptionally active promoter. *Nature* 452: 45–50
83. Gjerset RA, Martin DW, Jr. 1982. Presence of a DNA demethylating activity in the nucleus of murine erythroleukemic cells. *J Biol Chem* 257: 8581–3
84. Szyf M, Theberge J, Bozovic V. 1995. Ras induces a general DNA demethylation activity in mouse embryonal P19 cells. *J Biol Chem* 270: 12690–6
85. Ramchandani S, Bhattacharya SK, Cervoni N, Szyf M. 1999. DNA methylation is a reversible biological signal. *Proc Natl Acad Sci U S A* 96: 6107–12
86. Patra SK, Patra A, Zhao H, Dahiya R. 2002. DNA methyltransferase and demethylase in human prostate cancer. *Mol Carcinog* 33: 163–71

87. Mastronardi FG, Noor A, Wood DD, Paton T, Moscarello MA. 2007. Peptidyl argininedeiminase 2 CpG island in multiple sclerosis white matter is hypomethylated. *J Neurosci Res* 85: 2006–16

88. Jost JP. 1993. Nuclear extracts of chicken embryos promote an active demethylation of DNA by excision repair of 5-methyldeoxycytidine. *Proc Natl Acad Sci U S A* 90: 4684–8

89. Zhu B, Zheng Y, Hess D, Angliker H, Schwarz S, et al. 2000. 5-methylcytosine-DNA glycosylase activity is present in a cloned G/T mismatch DNA glycosylase associated with the chicken embryo DNA demethylation complex. *Proc Natl Acad Sci U S A* 97: 5135–9

90. Bhattacharya SK, Ramchandani S, Cervoni N, Szyf M. 1999. A mammalian protein with specific demethylase activity for mCpG DNA [see comments]. *Nature* 397: 579–83

91. Hendrich B, Guy J, Ramsahoye B, Wilson VA, Bird A. 2001. Closely related proteins MBD2 and MBD3 play distinctive but interacting roles in mouse development. *Genes Dev* 15: 710–23.

92. Sansom OJ, Berger J, Bishop SM, Hendrich B, Bird A, Clarke AR. 2003. Deficiency of Mbd2 suppresses intestinal tumorigenesis. *Nat Genet* 34: 145–7

93. Goel A, Mathupala SP, Pedersen PL. 2003. Glucose Metabolism in Cancer. EVIDENCE THAT DEMETHYLATION EVENTS PLAY A ROLE IN ACTIVATING TYPE II HEXOKINASE GENE EXPRESSION. *J Biol Chem* 278: 15333–40

94. Slack A, Bovenzi V, Bigey P, Ivanov MA, Ramchandani S, et al. 2002. Antisense MBD2 gene therapy inhibits tumorigenesis. *J Gene Med* 4: 381–9

95. Campbell PM, Bovenzi V, Szyf M. 2003. Methylated DNA binding protein 2 antisense inhibitors suppress tumorigenesis of human cancer lines in vitro and in vivo. *Carcinogenesis*

96. Pakneshan P, Szyf M, Rabbani SA. 2004. Methylation and inhibition of uPA expression by RAS oncogene: divergence of growth control and invasion in breast cancer cells. *Carcinogenesis*

97. Shukeir N, Pakneshan P, Chen G, Szyf M, Rabbani SA. 2006. Alteration of the Methylation Status of Tumor-Promoting Genes Decreases Prostate Cancer Cell Invasiveness and Tumorigenesis In vitro and In vivo. *Cancer Res* 66: 9202–10

98. Barreto G, Schafer A, Marhold J, Stach D, Swaminathan SK, et al. 2007. Gadd45a promotes epigenetic gene activation by repair-mediated DNA demethylation. Nature

99. Jin SG, Guo C, Pfeifer GP. 2008. GADD45A does not promote DNA demethylation. *PLoS Genet* 4: e1000013

100. Kangaspeska S, Stride B, Metivier R, Polycarpou-Schwarz M, Ibberson D, et al. 2008. Transient cyclical methylation of promoter DNA. *Nature* 452: 112–5

101. Peinado H, Ballestar E, Esteller M, Cano A. 2004. Snail mediates E-cadherin repression by the recruitment of the Sin3A/histone deacetylase 1 (HDAC1)/HDAC2 complex. *Mol Cell Biol* 24: 306–19

102. Cameron EE, Bachman KE, Myohanen S, Herman JG, Baylin SB. 1999. Synergy of demethylation and histone deacetylase inhibition in the re- expression of genes silenced in cancer. *Nat Genet* 21: 103–7

103. Kuendgen A, Lubbert M. 2008. Current status of epigenetic treatment in myelodysplastic syndromes. Ann Hematol

104. Banine F, Bartlett C, Gunawardena R, Muchardt C, Yaniv M, et al. 2005. SWI/SNF chromatin-remodeling factors induce changes in DNA methylation to promote transcriptional activation. *Cancer Res* 65: 3542–7

105. Gibbons RJ, McDowell TL, Raman S, O'Rourke DM, Garrick D, et al. 2000. Mutations in ATRX, encoding a SWI/SNF-like protein, cause diverse changes in the pattern of DNA methylation. *Nat Genet* 24: 368–71

106. Fuks F, Burgers WA, Brehm A, Hughes-Davies L, Kouzarides T. 2000. DNA methyltransferase Dnmt1 associates with histone deacetylase activity. *Nat Genet* 24: 88–91

107. Fuks F, Burgers WA, Godin N, Kasai M, Kouzarides T. 2001. Dnmt3a binds deacetylases and is recruited by a sequence-specific repressor to silence transcription. *Embo J* 20: 2536–44

108. Cervoni N, Detich N, Seo SB, Chakravarti D, Szyf M. 2002. The oncoprotein Set/TAF-1beta, an inhibitor of histone acetyltransferase, inhibits active demethylation of DNA, integrating DNA methylation and transcriptional silencing. *J Biol Chem* 277: 25026–31

109. Ou JN, Torrisani J, Unterberger A, Provencal N, Shikimi K, et al. 2007. Histone deacetylase inhibitor Trichostatin A induces global and gene-specific DNA demethylation in human cancer cell lines. *Biochem Pharmacol* 73: 1297–307

Chapter 10 / DNA Methylation in Breast Cancer

173

110. Milutinovic S, D'Alessio AC, Detich N, Szyf M. 2007. Valproate induces widespread epigenetic reprogramming which involves demethylation of specific genes. *Carcinogenesis* 28: 560–71

111. Nass SJ, Ferguson AT, El-Ashry D, Nelson WG, Davidson NE. 1999. Expression of DNA methyltransferase (DMT) and the cell cycle in human breast cancer cells. *Oncogene* 18: 7453–61

112. Detich N, Ramchandani S, Szyf M. 2001. A conserved 3'-untranslated element mediates growth regulation of DNA methyltransferase 1 and inhibits its transforming activity. *J Biol Chem* 276: 24881–90.

113. Szyf M, Bozovic V, Tanigawa G. 1991. Growth regulation of mouse DNA methyltransferase gene expression. *J Biol Chem* 266: 10027–30

114. Szyf M, Kaplan F, Mann V, Giloh H, Kedar E, Razin A. 1985. Cell cycle-dependent regulation of eukaryotic DNA methylase level. *J Biol Chem* 260: 8653–6

115. MacLeod AR, Rouleau J, Szyf M. 1995. Regulation of DNA methylation by the Ras signaling pathway. *J Biol Chem* 270: 11327–37

116. Rouleau J, MacLeod AR, Szyf M. 1995. Regulation of the DNA methyltransferase by the Ras-AP-1 signaling pathway. *J Biol Chem* 270: 1595–601

117. Bigey P, Ramchandani S, Theberge J, Araujo FD, Szyf M. 2000. Transcriptional regulation of the human DNA Methyltransferase (dnmt1) gene. *Gene* 242: 407–18

118. Slack A, Cervoni N, Pinard M, Szyf M. 1999. DNA methyltransferase is a downstream effector of cellular transformation triggered by simian virus 40 large T antigen. *J Biol Chem* 274: 10105–12

119. Torrisani J, Unterberger A, Tendulkar SR, Shikimi K, Szyf M. 2007. AUF1 cell cycle variations define genomic DNA methylation by regulation of DNMT1 mRNA stability. *Mol Cell Biol* 27: 395–410

120. Chuang LS, Ian HI, Koh TW, Ng HH, Xu G, Li BF. 1997. Human DNA-(cytosine-5) methyltransferase-PCNA complex as a target for p21WAF1. *Science* 277: 1996–2000

121. Knox JD, Araujo FD, Bigey P, Slack AD, Price GB, et al. 2000. Inhibition of DNA methyltransferase inhibits DNA replication. *J Biol Chem* 275: 17986–90

122. Milutinovic S, Brown SE, Zhuang Q, Szyf M. 2004. DNA methyltransferase 1 knock down induces gene expression by a mechanism independent of DNA methylation and histone deacetylation. *J Biol Chem* 279: 27915–27

123. Milutinovic S, Zhuang Q, Niveleau A, Szyf M. 2003. Epigenomic stress response. Knockdown of DNA methyltransferase 1 triggers an intra-S-phase arrest of DNA replication and induction of stress response genes. *J Biol Chem* 278: 14985–95

124. Unterberger A, Andrews SD, Weaver IC, Szyf M. 2006. DNA methyltransferase 1 knockdown activates a replication stress checkpoint. *Mol Cell Biol* 26: 7575–86

125. Linhart HG, Lin H, Yamada Y, Moran E, Steine EJ, et al. 2007. Dnmt3b promotes tumorigenesis in vivo by gene-specific de novo methylation and transcriptional silencing. *Genes Dev* 21: 3110–22

126. Piva R, Rimondi AP, Hanau S, Maestri I, Alvisi A, et al. 1990. Different methylation of oestrogen receptor DNA in human breast carcinomas with and without oestrogen receptor. *Br J Cancer* 61: 270–5

127. Fujii H, Biel MA, Zhou W, Weitzman SA, Baylin SB, Gabrielson E. 1998. Methylation of the HIC-1 candidate tumor suppressor gene in human breast cancer. *Oncogene* 16: 2159–64

128. Guo Y, Pakneshan P, Gladu J, Slack A, Szyf M, Rabbani SA. 2002. Regulation of DNA methylation in human breast cancer. Effect on the urokinase-type plasminogen activator gene production and tumor invasion. *J Biol Chem* 277: 41571–9

129. Pakneshan P, Szyf M, Farias-Eisner R, Rabbani SA. 2004. Reversal of the hypomethylation status of urokinase (uPA) promoter blocks breast cancer growth and metastasis. *J Biol Chem* 279: 31735–44

130. Narayan A, Ji W, Zhang XY, Marrogi A, Graff JR, et al. 1998. Hypomethylation of pericentromeric DNA in breast adenocarcinomas. *Int J Cancer* 77: 833–8

131. Baylin SB, Esteller M, Rountree MR, Bachman KE, Schuebel K, Herman JG. 2001. Aberrant patterns of DNA methylation, chromatin formation and gene expression in cancer. *Hum Mol Genet* 10: 687–92.

132. Feinberg AP, Gehrke CW, Kuo KC, Ehrlich M. 1988. Reduced genomic 5-methylcytosine content in human colonic neoplasia. *Cancer Res* 48: 1159–61

133. Huang TH, Perry MR, Laux DE. 1999. Methylation profiling of CpG islands in human breast cancer cells. *Hum Mol Genet* 8: 459–70
134. Brehmer B, Biesterfeld S, Jakse G. 2003. Expression of matrix metalloproteinases (MMP-2 and -9) and their inhibitors (TIMP-1 and -2) in prostate cancer tissue. *Prostate Cancer Prostatic Dis* 6: 217–22
135. Herman JG, Merlo A, Mao L, Lapidus RG, Issa JP, et al. 1995. Inactivation of the CDKN2/p16/MTS1 gene is frequently associated with aberrant DNA methylation in all common human cancers. *Cancer Res* 55: 4525–30
136. Silva J, Silva JM, Dominguez G, Garcia JM, Cantos B, et al. 2003. Concomitant expression of p16INK4a and p14ARF in primary breast cancer and analysis of inactivation mechanisms. *J Pathol* 199: 289–97
137. Hu XC, Wong IH, Chow LW. 2003. Tumor-derived aberrant methylation in plasma of invasive ductal breast cancer patients: clinical implications. *Oncol Rep* 10: 1811–5
138. Niwa Y, Oyama T, Nakajima T. 2000. BRCA1 expression status in relation to DNA methylation of the BRCA1 promoter region in sporadic breast cancers. *Jpn J Cancer Res* 91: 519–26
139. Rice JC, Ozcelik H, Maxeiner P, Andrulis I, Futscher BW. 2000. Methylation of the BRCA1 promoter is associated with decreased BRCA1 mRNA levels in clinical breast cancer specimens. *Carcinogenesis* 21: 1761–5
140. Murata H, Khattar NH, Kang Y, Gu L, Li GM. 2002. Genetic and epigenetic modification of mismatch repair genes hMSH2 and hMLH1 in sporadic breast cancer with microsatellite instability. *Oncogene* 21: 5696–703
141. Widschwendter M, Berger J, Hermann M, Muller HM, Amberger A, et al. 2000. Methylation and silencing of the retinoic acid receptor-beta2 gene in breast cancer. *J Natl Cancer Inst* 92: 826–32
142. Graff JR, Gabrielson E, Fujii H, Baylin SB, Herman JG. 2000. Methylation patterns of the E-cadherin 5' CpG island are unstable and reflect the dynamic, heterogeneous loss of E-cadherin expression during metastatic progression. *J Biol Chem* 275: 2727–32
143. Bachman KE, Herman JG, Corn PG, Merlo A, Costello JF, et al. 1999. Methylation-associated silencing of the tissue inhibitor of metalloproteinase-3 gene suggest a suppressor role in kidney, brain, and other human cancers. *Cancer Res* 59: 798–802
144. Lehmann U, Hasemeier B, Christgen M, Muller M, Romermann D, et al. 2008. Epigenetic inactivation of microRNA gene hsa-mir-9-1 in human breast cancer. *J Pathol* 214: 17–24
145. Roll JD, Rivenbark AG, Jones WD, Coleman WB. 2008. DNMT3b overexpression contributes to a hypermethylator phenotype in human breast cancer cell lines. *Mol Cancer* 7: 15
146. Ferguson AT, Lapidus RG, Baylin SB, Davidson NE. 1995. Demethylation of the estrogen receptor gene in estrogen receptor- negative breast cancer cells can reactivate estrogen receptor gene expression. *Cancer Res* 55: 2279–83
147. Langley B, D'Annibale MA, Suh K, Ayoub I, Tolhurst A, et al. 2008. Pulse inhibition of histone deacetylases induces complete resistance to oxidative death in cortical neurons without toxicity and reveals a role for cytoplasmic p21(waf1/cip1) in cell cycle-independent neuroprotection. *J Neurosci* 28: 163–76
148. Adams PD, Cairns P. 2003. Induction of the estrogen receptor by ablation of DNMT1 in ER-negative breast cancer cells. *Cancer Biol Ther* 2: 557–8
149. Yang Q, Shan L, Yoshimura G, Nakamura M, Nakamura Y, et al. 2002. 5-aza-2'-deoxycytidine induces retinoic acid receptor beta 2 demethylation, cell cycle arrest and growth inhibition in breast carcinoma cells. *Anticancer Res* 22: 2753–6
150. Szyf M. 2001. Towards a pharmacology of DNA methylation. *Trends Pharmacol Sci* 22: 350–4.
151. Chandler LA, Jones PA. 1985. Hypomethylation of DNA in the regulation of gene expression. *Dev Biol (N Y* 5: 335–49
152. Ramchandani S, MacLeod AR, Pinard M, von Hofe E, Szyf M. 1997. Inhibition of tumorigenesis by a cytosine-DNA, methyltransferase, antisense oligodeoxynucleotide. *Proc Natl Acad Sci U S A* 94: 684–9
153. Milutinovic S, Knox JD, Szyf M. 2000. DNA methyltransferase inhibition induces the transcription of the tumor suppressor p21(WAF1/CIP1/sdi1). *J Biol Chem* 275: 6353-9
154. Oki Y, Aoki E, Issa JP. 2007. Decitabine–bedside to bench. *Crit Rev Oncol Hematol* 61: 140–52

Chapter 10 / DNA Methylation in Breast Cancer 175

155. Weiss AJ, Metter GE, Nealon TF, Keanan JP, Ramirez G, et al. 1977. Phase II study of 5-azacytidine in solid tumors. *Cancer Treat Rep* 61: 55–8
156. Soriano AO, Yang H, Faderl S, Estrov Z, Giles F, et al. 2007. Safety and clinical activity of the combination of 5-azacytidine, valproic acid and all-trans retinoic acid in acute myeloid leukemia and myelodysplastic syndrome. Blood
157. Soares J, Pinto AE, Cunha CV, Andre S, Barao I, et al. 1999. Global DNA hypomethylation in breast carcinoma: correlation with prognostic factors and tumor progression. *Cancer* 85: 112–8
158. Bernardino J, Roux C, Almeida A, Vogt N, Gibaud A, et al. 1997. DNA hypomethylation in breast cancer: an independent parameter of tumor progression? *Cancer Genet Cytogenet* 97: 83–9
159. Alves G, Tatro A, Fanning T. 1996. Differential methylation of human LINE-1 retrotransposons in malignant cells. *Gene* 176: 39–44
160. Weber J, Salgaller M, Samid D, Johnson B, Herlyn M, et al. 1994. Expression of the MAGE-1 tumor antigen is up-regulated by the demethylating agent 5-aza-2'-deoxycytidine. *Cancer Res* 54: 1766–71
161. De Smet C, De Backer O, Faraoni I, Lurquin C, Brasseur F, Boon T. 1996. The activation of human gene MAGE-1 in tumor cells is correlated with genome-wide demethylation. *Proc Natl Acad Sci U S A* 93: 7149–53
162. De Smet C, Lurquin C, Lethe B, Martelange V, Boon T. 1999. DNA methylation is the primary silencing mechanism for a set of germ line- and tumor-specific genes with a CpG-rich promoter. *Mol Cell Biol* 19: 7327–35
163. Serrano A, Garcia A, Abril E, Garrido F, Ruiz-Cabello F. 1996. Methylated CpG points identified within MAGE-1 promoter are involved in gene repression. *Int J Cancer* 68: 464–70
164. Kavalar R, Sarcevic B, Spagnoli GC, Separovic V, Samija M, et al. 2001. Expression of MAGE tumour-associated antigens is inversely correlated with tumour differentiation in invasive ductal breast cancers: an immunohistochemical study. *Virchows Arch* 439: 127–31
165. Fisher JL, Field CL, Zhou H, Harris TL, Henderson MA, Choong PF. 2000. Urokinase plasminogen activator system gene expression is increased in human breast carcinoma and its bone metastases–a comparison of normal breast tissue, non-invasive and invasive carcinoma and osseous metastases. *Breast Cancer Res Treat* 61: 1–12
166. Lu A, Gupta A, Li C, Ahlborn TE, Ma Y, et al. 2001. Molecular mechanisms for aberrant expression of the human breast cancer specific gene 1 in breast cancer cells: control of transcription by DNA methylation and intronic sequences. *Oncogene* 20: 5173–85
167. Gupta A, Godwin AK, Vanderveer L, Lu A, Liu J. 2003. Hypomethylation of the synuclein gamma gene CpG island promotes its aberrant expression in breast carcinoma and ovarian carcinoma. *Cancer Res* 63: 664–73
168. Girault I, Tozlu S, Lidereau R, Bieche I. 2003. Expression analysis of DNA methyltransferases 1, 3A, and 3B in sporadic breast carcinomas. *Clin Cancer Res* 9: 4415–22
169. Pakneshan P, Szyf M, Rabbani SA. 2005. Methylation and inhibition of expression of uPA by the RAS oncogene: divergence of growth control and invasion in breast cancer cells. *Carcinogenesis* 26: 557–64
170. Bachman KE, Park BH, Rhee I, Rajagopalan H, Herman JG, et al. 2003. Histone modifications and silencing prior to DNA methylation of a tumor suppressor gene. *Cancer Cell* 3: 89–95
171. Ateq B, Unterberger A, Rabbani SA, Szyf M. 2008. Pharmacological Inhibition of DNA Methylation Induces Proinvasive and Prometastatic Genes In Vitro and In Vivo. *Neoplasia* 10: 1–13
172. Goffin J, Eisenhauer E. 2002. DNA methyltransferase inhibitors-state of the art. *Ann Oncol* 13: 1699–716
173. Winquist E, Knox J, Ayoub JP, Wood L, Wainman N, et al. 2006. Phase II trial of DNA methyltransferase 1 inhibition with the antisense oligonucleotide MG98 in patients with metastatic renal carcinoma: a National Cancer Institute of Canada Clinical Trials Group investigational new drug study. *Invest New Drugs* 24: 159–67
174. Campbell PM, Bovenzi V, Szyf M. 2004. Methylated DNA-binding protein 2 antisense inhibitors suppress tumourigenesis of human cancer cell lines in vitro and in vivo. *Carcinogenesis* 25: 499–507

11

Signal Transduction Inhibitors in the Treatment of Breast Cancer

Monica R. Maiello, Antonella De Luca, Marianna Gallo, Amelia D'Alessio, Pietro Carotenuto, and Nicola Normanno

SUMMARY

Current systemic therapies for breast cancer are often limited by their non-specific mechanism of action, unwanted toxicities on normal tissues and short-term efficacy due to the emergence of drug resistance. Identification of the molecular alterations in key proteins involved in breast cancer cell proliferation and survival resulted in development of various signal transduction inhibitors as new treatment strategy. Preclinical data support the use of these agents in breast cancer, including estrogen receptor positive breast cancer patients in which signalling inhibitors might prevent or treat resistance to endocrine therapy. These compounds have generally shown an acceptable toxicity profile. However, little clinical activity of signalling inhibitors as monotherapy in breast cancer patients has been reported up to now. Furthermore, the preliminary results of clinical trials of combinations of signalling inhibitors and endocrine therapies published to day are rather disappointing. These negative findings are likely due to the occurrence of mechanisms of resistance to these drugs.

Key Words: Breast cancer; Signal transduction; Tyrosine kinase; EGFR; Endocrine therapy; Resistance

From: *Current Clinical Oncology: Breast Cancer in the Post-Genomic Era,*
Edited by: A. Giordano and N. Normanno, DOI: 10.1007/978-1-60327-945-1_11,
© Humana Press, a part of Springer Science + Business Media, LLC 2009

1. INTRODUCTION

Breast cancer is a complex and heterogeneous disease in which several different molecular alterations are involved in its pathogenesis and progression. The development of high-throughput technologies has recently underscored such complexity by revealing the existence of different subtypes of breast carcinoma that are characterized by specific gene expression profiles (1). More importantly, the identification of the mechanisms that regulate proliferation and survival of tumour cells is leading to the development of novel therapeutic approaches. Several different agents, directed against specific signalling molecules expressed in tumour cells, have been developed. In most of the cases, the targets of these agents are also expressed in normal cells. However, the toxicity profile of these molecules is generally acceptable, and the side effects are much more tolerable as compared with conventional cytotoxic agents.

Drugs directed against molecular alterations of specific subtypes of breast carcinoma have long been approved for clinical use. As a matter of fact, the anti-estrogen tamoxifen is the first target-based agent developed in breast cancer. More recently, other endocrine therapies (aromatase inhibitors, fulvestrant) have been approved for treatment of estrogen receptor positive (ER+) breast cancer (2). The anti-ErbB-2 monoclonal antibody trastuzumab has shown significant clinical activity in patients with either advanced or early breast cancer that overexpresses the ErbB-2 receptor (3). More recently, the dual EGFR/ErbB-2 tyrosine kinase inhibitor (TKI) lapatinib has been approved for treatment of patients with metastatic breast cancer (3).

A number of novel agents directed against molecular targets are in clinical development in breast cancer. In this regard, we will limit our discussion to signalling inhibitors that are in early phase of clinical development, since drugs that are in advanced phase of clinical studies or that have already been approved for treatment of breast cancer patients will be addressed in a different chapter. We will also focus our discussion on trials of signalling inhibitors in monotherapy or in combination with endocrine therapy. Before discussing the preclinical and clinical findings obtained with these agents, we will briefly summarize the current knowledge on the role of different signalling pathways in the pathogenesis and progression of breast cancer. The potential mechanisms of de novo or acquired resistance to target-based agents will be discussed for each drug. Finally, the therapeutic strategies in which these novel drugs might be employed to prevent or to treat resistance to anti-estrogen agents will be discussed.

2. MOLECULAR TARGETS IN BREAST CANCER

The growth and survival of breast cancer cells is sustained by different growth factor receptor-driven signalling pathways. Among these, the role of the epidermal growth factor receptor (EGFR) family of tyrosine kinase receptors in the pathogenesis of breast cancer has long been established. The EGFR family includes four different receptor tyrosine kinases: EGFR (ErbB-1), ErbB-2, ErbB-3 and ErbB-4 (4). Each of these proteins possesses an extracellular ligand-binding domain, a single hydrophobic transmembrane domain and a cytoplasmic tyrosine kinase-containing domain (5). The receptors of the ErbB family are activated following binding to peptide growth factors of the EGF-family (Table 1). Upon ligand binding, the ErbB receptors form either homo- or hetero-dimers. Following dimerization, auto- and trans-phosphorylation in tyrosine residues of the ErbB receptors occurs (5).

The expression of the EGFR has been reported in 14–91% of breast carcinomas (Table 2) (6,7). Overexpression of the EGFR has been linked to a more aggressive breast tumour phenotype, with increased potential for invasiveness and metastasis (4,6,7). In this regard, EGFR expression has been related to poorer patient prognosis although the results are discordant.

Chapter 11 / Signal Transduction Inhibitors in the Treatment of Breast Cancer 179

Table 1
The ErbB receptors and their cognate ligands

ErbB receptor	Ligand
EGFR	Epidermal growth factor (EGF)
	Transforming growth factor α (TGF-α)
	Amphiregulin (AR)
	Epigen
EGFR and ErbB-4	Betacellulin (BTC)
	Heparin-binding growth factor (HB-EGF)
	Epiregulin (EPR)
ErbB-2	None
ErbB-3 and ErbB-4	Neuregulin 1 (NRG 1)
	Neuregulin 2 (NRG 2)
ErbB-4	Neuregulin 3 (NRG 3)
	Neuregulin 4 (NRG 4)
	Tomoregulin

Table 2
Frequency of expression of ErbB receptors in breast cancer

ErbB receptor	Percentage of expression
EGFR	14–91%
ErbB-2	9–39%
ErbB-3	22–90%
ErbB-4	82%

In fact, the prognostic significance of EGFR in breast cancer has been shown in studies with short follow-up, whereas it was not confirmed in studies with longer follow-up, suggesting that EGFR expression could be associated with early relapse of the disease *(4,6,7)*. More recently, it has been shown that the 'triple negative' or 'basal' breast cancer subtype expresses the EGFR at higher frequency as compared with other subtypes *(8)*. Expression of ErbB-2 is more restricted and occurs in approximately 30% of human primary breast carcinomas. High levels of expression of this receptor generally correlate with poor prognosis, although mixed results have also been reported *(4,6,7)*. ErbB-3 and ErbB-4 expression has been also demonstrated to occur at high frequency in breast cancer patients *(4,6,7)*. Co-expression of two or more ErbB receptors has been frequently found in breast carcinoma *(4,7)*. In this regard, expression of phosphorylated ErbB-2 or co-expression of ErbB-2 and EGFR was associated with the shortest survival in breast cancer patients *(9)*. In agreement with these findings, co-expression of EGFR, ErbB-2 and ErbB-3 was found to have a negative synergistic effect on patient outcome, independent of tumour size or lymph node status *(10)*. Taken together, these findings support that different ErbB receptors cooperate in sustaining the growth of breast carcinoma. The redundancy of expression is not limited to the ErbB receptors but it also occurs for EGF-like peptides, such as TGF-α, AR and/or NRG *(11)*. Finally, ErbB receptors and EGF-like peptides are generally expressed at higher levels in estrogen receptor negative (ER−) breast carcinomas as compared with ER+ tumours *(11)*.

However, a progressive increase in the levels of expression and of activation of EGFR and ErbB-2 has been described in ER+ breast cancer cells that develop resistance to anti-estrogen therapy *(2,12)*.

Following ligand-induced activation, the tyrosine-phosphorylated receptors become able to interact with adaptor proteins that couple the receptors to intracellular signalling pathways *(5)*. Indeed, the ErbB receptors can activate different intracellular signalling cascades, including the phosphatidylinositol 3-kinase PI3K/AKT and the ras/raf/MEK/mitogen-activated protein kinase (MAPK) pathways. However, these pathways might also be activated in an ErbB-independent manner by molecular alterations of signalling proteins or by tyrosine kinase receptors other than the ErbB receptors expressed in tumour cells. As we will discuss later, these phenomena might be involved in the resistance of breast cancer cells to anti-EGFR agents.

The Ras/Raf/MEK/MAPK pathway is activated by tyrosine kinase receptors through either Grb2 and Sos or Shc adaptor proteins *(13)*. In turn, Ras activates Raf-1 that, through intermediate steps, leads to phosphorylation of p42/44 MAPK *(13)*. Several studies have demonstrated that MAPK signalling promotes proliferation and survival of breast cancer cells *(14)*. Furthermore, as we will discuss in detail in the next paragraphs, activation of MAPK signalling has been associated with resistance to both EGFR targeting agents and endocrine therapy in breast carcinoma. Mutations of Ras and B-Raf genes lead to abnormal activation of this pathway in human cancer. However, Ras mutations have been rarely identified in human primary breast cancer *(15)*. Surprisingly, Ras mutations have been recently described in 18% of human breast cancer cell lines *(16)*. Similarly, B-Raf mutations have been identified in 10% of breast cancer cell lines whereas they have been found at much lower frequency in primary breast tumours *(16)*. Taken together, these findings suggest that Ras or Raf mutations might occur in a late stage of breast tumour progression, and that they might provide a growth advantage to clones of cells that can be therefore isolated as continuous cell lines.

The PI3K/AKT pathway is involved in different functions that play an important role in tumour progression, such as cell growth, survival, invasion and migration *(17)*. A mechanism for abnormal PI3K activation in cancer is through somatic mutations in the genes that encode positive and negative effectors of this pathway *(18)*. In particular, loss of expression or functional loss of PTEN, a powerful negative regulator of PI3K signalling, occurs in different cancer types, including breast cancer, and results in constitutive AKT activation *(19,20)*. Reconstitution of PTEN expression in PTEN-null cells has been shown to repress AKT, inhibit tumour growth via induction of apoptosis or repression of cell proliferation, and restore sensitivity to anti-EGFR agents *(21,22)*. However, the frequency of PTEN mutations in human primary breast carcinoma is approximately 6% *(23)*. More recently, activating mutations of the *PIK3CA* gene, which encodes for the PI3K p110 catalytic subunit, were found in approximately 25% of primary breast tumours *(24)*.

One of the main targets of the PI3K/AKT cascade is the mammalian target of rapamycin (mTOR) *(17)*. Activation of mTOR, in turn, regulates translation initiation through activation of ribosomal p70S6 kinase (S6K1) and inactivation of the 4E-BP1 suppressor protein *(17)*. The *RPS6KB1* gene, which encodes the mTOR effector S6K1, is amplified in approximately 10% of breast cancer *(25)*. *RPS6KB1* gene amplification correlates with ErbB-2 overexpression in breast tumours, possibly due to coamplification of RPS6KB1with ErbB-2 *(25)*. It is important to underline that the PI3K/AKT pathway is activated by different receptor tyrosine kinases, and that it plays an important role in the survival of tumour cells even in absence of mutations or amplifications of genes that are involved in its signalling.

Increasing evidence suggests a role of Src in breast cancer progression. Src is the prototype of a large family of non-receptor protein tyrosine kinases, known as the Src family kinases (SFKs) *(26)*. The 60-kDa Src protein is composed of a C-terminal tail containing a

Chapter 11 / Signal Transduction Inhibitors in the Treatment of Breast Cancer 181

negative-regulatory tyrosine residue, four SRC homology (SH) domains and a unique amino-terminal domain, which play different functions in the activation of this kinase *(26)*. Src can be activated by cytoplasmic proteins, such as focal adhesion kinase (FAK) or its molecular partner Crk-associated substrate (CAS), which play a prominent role in integrin signalling, and by ligand activated-receptor tyrosine kinases of cell surface receptors, including EGFR and ErbB-2 *(26)*. Src is able to activate several different intracellular signalling pathways, including the PI3K/AKT and the Ras/Raf/MEK/MAPK pathways. Src is overexpressed and highly activated in a wide variety of human cancers, including breast carcinoma *(27)*. In particular, in human mammary carcinomas Src kinase activity from 4 to 20-fold higher than normal tissues has been described *(27)*. A cooperation between Src and EGFR in breast cancer tumorigenesis has also been hypothesized *(28,29)*. Src might also play an important role in epithelial to mesenchymal transition (EMT) that enhances the metastatic potential of tumour cells *(30)*.

Finally, angiogenesis, the formation of new blood vessels from the existing vasculature, is essential for the growth of the primary tumour and for the formation of metastasis. One of the key molecules responsible for the regulation of tumour-associated neoangiogenesis is vascular endothelial growth factor-A (VEGF-A, from now referred as VEGF), although additional growth factors, such as interleukin-8 (IL-8), basic fibroblast growth factor (bFGF) and the EGFR ligands EGF and TGF-α, might play a role in this phenomenon *(31–33)*. VEGF binds two related receptor tyrosine kinases: VEGFR-1 (Flt-1) and VEGFR-2 (Flk/KDR) *(31)*. VEGFR-1 is a potent, positive regulator of physiologic and developmental angiogenesis and is thought to be important for endothelial cell migration and differentiation. VEGFR-2 mediates the majority of the downstream effects of VEGF, including vascular permeability, endothelial cell proliferation, invasion, migration and survival. An additional VEGFR related receptor (VEGFR-3) is involved in lymphangiogenesis *(34)*.

Increased VEGF expression has been observed in breast cancer patients. Although a clear correlation between levels of VEGF and tumour progression has not been established yet, several studies suggested that a correlation might exist between high VEGF expression and poor clinical outcome in breast cancer *(35)*. High VEGF levels have also been linked with a lack of response to radiotherapy and chemotherapy *(35)*. These observations support the rationale for the use of anti-VEGF agents in breast cancer.

3. ANTI-EGFR DRUGS IN BREAST CANCER

In the past two decades several agents direct against the EGFR have been explored for their anti-tumour activity. Monoclonal antibodies that block the interaction between the EGFR and its ligands and TKIs, which directly inhibit tyrosine kinase phosphorylation by physical interaction with either the ATP and/or the enzyme substrate binding site, are in advanced phase of clinical development in different tumour types *(7)*. We will focus our discussion on the EGFR-TKIs gefitinib and erlotinib, for which preclinical and clinical data in breast cancer are available (Table 3).

Gefitinib (ZD1839/Iressa) is an orally active, specific EGFR tyrosine kinase inhibitor. This drug is able to block the in vitro and in vivo growth of a wide range of EGFR-expressing human cancer cell lines, including breast cancer cells *(36–39)*. The activity of this molecule is generally cytostatic, although it was shown to induce apoptosis in several cancer cell lines *(37–40)*. The anti-tumour activity of gefitinib does not depend on the levels of expression of the EGFR but it might be correlated with the total levels of expression of the different ErbB receptors *(38)*.

Several phase II clinical trials with gefitinib as single agents in breast cancer patients have been reported (Table 4) *(41)*. These studies showed that gefitinib is well tolerated at daily

Table 3
Signal transduction inhibitors in early phase of clinical development in breast cancer

Target	Drug	Other sites of action(s)
EGFR	Gefitinib	None
	Erlotinib	ErbB-2
VEGFR1	Sorafenib	VEGFR2, VEGFR3, PDGFR-β, KIT
	Sunitinib	VEGFR1, VEGFR2, VEGFR3, PDGFR-α and -β, KIT, RET, FLT3, CSF-1R
	Vandetanib	VEGFR2, EGFR, RET
Farnesyltransferase	Tipifarnib	For all FTIs:
	Lonafarnib	lamin A, PxF, RhoB, cyclic guanosine monophosphate phosphodiesterase α, rhodopsin kinase, transducin
	AZD3409	geranylgeranyl transferase
Src	Dasatinib	Abl
	AZD0530	Abl
	Bosutinib	Abl
MEK 1/2	AZD6244	None

Abbreviations: CSF-1R, colony-stimulating factor 1 receptor; FLT3, FMS-like tyrosine kinase 3, PDGFR, platelet-derived growth factor receptor; PxF, human perioxisomal farnesylated protein

doses of 500 mg. Skin rashes and diarrhoea were the most frequent adverse effects. The majority of events were mild to moderate in severity and reversible on cessation of treatment. However, gefitinib did not show significant activity in these studies. Albain and co-workers enrolled 63 patients with metastatic breast cancer in a trial of daily administration of gefitinib (500 mg/die) *(42)*. Of the 63 patients, 27 (43%) expressed ER and 17 (27%) had high levels of ErbB-2 expression. The majority of the patients were heavily pretreated with several lines of chemotherapy and/or hormonal therapy. All ErbB-2 positive patients had been previously treated with the anti-ErbB-2 antibody trastuzumab. Only one patient had partial remission (PR), whereas stabilization of the disease (SD) lasting at least 4 months was observed in five patients. In the study by von Minckwitz et al. *(43)*, 58 patients with advanced breast cancer were enrolled. One patient (1.7%) had PR, and 51 patients (98.3%) had progressive disease (PD). No significant clinical activity of gefitinib in pretreated advanced breast cancer patients was also reported by Baselga et al. *(44)* and Robertson et al. *(45)*. However, in the latter study, a disease control rate of 66.6% was observed in a small cohort of ER+ tamoxifen resistant patients. Pharmacodynamic studies in breast cancer patients treated with gefitinib showed that EGFR phosphorylation was successfully inhibited in tumour biopsies in all patients *(44)*. This observation suggests that lack of clinical response is due to lack of tumour dependence upon EGFR rather than incomplete receptor blockade. Furthermore, no correlation between receptor expression and response was observed in these studies.

The above summarized findings suggest that resistance to anti-EGFR agents is a common phenomenon in breast cancer patients. In this regard, different preclinical studies suggested that high levels of activation of MAPK and AKT might mediate resistance to gefitinib *(36,39,46)*. The PI3K/AKT pathway was accounted as the main mediator of the resistance of breast cancer cells to EGFR-TKIs *(36,39)*. In particular, PTEN-null breast cancer cells, which have high constitutive levels of activation of AKT, were found to be resistant to the growth inhibitory effect of gefitinib *(36,39)*. Furthermore, as above described, reconstitution

Table 4
Summary of clinical phase II trials of selected target-based agents as monotherapy in breast cancer

Drug	Dose (mg/die)	N. pts	ORR (%)	CBR (%)	Reference	Notes
Gefitinib	500	63	1.6	9.5	(42)	MBC
Gefitinib	500	58	1.7	1.7	(43)	MBC
Gefitinib	500	31	0	9.7	(44)	MBC
Gefitinib	500	18	5.5	11	(45)	ER
Gefitinib	500	9	11.1	66.6	(45)	ER+
Erlotinib	150	69	2.9	14.5	(54)	MBC or LABC
Sorafenib	400	23	5	10	(56)	MBC
Sorafenib	400/twice daily	54	1.8	38.8	(57)	MBC
Sunitinib	50	64	11	16	(61)	MBC
Vandetanib	100	22	0	0	(65)	MBC
Vandetanib	300	24	0	4.2	(65)	MBC
Tipifarnib	CD 300 or 400 b.i.d.	41	10	24	(70)	MBC
Tipifarnib	ID 300 b.i.d.	35	14	23	(70)	MBC

Abbreviations: CD, continuous dosing; ID intermittent dosing; CBR, clinical benefit rate; MBC, metastatic breast cancer; LABC, locally advanced breast cancer; ORR, objective response rate

of PTEN function in these cells restored sensitivity to gefitinib and re-established EGFR-stimulated AKT signalling *(21,22)*. In agreement with these findings, gefitinib was found to inhibit MAPK but not AKT activation in tumour biopsies obtained from patients treated with this drug *(44)*. Activation of the insulin-like growth factor type 1 receptor (IGF-1R), a tyrosine kinase receptor that is a powerful activator of PI3K/AKT signalling, has also been associated with both de novo and acquired resistance to gefitinib *(47, 48)*. In fact, Camirand et al. *(48)* showed that blockade of IGF-1R increased the anti-tumour effects of gefitinib in breast cancer cells. Furthermore, prolonged treatment with gefitinib of tamoxifen-resistant MCF-7 breast cancer cells generated cells with acquired resistance to gefitinib (TAM/TKI-R) *(47)*. The resistance to this drug was associated with no detectable basal EGFR activity and minimal MAPK activity, but with significantly high levels of IGF-1R and AKT activity as compared with parental TAM-R cells. It has also been recently shown that breast cancer cells that co-express EGFR, ErbB-2 and ErbB-3, such as SK-Br-3 cells, escape the activity of EGFR-TKIs through ErbB-2-dependent activation of the ErbB-3/PI3K/AKT pathway *(49)*. However, this mechanism of resistance developed following short treatment with EGFR-TKIs (up to 96 h), whereas breast cancer patients have been treated for much longer periods in clinical trials of gefitinib *(41)*.

Evidence suggests that MAPK signalling might also be involved in the resistance of breast cancer cells to gefitinib. Indeed, gefitinib was not able to efficiently down-regulate the activation of both the MEK/MAPK and the PI3K/AKT pathways in breast cancer cells with relative resistance to this drug, such as the MDA-MB-468 cell line *(46)*. The growth of these cells was significantly inhibited by treatment with either the PI3K-inhibitor LY294002 or the MEK-inhibitor PD98059 and a synergistic anti-tumour effect was observed when this cell line was treated with a combination of gefitinib and both MEK and PI3K inhibitors *(46)*.

These findings suggest that both pathways are involved in the intrinsic resistance of these cells to gefitinib. In addition, persistent EGFR-independent activation of MAPK was observed in three different gefitinib-resistant breast cancer cell lines that were generated by exposing cells for long term (5–8 months) to the drug *(50)*. In particular, gefitinib-resistant SK-Br-3 cells showed an increased sensitivity to the MEK inhibitor PD98059 as compared with wild-type SK-Br-3 cells, and a synergistic anti-tumour effect was observed when resistant cells were treated with a combination of gefitinib and PD98059 *(50)*.

An unexpected activity of gefitinib on bone pain in breast cancer patients has been reported. In particular, Albain et al. *(42)* enrolled in their study of gefitinib in breast cancer 12 patients with bone metastasis and bone pain. Surprisingly, 5 out of 12 patients had a significant relief of bone pain, leading to the complete withdrawal of all scheduled narcotics in several cases. Due to the impressive effects on bone pain palliation, two patients were maintained on gefitinib despite objective progression of the disease. A significant improvement in bone pain was also reported in a patient enrolled in the study by von Minckwitz *(43)*. In this regard, we have shown that gefitinib affects the ability of bone marrow stromal cells to secrete pro-osteoclastogenic factors such as macrophage colony stimulating factor (M-CSF), which induces proliferation and differentiation of pre-osteoclast cells, and receptor activator of NF-kB ligand (RANKL) that is involved in fusion and activation of these cells *(51)*. Accordingly, treatment with gefitinib reduced the ability of MSC-like cells to induce osteoclast differentiation *(51)*.

Erlotinib (OSI-774/Tarceva) is an orally available, reversible inhibitor of the EGFR tyrosine kinase. This drug is able to specifically block the kinase activity of purified EGFR and EGFR autophosphorylation in intact cells with IC50 values of 2 and 20 nM, respectively *(7)*. In preclinical studies erlotinib has shown a potent anti-tumour activity in many cell lines, including breast cancer cells *(7)*. It has been suggested that erlotinib is also able to block ErbB-2 kinase in intact cells through direct interaction with ErbB-2 *(52)*. However, this drug is 12-fold less active against ErbB-2 kinase if compared with the EGFR kinase. In agreement with these findings, Guix et al. *(53)* showed that erlotinib at the concentration of 3 μM was able to directly inhibit ErbB-2 activation in cells engineered to express only this receptor, whereas 0.1 μM of the drug was sufficient to block the activation of the EGFR. Interestingly, 1 μM erlotinib was able to block EGFR-dependent ErbB-2 activation in cells expressing both receptors.

In a phase II clinical trial 69 patients with locally advanced or metastatic breast cancer were enrolled and treated with erlotinib (150 mg/die) as monotherapy (Table 4) *(54)*. The patients were divided in 2 arms. Arm 1 included 47 patients who had received previous anthracycline, taxane and capecitabine therapy. In this arm, one patient had PR and six patients had SD longer than 12 weeks. Arm 2 included 22 patients who had received different previous treatment for metastatic breast cancer. In this group, one patient had PR and two patients had SD longer than 8 weeks. The most common side effects were skin rashes (78%) and diarrhoea (59%).

In the study of Guix et al. *(53)*, 52 patients with untreated operable breast cancer (stage I to IIIA) were enrolled. They received erlotinib (150 mg/die) orally for 6–10 days until approximately 24 h before surgery. Of 52 patients, 41 completed treatment. The most common adverse effect was rash. Immunohistochemical analysis revealed that only 5 tumours were EGFR positive, 20 were ER+/progesterone receptor (PR)+ and 3 tumours were ER+/PR–. Moreover, nine patients expressed ErbB-2 and nine patients were triple negative. Some tumours exhibited detectable pEGFR ($n = 5$) and pErbB-2 ($n = 9$) in pretherapy specimens, which were markedly reduced after treatment. Erlotinib also induced a statistically significant reduction of AKT and MAPK phosphorylation. In ER+ breast carcinomas, a reduction in the levels of ER phosphorylation at ser118 was also observed following treatment with this drug. A complete cell cycle response, as defined by a <1% Ki67 index after neoadjuvant therapy, was observed in 17 patients, 16 of which were ER+.

In conclusion, phase II studies have suggested that the EGFR TKIs gefitinib and erlotinib as monotherapy do not have a significant efficacy in a non-selected, heavily pretreated population of patients with metastatic breast cancer. In addition, no data have been reported up to now to support the use of combinations of EGFR-TKIs and chemotherapy in breast cancer patients.

4. VEGFR SIGNALLING INHIBITORS IN BREAST CANCER

Several therapeutic agents that block VEGFR signalling have been developed and are in clinical development *(34)*. In particular, the monoclonal antibody bevacizumab that blocks VEGF has been recently approved for treatment of breast cancer patients. The preclinical and clinical findings with this compound are described in a different chapter. Several different tyrosine kinase inhibitors that bind to and block the catalytic site of the tyrosine kinase domain of VEGFRs are in early clinical development in breast cancer, and the results obtained with these drugs are described (Tables 3 and 4).

Sorafenib (BAY 43-9006/Nexavar) is an orally active, multikinase inhibitor with a broad spectrum of anti-tumour activity on cancer cell proliferation and angiogenesis *(55)*. Preclinical studies demonstrated that sorafenib inhibited Raf kinase isoforms (Raf-1, wild-type B-Raf and mutant B-Raf). As an inhibitor of Raf kinase, this drug is able to decrease phosphorylation of p42/44 MAPK in tumour cell lines. Indeed, sorafenib treatment completely blocked activation of MAPK pathway in MDA-MB-231 breast cancer cells that carry mutation of both KRas and BRaf. However, sorafenib had no effect on AKT activation in MDA-MB-231 cells, thus demonstrating its selectivity for the inhibition of the MAPK pathway *(55)*. Biochemical assays showed that sorafenib also inhibits several receptor tyrosine kinases involved in angiogenesis such as VEGFR-2, VEGFR-3, platelet-derived growth factor receptors (PDGFR)- β, and stem-cell factor receptor (c-KIT). The inhibition of receptor tyrosine kinases autophosphorylation occurred at significantly lower drug concentration as compared with the blockade of the Raf/MEK/MAPK pathway, which might require inhibition of multiple Ras isoforms *(55)*. Once daily oral dosing of sorafenib demonstrated broad-spectrum anti-tumour activity in colon, breast and non–small-cell lung cancer xenograft models, with MDA-MB-231 breast cancer cells showing the highest sensitivity to sorafenib *(55)*. A close association between inhibition of tumour growth and inhibition of the Raf/MEK/MAPK pathway was demonstrated in some but not all models *(55)*. However, significant inhibition of neovascularization was found in all the xenograft models, suggesting that both the anti-tumour and the anti-angiogenic effects contribute to the growth inhibitory activity of sorafenib *(55)*.

Phase II clinical trials of sorafenib in patients with metastatic breast cancer have been reported. Moreno-Aspitia et al. *(56)* enrolled 23 patients with metastatic breast cancer in a trial in which sorafenib was administered at the dose of 400 mg twice daily on days 1–28 of each 4-week cycle. The dose was reduced to 400 mg/die due to skin toxicity, hypertension, and cramps. The majority of patients had previously received an anthracycline and/or taxane treatment in neoadjuvant, adjuvant or metastatic setting. The most frequent side effects were grade 3 acne, skin reaction, neutropenia, cough and prolonged PTT. Of 20 eligible patients, only 1 (5%) had PR with duration of 3.6 months and 1 had SD for almost 6 months. At 6 months, the overall survival (OS) rate was 81% and the progression-free survival (PFS) rate was 6% with a median time to progression of 2 months. In the study of Bianchi et al. *(57)*, 54 patients with metastatic breast cancer, who had failed almost one prior chemotherapy, received a dose of 400 mg twice daily until tumour progression or unacceptable toxicity.

Most of patients had ER+/PR+ tumours. The most frequent side effect was grade 4 increase of γGT. Of 54 patients, only 1 (1.8%) patient had PR, whereas 20 (37%) patients had SD, with prolonged stabilization for 4 and 6 months occurring in 22% and 11% of the patients, respectively. Higher circulating ErbB-2 levels and/or higher baseline serum VEGF levels were associated with shorter time to progression. Studies of sorafenib in combination with chemotherapeutic agents are underway in metastatic breast cancer patients.

Sunitinib (SU11248, Sutent) is an oral, multitarget receptor tyrosine kinase inhibitor of VEGFR1, VEGFR2 and VEGFR3, PDGFRs-α and -β, c-KIT, glial cell line-derived neurotrophic factor receptor (REarranged during Transfection; RET), FMS-like tyrosine kinase 3 (FLT3), and colony-stimulating factor 1 receptor (CSF-1R) *(34)*.

In breast cancer tumour xenograft models sunitinib demonstrated effective anti-tumour activity *(58)*. Moreover, activity of sunitinib has been demonstrated in an in vivo model of breast cancer bone metastases and tumour-associated osteolysis *(59)*. In phase I studies of Sunitinib in patients with solid tumours, various schedules were used, including a 3-week cycle consisting of treatment for 2 weeks followed by a 1-week rest period (schedule 2/1), a 4-week cycle comprising treatment for 2 weeks followed by a 2-week rest period (schedule 2/2), or a 6-week cycle of treatment for 4 weeks followed by a 2-week rest period (schedule 4/2). These schedules explored both daily and every other day administration, and incorporated planned rest periods due to the prolonged half-life of the compound and evidence of accumulation with continuous daily dosing. Dose-limiting toxicities of fatigue, asthenia and thrombocytopenia occurred at 75 mg/die on all the schedules, thereby establishing the recommended phase II dose of 50 mg/die *(60)*. A phase II study of sunitinib in patients with anthracycline-resistant and taxane-resistant metastatic breast cancer was recently reported *(61)*. Sixty-four patients received sunitinib at dose 50 mg/die (schedule 4/2). The overall response rate (ORR) was 11%, with seven patients achieving a PR. Three additional patients (5%) had SD for at least 6 months yielding a clinical benefit rate of 16%. Interestingly, among the triple negative patients, the response rate was 15% and in ErbB2-positive, trastuzumab-treated patients, the response rate was 25%. The most frequently reported adverse effects were fatigue, followed by nausea, diarrhoea, mucosal inflammation and anorexia. Most adverse effects were mild to moderate (grades 1 to 2) in severity. Grade 3/4, transient neutropenia was experienced by 34% of patients. The higher incidence of neutropenia reported here may be due to the heavily pretreated nature of the study population. Fifty-six percent of patients had their dose interrupted or reduced as a result of an adverse effect, but none was considered to have discontinued treatment due to an adverse effect.

Phase II and phase III clinical trials of sunitinib in combination with chemotherapeutic agents or target-based agents (bevacizumab or trastuzumab) are ongoing.

Vandetanib (ZD6474, Zactima) is a small molecule receptor tyrosine kinase inhibitor that inhibits VEGFR2, EGFR and RET *(34)*. Vandetanib has shown anti-tumour activity in a broad range of preclinical models *(62–64)*. Phase I studies of vandetanib in patients with advanced solid tumours have demonstrated that the once daily oral administration at 100–300 mg/die is well tolerated *(34)*. In a phase II clinical trial 46 patients with metastatic breast cancer, who had received prior treatment with an anthracycline and taxane, were treated orally with vandetanib as single agent *(65)*. Patients were randomized in two groups that received respectively 100 or 300 mg/die of vandetanib. Diarrhoea and rash were the most frequent adverse effects and increased with dose. Rash was reported by 26% of patients overall but was never worse than grade 2. No objective responses were observed; one patient in the 300 mg group had SD for ≥24 weeks. Studies of vandetanib in combination with chemotherapeutics agents in breast cancer are underway. In this regard, a randomized phase II study of the combination of vandetanib plus docetaxel versus docetaxel plus placebo as second line treatment for advanced breast cancer failed to demonstrate any advantage for the combination *(66)*.

5. INHIBITORS OF INTRACELLULAR SIGNAL TRANSDUCTION PATHWAYS

A number of drugs targeting intracellular signal transduction pathways are being explored in breast cancer patients. In particular, agents directed against the PI3K/AKT, the ras/raf/MAPK and the Src pathways have shown anti-tumour activity in preclinical models of breast cancer (Table 3). Up to now, the encouraging preclinical findings have not been confirmed for the majority of these agents in clinical trials in breast cancer patients. The main preclinical and clinical results of studies conducted with inhibitors of intracellular signalling pathways in early phase of clinical development are summarized in this paragraph. Drugs in phase III clinical trials (temsirolimus and everolimus) are described in a different chapter.

Ras proteins undergo several post-translational modifications that facilitate their attachment to the inner face of the plasma membrane. Among these, the most crucial modification is the covalent attachment of a farnesyl isoprenoid lipid to a cysteine residue in the COOH-terminal of Ras proteins that is catalysed by the enzyme farnesyl transferase *(13)*. Farnesyl transferase inhibitors (FTIs) are potent inhibitors of this enzyme. However, many potential substrates for FTIs independent of Ras have been identified, such as lamin A and human perioxisomal farnesylated protein (PxF), both of which have been used as surrogate markers of farnesylation, RhoB, cyclic guanosine monophosphate phosphodiesterase a, rhodopsin kinase and the g subunit of the retinal protein, transducin *(67)*.The FTIs currently in clinical development are the orally active compounds tipifarnib, lonafarnib and AZD3409.

Tipifarnib (R115777, Zarnestra) has shown anti-tumour activity in breast cancer preclinical models in vitro and in vivo *(68)*. In particular, tipifarnib inhibited the growth of MCF-7 cells, which express wild-type Ras, at submicromolar concentration. In addition, in mice bearing MCF-7 xenografts treatment with this drug slowed the rate of tumour growth with a cytostatic effect *(68)*. More recently, a synergistic anti-tumour effect of combination of tipifarnib and 4-hydroxy-tamoxifen was observed in MCF-7 cells *(69)*. Several phase I studies of tipifarnib in cancer patients have been performed with different dosing schedules *(67)*. Continuous dosing was associated with severe toxicities. Dose-related diarrhoea, nausea, vomiting, renal dysfunction and myelosuppression were observed. A phase II study of tipifarnib, as single agent, in endocrine therapy, and/or chemotherapy-resistant patients with metastatic breast cancer, has shown encouraging results (Table 4) *(70)*. A total of 76 patients were treated with tipifarnib, either as a continuous dose of 300 or 400 mg b.i.d. ($n = 41$) or an intermittent dose of 300 mg b.i.d. for 21 days followed by 7 days of therapy ($n = 35$). In the continuous treatment arm, there were four PR (10%) lasting 4–12 months and six patients with SD (15%) for at least 6 months. In the intermittent treatment arm, there were five PR (14%) and three patients with SD (9%). However, the incidence of hematologic and neurologic toxicities was significantly higher in the continuous treatment arm as compared with the intermittent arm. Phase II studies of tipifarnib in combination with chemotherapeutic agents are ongoing.

Lonafarnib (SCH66336, Sarazar) has shown to inhibit the in vitro anchorage-independent growth of many human tumour cell lines and the growth of a number of human xenografts in a dose-dependent manner *(71)*. In phase I trials of Lonafarnib in solid tumours various dosing schedules were examined, but continuous dosing was associated with intolerable toxicities *(67)*. The dose limiting toxicity was usually gastrointestinal. Fatigue, which was severe at higher doses, and myelosuppression, generally brief durations of leucopenia and neutropenia, were noted. Reversible renal dysfunction was also seen, but only in patients with diarrhoea and/or nausea and vomiting, and was likely to be due to dehydration. Occasional responses were observed in phase I trials *(67)*. Phase II studies of Lonafarnib in combination with aromatase inhibitors (anastrozole) or trastuzumab plus chemotherapeutic agents (paclitaxel) are ongoing.

AZD3409 is a novel prenyl transferase inhibitor that was designed to mimic the C-terminal CAAX (CVIM:cysteine, valine, isoleucine, methionine) sequence of KRas 4B, the Ras isoform most commonly mutated in human cancers *(72,73)*. This compound has shown activity against both farnesyl transferase and geranylgeranyl transferase I in isolated enzyme studies. AZD3409 was able to inhibit the growth of tumour cells carrying either mutated or wild-type Ras *(72,74)*. Interestingly, in preclinical studies it has been demonstrated that AZD3409 significantly affected the growth of breast cancer cells with intrinsic resistance to gefitinib *(75)*. In particular, the combined treatment with AZD3409 and gefitinib of gefitinib-resistant breast cancer cells resulted in a synergistic anti-tumour effect *(75)*.

Results of a phase I trial of AZD3409 in patients with advanced solid malignancies were recently published *(76)*. Twenty-nine patients were treated at seven dose levels, starting from 500 mg AZD3409 once daily. The MTD was defined as 750 mg b.i.d. in the fasted state. Adverse events were mainly gastrointestinal and the severity was on average mild to moderate and reversible. The dose-limiting toxicities were vomiting, diarrhoea and uncontrolled nausea. Pharmacodynamic studies also showed that farnesyltransferase was inhibited at all dose levels.

Several inhibitors of Src are in clinical development in different tumour types, including breast cancer.

Dasatinib (BMS-354825) is a novel orally active small molecule kinase inhibitor of both SRC and Abl proteins. Dasatinib competes with ATP in binding to these kinases, and inhibits their autophosphorylation with IC50s value of 0.55 and 3.0 nM, respectively *(77)*. Preclinical studies demonstrated that dasatinib significantly inhibits the growth of different breast cancer cell lines with IC50s ranging between 5.5 and 600 nM *(78,79)*. Analysis of a wide panel of breast cancer cell lines revealed a significant relationship between breast cancer subtype and sensitivity to dasatinib *(79)*. In fact, breast cancer cell lines belonging to the basal-subtype or that have undergone epithelial to mesenchymal transition (EMT) were found to be the most sensitive to this drug *(79)*. Interestingly, a set of three genes, moesin, caveolin-1 and YAP-1, whose elevated expression is associated with response to dasatinib, was identified *(79)*. A six gene signature, including caveolin 1 and 2, annexin A1, EPH receptor A2, polymerase I and transcript release factor and insulin-like growth factor binding protein 2, was also found to predict sensitivity to dasatinib *(78)*. Interestingly, this gene signature was observed in basal-like breast tumours, thus confirming the potential sensitivity of this subtype for dasatinib *(78)*. Following these findings, a phase II clinical trial of dasatinib in recurrent or locally advanced triple negative breast cancer has been planned. Results from phase I clinical trial of dasatinib in solid tumours have been reported. In a dose-escalation study, 19 patients with solid tumours, including 1 breast cancer patient, were enrolled *(80)*. Patients received dasatinib as oral dose of 35, 50 or 70 mg b.i.d. for 5 days followed by 2 days break, every week. Toxicity included grade 3 lymphopenya, anorexia and elevation of alkaline phosphatase; no dose-limiting toxicity was observed. Of 19 evaluable patients, 5 had SD for a median duration of 3 months whereas no objective response was observed. A pharmacodynamic study showed that, on the b.i.d. regimen, Src phosphorylation was inhibited in a dose-dependent manner, by assessing Src activation in peripheral blood mononuclear cells *(81)*. A phase I study of dasatinib and capecitabine in patients with advanced breast cancer is ongoing.

AZD0530 is a novel, orally active anilinoquinazoline with a high affinity and specificity for the tyrosine kinase domain of Src and Abl, which are inhibited at low nanomolar concentrations of the drug *(82)*. In preclinical studies, AZD0530 was able to inhibit the anchorage-independent growth of MCF-7 breast cancer cells wild-type or stably expressing a mutant

Chapter 11 / Signal Transduction Inhibitors in the Treatment of Breast Cancer 189

ER with increased sensitivity to estrogen *(83)*. However, these effects were reversed by estrogen. A cooperative inhibitory effect was observed when ER+ breast cancer cells were treated with a combination of AZD0530 and tamoxifen, suggesting that therapeutic use of this drug in ER+ breast cancer patients might require blockade of ER signalling *(83)*. Interestingly, AZD0530 also reduced motility and invasion of MCF-7 cells with acquired resistance to tamoxifen *(84)*. MCF-7 cells resistant to tamoxifen display increased levels of EGFR expression as compared with wild-type cells, and an additive effect in inhibition of cell motility and invasion was observed following treatment with a combination of AZD0530 and gefitinib *(84)*. Furthermore, combined treatment of MCF-7 cells with AZD0530 and tamoxifen was found to prevent the emergence of clones with acquired resistance to anti-estrogen therapy *(85)*. Taken together, these findings provide a strong rationale for the development of AZD0530 in ER+ breast cancer patients.

The results of a phase I and pharmacodynamic study of AZD0530 have been recently reported *(86)*. Patients received daily doses of AZD0530 ranging from 50 to 250 mg. The daily dose of 175 mg/die was defined as the maximum tolerated dose. Dose limiting toxicities (DLTs) occurred in three patients at 250 mg [leukopenia; septic shock (grd5) with renal failure; asthenia] and in two patients at 200 mg (febrile neutropenia; dyspnea). Thirteen patients were treated for 12 weeks or more. In agreement with preclinical findings, a consistent modulation of phosphorylation and/or cellular localization of tumour paxillin and FAK, two targets of Src tyrosine kinase, was observed in patients treated with AZD0530. Finally, AZD0530 therapy produced a significant decrease in markers of osteoclast-mediated bone resorption with a dose response trend.

Bosutinib (SKI-606) is an orally active inhibitor of Abl and Src kinases. Treatment of MDA-MB-231 breast cancer cells with bosutinib produced a marked inhibition of cell proliferation, invasion and migration, as well as a significant inhibition of MAPK and AKT activation *(87)*. Bosutinib also efficiently blocked the in vivo growth of MDA-MB-231 cells, and this phenomenon was associated with significant reduction in Src phosphorylation at Tyr416 *(87)*. In a phase I study of bosutinib, the MTD was found at 500 mg/die once daily *(88)*. However, the recommended dose for phase II studies was 400 mg, due to significant grade 2 gastrointestinal toxicity observed in patients treated with 500 mg. The most frequent adverse effects were nausea, diarrhoea, anorexia, asthenia and vomiting. Stabilization of the disease for more than 24 weeks was observed in 3/51 patients, including one breast cancer patient. Bosutinib as monotherapy is currently in phase II study in patients with advanced or metastatic breast cancer.

A number of MEK inhibitors are in preclinical and clinical development in different tumour types. Data in breast cancer are available only for *AZD6244 (ARRY-142886)*, a highly specific MEK 1/2 inhibitor *(89)*. This drug binds to the allosteric inhibitor binding site and locks MEK 1/2 in an inactive conformation. The IC50 value of AZD6244 against purified constitutively activated MEK 1 and 2 is about 14 nM *(89)*. This drug has no inhibitory effects on several serine/threonine and tyrosine kinases up to doses of 10 μM *(89)*. Preclinical studies have evaluated the sensitivity of a wide panel of cancer cell lines, including breast cancer cells, to AZD6244 *(89,90)*. Tumour cells carrying activating Ras and/or B-Raf mutations were found to be more sensitive to AZD6244 as compared with those possessing wild-type genes. For example, SK-Br-3, MDA-MB-468, BT-474 and Zr-75-1 breast cancer cells that have Ras and Raf wild-type genes are relatively resistant to AZD6244, whereas MDA-MB-231 cells, which carries KRas and B-Raf mutations, are moderately sensitive *(89,90)*. However, AZD6244 was found to inhibit the in vivo growth of ZR-75-1 xenografts despite little effects on cell viability in vitro. The efficacy of AZD6244 observed in this tumour models might be due, in part, to in vivo inhibition of angiogenesis *(89)*. It is also possible that in vivo tumour growth is more sensitive to MEK inhibition due to the interactions between tumour and host factors that might affect the levels of activation and the role of MEK 1/2 in tumour growth.

In a phase I clinical trial, 57 patients with solid tumour, including breast cancer, were enrolled *(91)*. Most of the patients had received prior chemotherapic treatments, radiation or surgery. Patients were treated with AZD6244 as oral doses of 50, 100, 200 and 300 mg b.i.d./ die. The most frequent side effects were acne-form rash, diarrhoea, nausea and fatigue. The toxicity was dose dependent and resolution occurred with dose reduction and/or interruption of treatment. AZD6244 was well tolerated up to 100 mg b.i.d.. Complete inhibition of MAPK phosphorylation in peripheral blood mononuclear cells (PBMCs) was observed 1 h after drug administration. Up to 90% inhibition of MAPK phosphorylation was seen in the samples on day 15 or 22, indicating that target inhibition was maintained throughout the b.i.d. dosing regimen and suggesting that PBMC pMAPK might be a biomarker of MEK1/2 inhibition. Analyses of paired tumour samples collected before and after treatment showed that treatment with AZD6244 produced a significant inhibition of MAPK phosphorylation in tumour tissue. Ki-67 labelling index was also reduced in these samples but not as consistently as pMAPK. The best clinical response was SD, lasted for 5 or more months in nine patients (16%). In this small cohort of patients no correlation was found between activity of AZD6244 and mutational status of Ras or Raf. Phase II clinical trials are ongoing.

6. ENDOCRINE THERAPY IN COMBINATION WITH SIGNALLING INHIBITORS

Despite improvements in the efficacy of endocrine therapy for breast cancer, the occurrence of de novo or acquired endocrine resistance represents the major limit of this therapeutic approach. Preclinical and clinical studies have demonstrated that activation of growth factor-driven signalling pathways mediates both the intrinsic and acquired resistance to endocrine agents. These mechanisms have been extensively reviewed by our group in a recent publication and therefore they will be briefly summarized in the next paragraphs *(2)*. More importantly, the results of preclinical studies provided the rationale for clinical investigation of combinations of different inhibitors with anti-estrogen agents with the aim to prevent the emergence of resistance or to restore anti-hormone responsiveness in resistant cells. The results of some of these trials have been recently reported and these findings are commented (Table 5).

Increased levels of expression of EGFR and/or ErbB-2 and increased sensitivity to anti-EGFR agents have been found in breast cancer cell lines with acquired resistance to tamoxifen and to fulvestrant, as well as in estrogen-dependent cells cultured for long term in absence of estrogen, an in vitro condition that resembles anti-estrogen therapy in vivo *(92,93)*. Breast cancer xenografts in immunocompromised mice with acquired resistance to letrozole have been recently established *(94)*. These tumours also showed increased EGFR/ ErbB-2 signalling and increased response to the EGFR-TKI gefitinib *(94)*. In addition, it has been shown that treatment of breast cancer cells with combinations of anti-EGFR and/or anti-ErbB-2 drugs and endocrine agents prevents the occurrence of resistant clones *(95,96)*. Finally, increased levels of EGFR and/or ErbB-2 have been shown to be associated with reduced effects of tamoxifen, particularly in the ER+/PR-subgroup of breast cancer patients *(97)*. A number of trials of gefitinib and erlotinib in combination with anti-estrogen agents in breast cancer patients have been planned.

Two trials of preoperative gefitinib in combination with anastrozole have been reported. In a randomized phase II clinical trial, Polychronis et al. *(98)* enrolled 56 postmenopausal patients with ER+ and EGFR+ primary untreated breast cancer. Of 56 patients, 29 received

Table 5
Summary of clinical trials of EGFR-TKIs in combination with endocrine therapy in breast cancer

Drug	Trial design	N. pts	ORR (%)	CBR (%)	PFS (months)	Reference	Notes
Gefitinib	Gefitinib + anastrozole vs. gefitinib + placebo	56	50			(98)	Preoperative
			54				
	(A) gefitinib + anastrozole for 16 weeks	206	48 (A + B)			(99)	Preoperative
	(B) placebo + anastrozole for 2 weeks then gefitinib + anastrozole for 14 weeks						
	(C) placebo + anastrozole for 16 weeks		61 (C)				
	Gefitinib + anastrozole	15	0			(100)	MBC
	Gefitinib + anastrozole vs. placebo + anastrozole	93	2	49	14.5[a]	(101)	MBC
			12	34	8.2		
	Gefitinib + tamoxifen vs. placebo + tamoxifen	206[b]	12.4	50.5	10.9	(102)	MBC
		84[c]	14.9	45.5	8.8		
			0	29.2	5.7		
			0	31.4	7.0		
Erlotinib	Erlotinib + letrozole	22	25	55	13[d]	(103)	MBC

Abbreviations: CBR, clinical benefit rate; MBC, metastatic breast cancer; ORR, objective response rate; PFS, median progression-free survival
[a]Hazard ratio 0.55, 95% CI 0.32–0.94
[b]Patients with newly diagnosed metastatic breast cancer or completed adjuvant tamoxifen at least 1 year before study entry
[c]Metastatic breast cancer following adjuvant aromatase inhibitor or failed first-line aromatase inhibitor treatment
[d]TTP, median time to progression

once daily administration of gefitinib (250 mg) and anastrozole (1 mg), and 27 received once daily administration of gefitinib (250 mg) and placebo. Treatment was given for 4–6 weeks or until disease progression, unacceptable toxic effects or withdrawal of consent. Treatment was well tolerated in both groups. Patients assigned to receive gefitinib and anastrozole had a greater reduction of Ki67 labelling index as compared with those receiving gefitinib and placebo. Ultrasonography revealed a significant decrease of tumour mass (PR) in 50% of patients treated with gefitinib and anastrozole, and in 54% of patients who received gefitinib as single agent. The activation of EGFR and MAPK and the levels of ser118 phosphorylation of ER were also significantly reduced in both groups.

In contrast, in a neoadjuvant randomized phase II clinical trial, Smith et al. *(99)* enrolled 206 patients with stage from I to IIIB breast cancer and ER+ and/or PR+ tumours. All patients received daily anastrozole (1 mg) for 16 weeks. Patients were divided in three arms: arm A (*n* = 31) also received daily gefitinib (250 mg); arm B (*n* = 90) received placebo for 2 weeks followed by gefitinib (250 mg) for 14 weeks; arm C (*n* = 85) received placebo for 16 weeks. About 13% and 2% of patients, receiving gefitinib and anastrozole or anastrozole alone, respectively, discontinued treatment because of adverse events. Neither biological nor clinical activity of anastrozole was enhanced by the addition of gefitinib. There was no significant change of Ki67 labelling index in patients who received anastrozole and gefitinib as compared with those treated with anastrozole alone. Moreover, the addition of gefitinib after 2 weeks of anastrozole did not further suppress Ki67 labelling index. The overall objective response rate for anastrozole and gefitinib was 48% compared with 61% for anastrozole alone. It must be emphasized that this trial, in contrast to Polychronis' study, did not require EGFR positivity as inclusion criteria. Post-study evaluation of EGFR revealed that only one of the patients enrolled in the trial expressed low levels of EGFR protein.

A phase II study of gefitinib plus anastrozole in patients with ER+ advanced breast cancer, who had previously failed hormonal therapy, found no clinical benefit of the combination *(100)*. Of 15 patients receiving once daily gefitinib (250 mg) and anastrozole (1 mg), none showed a strong anti-tumour activity lasting more than 6 months. In contrast, positive findings of the gefitinib/anastrozole combination as first line treatment of metastatic breast cancer were recently reported. A phase II randomized trial of anastrozole plus gefinitib versus anastrozole plus placebo enrolled a total of 94 women with newly diagnosed metastatic breast cancer *(101)*. Patients were randomized to receive anastrozole 1 mg/die and either gefitinib 250 mg/die or placebo. A significant increase in progression-free survival was seen for anastrozole plus gefitinib over the anastrozole plus placebo arm (hazard ratio 0.55, 95% CI 0.32–0.94, median 14.5 m vs. 8.2 m). An advantage in the clinical benefit rate was also observed for anastrozole plus gefitinib (49% vs. 34%). Treatment-related adverse events were reported in 79% of patients in the anastrozole plus gefitinib arm versus 38% in the anastrozole plus placebo arm and were mostly mild.

The results of a phase II, randomized, double-blind, stratified, multi-centre trial of gefitinib or placebo in combination with tamoxifen in ER+ and/or PR+ metastatic breast cancer patients have been reported *(102)*. Two patient populations were enrolled: in stratum 1 (S1), patients had newly diagnosed metastatic breast cancer or had completed adjuvant tamoxifen at least 1 year before study entry; patients in stratum 2 (S2) developed metastatic breast cancer following adjuvant aromatase inhibitor or had failed first-line aromatase inhibitor treatment. Two hundred six patients and eighty-four patients were enrolled in S1 and in S2, respectively. In S1, the PFS hazard ratio (HR) of gefitinib to placebo was 0.84 (95% confidence interval [CI] 0.59, 1.18; $p = 0.31$; median PFS 10.9 vs. 8.8 months). CBR were 50.5% (53/105) among patients treated with tamoxifen + gefitinib and 45.5% (46/101) in the tamoxifen + placebo group; objective response rates were 12.4% (13/105) and 14.9%

(15/101), respectively. In S2, CBR were 29.2% (14/48) for tamoxifen + gefitinib and 31.4% (11/35) for the tamoxifen + placebo (odds ratio 0.72, 95% CI 0.26, 1.95; $p = 0.52$) and no patient showed an objective response. In S2, the PFS HR for gefitinib to placebo was 1.16 (95% CI 0.69, 1.93; $p = 0.58$; median PFS 5.7 vs. 7.0 months). Patients treated with tamoxifen + gefitinib showed higher incidences of serious adverse events (26% vs. 15%) as compared with tamoxifen + placebo. Although the increase in PFS of S1 met the predefined success criteria (increase in PFS $\geq$ 5%), the overall results of this trial are definitely disappointing.

Finally, the combination of erlotinib and letrozole was evaluated as first or second line therapy in a phase II clinical trial that enrolled 22 metastatic breast cancer patients *(103)*. All patients received erlotinib (150 mg/die) and letrozole (2.5 mg/die) until disease progression. The treatment was well tolerated. Among the 20 evaluable patients, 1 had a complete response (CR), 4 had PR and 6 had SD for 13 months; 11 patients were still on treatment at the time the data were reported. EGFR status did not correlate with clinical response.

Trials of combinations of anti-ErbB-2 agents (herceptin and lapatinib) and endocrine therapies are ongoing. In a phase II clinical trial in patients with ER+/ErbB-2+ metastatic breast cancer, the combination of letrozole and trastuzumab produced a CBR (PR + SD) of 50%, which is similar to the efficacy of trastuzumab alone in previously untreated patients *(104)*. A phase III trial showed a significant improvement of the progression-free survival in metastatic breast cancer patients treated with the combination of herceptin plus anastrozole over anastrozole alone (4.8 vs. 2.4 months) *(105)*. No difference in overall survival were reported. This might be due to the cross-over of the patients who progressed in the anastrozole arm to the combination arm. However, these results have been questioned due to the low activity reported for anastrozole as single agent in this trial.

Preclinical studies have suggested that both farnesyltransferase inhibitors and mTOR inhibitors have a synergistic anti-tumour effect when combined with endocrine therapies *(69,106)*. However, phase II trials of FTIs plus letrozole versus letrozole alone in tamoxifen resistant tumours failed to demonstrate any advantage of the combination *(107)*. A phase II study of letrozole alone or in combination with temsirolimus 10 mg daily or 30 mg intermittently (daily for 5 days every 2 weeks) has also been reported *(108)*. Preliminary results suggested a benefit to the combination with intermittent temsirolimus in terms of median PFS (13.2 months vs. 11.6 months) and survival (90% vs. 76%). However, a large phase III randomized trial of letrozole +/− temsirolimus was terminated early after an interim analysis demonstrated a lack of benefit for the combination *(109)*.

Phase II trials of the anti-VEGF monoclonal antibody bevacizumab or anti-VEGFR tyrosine kinase inhibitors in combination with endocrine therapy are ongoing. Preliminary results of a phase II trial of bevacizumab and letrozole suggested a modest anti-tumour activity of this combination *(110)*.

7. CONCLUSIONS

Although preclinical studies have shown that different signalling inhibitors are able to efficiently block the in vitro and in vivo growth of breast cancer cells, clinical trials have demonstrated little activity of these drugs, at least when used as monotherapy. Similarly, evidence suggests that increased growth factor-driven signalling is involved in the de novo and acquired resistance of breast cancer cells to endocrine therapies. In particular, different preclinical studies have suggested that combination of endocrine therapy and signalling inhibitors can efficiently block the growth of breast cancer cells with resistance to endocrine agents. Based on these preclinical data, numerous clinical trials have been initiated including randomized trials. The preliminary results of these studies are rather disappointing with no clear improvement of the efficacy by adding signalling inhibitors to endocrine therapy.

Cancer is the result of several, different genetic and epigenetic alterations. Co-expression of different growth factors and growth factor receptors has been demonstrated in breast cancer. Furthermore, activation of different signalling pathways has been shown in breast cancer cells, and this phenomenon might be significantly altered by treatment with anti-cancer agents, including target-based agents and endocrine therapies. For example, we found that treatment of breast cancer cells with a combination of gefitinib and a MEK inhibitor induced in breast cancer cells a compensative response that led to increased activation of AKT and to MAPK-independent phosphorylation of BAD in serine 112 *(46)*. It has also been demonstrated that an ErbB-2/ErbB-3/AKT pathway is involved in the resistance of ErbB-2 overexpressing breast cancer cells to EGFR TKIs *(49)*. However, when these cells are exposed to EGFR TKIs for several weeks, the levels of activation of ErbB-3 start to decrease, the levels of activation of MAPK increase and breast cancer cells become more dependent on the MAPK pathway *(50)*. Furthermore, gene expression profiling of both fulvestrant- and tamoxifen-resistant breast cancer cells showed that in both cell lines resistance to endocrine therapy is characterized by significant upregulation of multiple growth-stimulatory pathways, a phenomenon that was more pronounced in fulvestrant resistant cells *(111)*. Interestingly, estrogen receptor signalling has been shown to mediate the resistance of cells that express both the estrogen receptor and ErbB-2 to the dual EGFR/ErbB-2 inhibitor lapatinib *(96)*. Finally, tamoxifen resistant cells have been shown to respond to the EGFR TKI gefitinib *(92)*. However, long-term exposure of these cells to gefitinib leads to resistance to EGFR TKIs through the activation of an IGF/PKC/AKT pathway *(47)*.

Taken together, the above mentioned findings clearly demonstrate that the redundancy of oncogenic pathways activated in cancer cells, the heterogeneity that has been found among primary tumours and cell lines, and the plasticity of tumour cells that are capable to adapt to different growth conditions, significantly hamper the efficacy of signalling inhibitors in breast cancer cells. In this respect, the molecular characterization of the tumours of each individual patient and the identification of biological markers that are associated with response or resistance to treatment are mandatory to improve the efficacy of target-based agents in breast cancer. The finding that the molecular profile of the tumour might change during the time under the pressure of therapeutic agents that select for clones of cells with acquired resistance, underscores the need to develop novel techniques to monitor the molecular profile of the tumour during the time. In conclusion, a comprehensive approach to the complex molecular alterations that characterize the different subtypes of breast carcinoma is necessary to improve the efficacy of target-based therapy.

REFERENCES

1. Sorlie T, Perou CM, Tibshirani R, et al. Gene expression patterns of breast carcinomas distinguish tumor subclasses with clinical implications. Proc Natl Acad Sci U S A 2001;98(19):10869–74.
2. Normanno N, Di Maio M, De Maio E, et al. Mechanisms of endocrine resistance and novel therapeutic strategies in breast cancer. Endocr Relat Cancer 2005;12(4):721–47.
3. Nanda R. Targeting the human epidermal growth factor receptor 2 (HER2) in the treatment of breast cancer: recent advances and future directions. Rev Recent Clin Trials 2007;2(2):111–6.

Chapter 11 / Signal Transduction Inhibitors in the Treatment of Breast Cancer   195

4. Normanno N, Bianco C, Strizzi L, et al. The ErbB receptors and their ligands in cancer: an overview. Curr Drug Targets 2005;6(3):243–57.
5. Olayioye MA, Neve RM, Lane HA, Hynes NE. The ErbB signaling network: receptor heterodimerization in development and cancer. Embo J 2000;19(13):3159–67.
6. Salomon DS, Brandt R, Ciardiello F, Normanno N. Epidermal growth factor-related peptides and their receptors in human malignancies. Crit Rev Oncol Hematol 1995;19(3):183–232.
7. Normanno N, Bianco C, De Luca A, Maiello MR, Salomon DS. Target-based agents against ErbB receptors and their ligands: a novel approach to cancer treatment. Endocr Relat Cancer 2003;10(1):1–21.
8. Reis-Filho JS, Tutt AN. Triple negative tumours: a critical review. Histopathology 2008;52(1):108–18.
9. DiGiovanna MP, Stern DF, Edgerton SM, Whalen SG, Moore D, 2nd, Thor AD. Relationship of epidermal growth factor receptor expression to ErbB-2 signaling activity and prognosis in breast cancer patients. J Clin Oncol 2005;23(6):1152–60.
10. Wiseman SM, Makretsov N, Nielsen TO, et al. Coexpression of the type 1 growth factor receptor family members HER-1, HER-2, and HER-3 has a synergistic negative prognostic effect on breast carcinoma survival. Cancer 2005;103(9):1770–7.
11. Normanno N, Bianco C, De Luca A, Salomon DS. The role of EGF-related peptides in tumor growth. Front Biosci 2001;6:D685–707.
12. Nicholson RI, Staka C, Boyns F, Hutcheson IR, Gee JM. Growth factor-driven mechanisms associated with resistance to estrogen deprivation in breast cancer: new opportunities for therapy. Endocr Relat Cancer 2004;11(4):623–41.
13. Downward J. Targeting RAS signalling pathways in cancer therapy. Nat Rev Cancer 2003;3(1):11–22.
14. Dunn KL, Espino PS, Drobic B, He S, Davie JR. The Ras-MAPK signal transduction pathway, cancer and chromatin remodeling. Biochem Cell Biol 2005;83(1):1–14.
15. Bos JL. ras oncogenes in human cancer: a review. Cancer Res 1989;49(17):4682–9.
16. Hollestelle A, Elstrodt F, Nagel JH, Kallemeijn WW, Schutte M. Phosphatidylinositol-3-OH kinase or RAS pathway mutations in human breast cancer cell lines. Mol Cancer Res 2007;5(2):195–201.
17. Liu W, Bagaitkar J, Watabe K. Roles of AKT signal in breast cancer. Front Biosci 2007;12:4011–9.
18. Crowder RJ, Ellis MJ. Treating breast cancer through novel inhibitors of the phosphatidylinositol 3'-kinase pathway. Breast Cancer Res 2005;7(5):212–4.
19. Ali IU, Schriml LM, Dean M. Mutational spectra of PTEN/MMAC1 gene: a tumor suppressor with lipid phosphatase activity. J Natl Cancer Inst 1999;91(22):1922–32.
20. Vivanco I, Sawyers CL. The phosphatidylinositol 3-Kinase AKT pathway in human cancer. Nat Rev Cancer 2002;2(7):489–501.
21. Bianco R, Shin I, Ritter CA, et al. Loss of PTEN/MMAC1/TEP in EGF receptor-expressing tumor cells counteracts the antitumor action of EGFR tyrosine kinase inhibitors. Oncogene 2003;22(18):2812–22.
22. She QB, Solit D, Basso A, Moasser MM. Resistance to gefitinib in PTEN-null HER-overexpressing tumor cells can be overcome through restoration of PTEN function or pharmacologic modulation of constitutive phosphatidylinositol 3'-kinase/Akt pathway signaling. Clin Cancer Res 2003;9(12):4340–6.
23. Forbes S, Clements J, Dawson E, et al. Cosmic 2005. Br J Cancer 2006;94(2):318–22.
24. Karakas B, Bachman KE, Park BH. Mutation of the PIK3CA oncogene in human cancers. Br J Cancer 2006;94(4):455–9.

25. Sinclair CS, Rowley M, Naderi A, Couch FJ. The 17q23 amplicon and breast cancer. Breast Cancer Res Treat 2003;78(3):313–22.
26. Yeatman TJ. A renaissance for SRC. Nat Rev Cancer 2004;4(6):470–80.
27. Irby RB, Yeatman TJ. Role of Src expression and activation in human cancer. Oncogene 2000;19(49):5636–42.
28. Maa MC, Leu TH, McCarley DJ, Schatzman RC, Parsons SJ. Potentiation of epidermal growth factor receptor-mediated oncogenesis by c-Src: implications for the etiology of multiple human cancers. Proc Natl Acad Sci U S A 1995;92(15):6981–5.
29. Dimri M, Naramura M, Duan L, et al. Modeling breast cancer-associated c-Src and EGFR overexpression in human MECs: c-Src and EGFR cooperatively promote aberrant three-dimensional acinar structure and invasive behavior. Cancer Res 2007;67(9):4164–72.
30. Larue L, Bellacosa A. Epithelial-mesenchymal transition in development and cancer: role of phosphatidylinositol 3' kinase/AKT pathways. Oncogene 2005;24(50):7443–54.
31. Ferrara N, Kerbel RS. Angiogenesis as a therapeutic target. Nature 2005;438 (7070):967–74.
32. Kowanetz M, Ferrara N. Vascular endothelial growth factor signaling pathways: therapeutic perspective. Clin Cancer Res 2006;12(17):5018–22.
33. De Luca A, Carotenuto A, Rachiglio A, et al. The role of the EGFR signaling in tumor microenvironment. J Cell Physiol 2008;214(3):559–67.
34. Morabito A, De Maio E, Di Maio M, Normanno N, Perrone F. Tyrosine kinase inhibitors of vascular endothelial growth factor receptors in clinical trials: current status and future directions. Oncologist 2006;11(7):753–64.
35. Marty M, Pivot X. The potential of anti-vascular endothelial growth factor therapy in metastatic breast cancer: clinical experience with anti-angiogenic agents, focusing on bevacizumab. Eur J Cancer 2008;44(7):912–20.
36. Moasser MM, Basso A, Averbuch SD, Rosen N. The tyrosine kinase inhibitor ZD1839 ('Iressa') inhibits HER2-driven signaling and suppresses the growth of HER2-overexpressing tumor cells. Cancer Res 2001;61(19):7184–8.
37. Normanno N, Campiglio M, De Luca A, et al. Cooperative inhibitory effect of ZD1839 (Iressa) in combination with trastuzumab (Herceptin) on human breast cancer cell growth. Ann Oncol 2002;13(1):65–72.
38. Campiglio M, Locatelli A, Olgiati C, et al. Inhibition of proliferation and induction of apoptosis in breast cancer cells by the epidermal growth factor receptor (EGFR) tyrosine kinase inhibitor ZD1839 ('Iressa') is independent of EGFR expression level. J Cell Physiol 2004;198(2):259–68.
39. Moulder SL, Yakes FM, Muthuswamy SK, Bianco R, Simpson JF, Arteaga CL. Epidermal growth factor receptor (HER1) tyrosine kinase inhibitor ZD1839 (Iressa) inhibits HER2/neu (erbB2)-overexpressing breast cancer cells in vitro and in vivo. Cancer Res 2001;61(24):8887–95.
40. Ciardiello F, Caputo R, Bianco R, et al. Antitumor effect and potentiation of cytotoxic drugs activity in human cancer cells by ZD-1839 (Iressa), an epidermal growth factor receptor-selective tyrosine kinase inhibitor. Clin Cancer Res 2000;6(5):2053–63.
41. Normanno N, De Luca A, Maiello MR, et al. Epidermal growth factor receptor (EGFR) tyrosine kinase inhibitors in breast cancer: current status and future development. Front Biosci 2005;10:2611–7.
42. Albain KS ER, Gradishar WJ, Hayes DF, Rowinsky E, Hudis C, Pusztai L, Tripathy D, Modi S, Rubi S. Open-label, phase II, multicenter trial of ZD1839 ('Iressa') in patients with advanced breast cancer. Breast Cancer Research and Treatment 2002;76:S33.

43. von Minckwitz G, Jonat W, Fasching P, et al. A multicentre phase II study on gefitinib in taxane- and anthracycline-pretreated metastatic breast cancer. Breast Cancer Res Treat 2005;89(2):165–72.
44. Baselga J, Albanell J, Ruiz A, et al. Phase II and tumor pharmacodynamic study of gefitinib in patients with advanced breast cancer. J Clin Oncol 2005;23(23):5323–33.
45. Robertson JFR, Gutteridge E, Cheung KL, et al. Gefitinib (ZD1839) is active in acquired tamoxifen (TAM)-resistant oestrogen receptor (ER)-positive and ER-negative breast cancer: Results from a phase II study. Proc Am Soc Clin Oncol 2003;22:abstr 23.
46. Normanno N, De Luca A, Maiello MR, et al. The MEK/MAPK pathway is involved in the resistance of breast cancer cells to the EGFR tyrosine kinase inhibitor gefitinib. J Cell Physiol 2006;207(2):420–7.
47. Jones HE, Goddard L, Gee JM, et al. Insulin-like growth factor-I receptor signalling and acquired resistance to gefitinib (ZD1839; Iressa) in human breast and prostate cancer cells. Endocr Relat Cancer 2004;11(4):793–814.
48. Camirand A, Zakikhani M, Young F, Pollak M. Inhibition of insulin-like growth factor-1 receptor signaling enhances growth-inhibitory and proapoptotic effects of gefitinib (Iressa) in human breast cancer cells. Breast Cancer Res 2005;7(4):R570–9.
49. Sergina NV, Rausch M, Wang D, et al. Escape from HER-family tyrosine kinase inhibitor therapy by the kinase-inactive HER3. Nature 2007;445(7126):437–41.
50. Normanno N, Campiglio M, Maiello MR, et al. Breast cancer cells with acquired resistance to the EGFR tyrosine kinase inhibitor gefitinib show persistent activation of MAPK signaling. Breast Cancer Res Treat 2007.
51. Normanno N, De Luca A, Aldinucci D, et al. Gefitinib inhibits the ability of human bone marrow stromal cells to induce osteoclast differentiation: implications for the pathogenesis and treatment of bone metastasis. Endocr Relat Cancer 2005;12(2):471–82.
52. Schaefer G, Shao L, Totpal K, Akita RW. Erlotinib directly inhibits HER2 kinase activation and downstream signaling events in intact cells lacking epidermal growth factor receptor expression. Cancer Res 2007;67(3):1228–38.
53. Guix M, Granja Nde M, Meszoely I, et al. Short preoperative treatment with erlotinib inhibits tumor cell proliferation in hormone receptor-positive breast cancers. J Clin Oncol 2008;26(6):897–906.
54. Dickler MN, Cobleigh MA, Miller KD, Klein PM, Winer EP. Efficacy and safety of erlotinib in patients with locally advanced or metastatic breast cancer. Breast Cancer Res Treat 2008.
55. Wilhelm SM, Carter C, Tang L, et al. BAY 43–9006 exhibits broad spectrum oral antitumor activity and targets the RAF/MEK/ERK pathway and receptor tyrosine kinases involved in tumor progression and angiogenesis. Cancer Res 2004;64(19):7099–109.
56. Moreno-Aspitia A, Hillman DW, Wiesenfeld M, et al. BAY 43-9006 as single oral agent in patients with metastatic breast cancer previously exposed to anthracycline and/or taxane. J Clin Oncol (Meeting Abstracts) 2006;24(18_suppl):577.
57. Bianchi GV, Loibl S, Zamagni C, et al. Phase II multicenter trial of sorafenib in the treatment of patients with metastatic breast cancer. In: Breast Cancer Symposium; 2007; Abstr. 164.
58. Abrams TJ, Murray LJ, Pesenti E, et al. Preclinical evaluation of the tyrosine kinase inhibitor SU11248 as a single agent and in combination with 'standard of care' therapeutic agents for the treatment of breast cancer. Mol Cancer Ther 2003;2(10):1011–21.
59. Murray LJ, Abrams TJ, Long KR, et al. SU11248 inhibits tumor growth and CSF-1R-dependent osteolysis in an experimental breast cancer bone metastasis model. Clin Exp Metastasis 2003;20(8):757–66.

60. Chow LQ, Eckhardt SG. Sunitinib: from rational design to clinical efficacy. J Clin Oncol 2007;25(7):884–96.
61. Burstein HJ, Elias AD, Rugo HS, et al. Phase II study of sunitinib malate, an oral multitargeted tyrosine kinase inhibitor, in patients with metastatic breast cancer previously treated with an anthracycline and a taxane. J Clin Oncol 2008;26(11):1810–6.
62. Wedge SR, Ogilvie DJ, Dukes M, et al. ZD6474 Inhibits Vascular Endothelial Growth Factor Signaling, Angiogenesis, and Tumor Growth following Oral Administration. Cancer Res 2002;62(16):4645–55.
63. Ciardiello F, Caputo R, Damiano V, et al. Antitumor Effects of ZD6474, a Small Molecule Vascular Endothelial Growth Factor Receptor Tyrosine Kinase Inhibitor, with Additional Activity against Epidermal Growth Factor Receptor Tyrosine Kinase. Clin Cancer Res 2003;9(4):1546–56.
64. Ciardiello F, Bianco R, Caputo R, et al. Antitumor activity of ZD6474, a vascular endothelial growth factor receptor tyrosine kinase inhibitor, in human cancer cells with acquired resistance to antiepidermal growth factor receptor therapy. Clin Cancer Res 2004;10(2):784–93.
65. Miller KD, Trigo JM, Wheeler C, et al. A Multicenter Phase II Trial of ZD6474, a Vascular Endothelial Growth Factor Receptor-2 and Epidermal Growth Factor Receptor Tyrosine Kinase Inhibitor, in Patients with Previously Treated Metastatic Breast Cancer. Clin Cancer Res 2005;11(9):3369–76.
66. Boer K, Lang I, Llombart-Cussac A, et al. Vandetanib with docetaxel as second-line treatment for advanced breast cancer: a double-blind, placebo-controlled, randomized Phase II study. San Antonio Breast Cancer Symposium 2007:Abstr 6081.
67. O'Regan RM, Khuri FR. Farnesyl transferase inhibitors: the next targeted therapies for breast cancer? Endocr Relat Cancer 2004;11(2):191–205.
68. Kelland LR, Smith V, Valenti M, et al. Preclinical antitumor activity and pharmacodynamic studies with the farnesyl protein transferase inhibitor R115777 in human breast cancer. Clin Cancer Res 2001;7(11):3544–50.
69. Martin LA, Head JE, Pancholi S, et al. The farnesyltransferase inhibitor R115777 (tipifarnib) in combination with tamoxifen acts synergistically to inhibit MCF-7 breast cancer cell proliferation and cell cycle progression in vitro and in vivo. Mol Cancer Ther 2007;6(9):2458–67.
70. Johnston SR, Hickish T, Ellis P, et al. Phase II study of the efficacy and tolerability of two dosing regimens of the farnesyl transferase inhibitor, R115777, in advanced breast cancer. J Clin Oncol 2003;21(13):2492–9.
71. Liu M, Bryant MS, Chen J, et al. Antitumor Activity of SCH 66336, an Orally Bioavailable Tricyclic Inhibitor of Farnesyl Protein Transferase, in Human Tumor Xenograft Models and Wap-ras Transgenic Mice. Cancer Res 1998;58(21):4947–56.
72. Stephens TC, Wardleworth MJ, Matusiak ZS, et al. AZD3409, a novel, oral, prenyl transferase inhibitor with promising preclinical antitumour activity. Proc Am Ass Cancer Res 2003;44:970.
73. Wakeling AE. Inhibitors of growth factor signalling. Endocr Relat Cancer 2005;12(Supplement_1):S183–7.
74. Khafagy R, Stephens T, Hart C, Ramani V, Brown M, Clarke N. In vitro effects of the prenyl transferase inhibitor AZD3409 on prostate cancer epithelial cells. J Clin Oncol (Meeting Abstracts) 2004;22(14_suppl):4744.
75. Maiello MR, D'Alessio A, De Luca A, et al. AZD3409 inhibits the growth of breast cancer cells with intrinsic resistance to the EGFR tyrosine kinase inhibitor gefitinib. Breast Cancer Res Treat 2007;102(3):275–82.

Chapter 11 / Signal Transduction Inhibitors in the Treatment of Breast Cancer   199

76. Appels NM, Bolijn MJ, Chan K, et al. Phase I pharmacokinetic and pharmacodynamic study of the prenyl transferase inhibitor AZD3409 in patients with advanced cancer. Br J Cancer 2008;98(12):1951–8.

77. Lombardo LJ, Lee FY, Chen P, et al. Discovery of N-(2-chloro-6-methyl- phenyl)-2-(6-(4-(2-hydroxyethyl)- piperazin-1-yl)-2-methylpyrimidin-4- ylamino)thiazole-5-carboxamide (BMS-354825), a dual Src/Abl kinase inhibitor with potent antitumor activity in preclinical assays. J Med Chem 2004;47(27):6658–61.

78. Huang F, Reeves K, Han X, et al. Identification of candidate molecular markers predicting sensitivity in solid tumors to dasatinib: rationale for patient selection. Cancer Res 2007;67(5):2226–38.

79. Finn RS, Dering J, Ginther C, et al. Dasatinib, an orally active small molecule inhibitor of both the src and abl kinases, selectively inhibits growth of basal-type/'triple-negative' breast cancer cell lines growing in vitro. Breast Cancer Res Treat 2007;105(3):319–26.

80. Evans TRJ, Morgan JA, van den Abbeele AD, et al. Phase I dose-escalation study of the SRC and multi-kinase inhibitor BMS-354825 in patients (pts) with GIST and other solid tumors. J Clin Oncol (Meeting Abstracts) 2005;23(16_suppl):3034.

81. Luo FR, Luo FR, Barrett Y, et al. Dasatinib (BMS-354825) pharmacokinetics correlate with pSRC pharmacodynamics in phase I studies of patients with cancer (CA180002, CA180003). J Clin Oncol (Meeting Abstracts) 2006;24(18_suppl):3046.

82. Hennequin LF, Allen J, Breed J, et al. N-(5-chloro-1,3-benzodioxol-4-yl)-7-[2-(4-methylpiperazin-1-yl)ethoxy]-5- (tetrahydro-2H-pyran-4-yloxy)quinazolin-4-amine, a novel, highly selective, orally available, dual-specific c-Src/Abl kinase inhibitor. J Med Chem 2006;49(22):6465–88.

83. Herynk MH, Beyer AR, Cui Y, et al. Cooperative action of tamoxifen and c-Src inhibition in preventing the growth of estrogen receptor-positive human breast cancer cells. Mol Cancer Ther 2006;5(12):3023–31.

84. Hiscox S, Morgan L, Green TP, Barrow D, Gee J, Nicholson RI. Elevated Src activity promotes cellular invasion and motility in tamoxifen resistant breast cancer cells. Breast Cancer Res Treat 2006;97(3):263–74.

85. Hiscox S, Green TP, Smith C, Jordan N, James M, Nicholson R. Effectiveness of the dual specific Src/Abl kinase inhibitor AZD0530 in combination with tamoxifen in preventing acquired anti-estrogen resistance in breast cancer cells. J Clin Oncol (Meeting Abstracts) 2007;25(18_suppl):14054.

86. Tabernero J, Cervantes A, Hoekman K, et al. Phase I study of AZD0530, an oral potent inhibitor of Src kinase: First demonstration of inhibition of Src activity in human cancers. J Clin Oncol (Meeting Abstracts) 2007;25(18_suppl):3520.

87. Jallal H, Valentino M-L, Chen G, Boschelli F, Ali S, Rabbani SA. A Src/Abl Kinase Inhibitor, SKI-606, Blocks Breast Cancer Invasion, Growth, and Metastasis In vitro and In vivo. Cancer Res 2007;67(4):1580–8.

88. Messersmith WA, Krishnamurthi S, Hewes BA, et al. Bosutinib (SKI-606), a dual Src/Abl tyrosine kinase inhibitor: Preliminary results from a phase 1 study in patients with advanced malignant solid tumors. J Clin Oncol (Meeting Abstracts) 2007;25(18_suppl):3552.

89. Yeh TC, Marsh V, Bernat BA, et al. Biological characterization of ARRY-142886 (AZD6244), a potent, highly selective mitogen-activated protein kinase kinase 1/2 inhibitor. Clin Cancer Res 2007;13(5):1576–83.

90. Davies BR, Logie A, McKay JS, et al. AZD6244 (ARRY-142886), a potent inhibitor of mitogen-activated protein kinase/extracellular signal-regulated kinase kinase 1/2 kinases: mechanism of action in vivo, pharmacokinetic/pharmacodynamic relationship, and potential for combination in preclinical models. Mol Cancer Ther 2007;6(8):2209–19.

91. Adjei AA, Cohen RB, Franklin W, et al. Phase I pharmacokinetic and pharmacodynamic study of the oral, small-molecule mitogen-activated protein kinase kinase 1/2 inhibitor AZD6244 (ARRY-142886) in patients with advanced cancers. J Clin Oncol 2008;26(13):2139–46.

92. Knowlden JM, Hutcheson IR, Jones HE, et al. Elevated levels of epidermal growth factor receptor/c-erbB2 heterodimers mediate an autocrine growth regulatory pathway in tamoxifen-resistant MCF-7 cells. Endocrinology 2003;144(3):1032–44.

93. Martin LA, Farmer I, Johnston SR, Ali S, Marshall C, Dowsett M. Enhanced estrogen receptor (ER) alpha, ERBB2, and MAPK signal transduction pathways operate during the adaptation of MCF-7 cells to long term estrogen deprivation. J Biol Chem 2003;278(33):30458–68.

94. Jelovac D, Sabnis G, Long BJ, Macedo L, Goloubeva OG, Brodie AM. Activation of mitogen-activated protein kinase in xenografts and cells during prolonged treatment with aromatase inhibitor letrozole. Cancer Res 2005;65(12):5380–9.

95. Gee JM, Harper ME, Hutcheson IR, et al. The antiepidermal growth factor receptor agent gefitinib (ZD1839/Iressa) improves antihormone response and prevents development of resistance in breast cancer in vitro. Endocrinology 2003;144(11):5105–17.

96. Xia W, Bacus S, Hegde P, et al. A model of acquired autoresistance to a potent ErbB2 tyrosine kinase inhibitor and a therapeutic strategy to prevent its onset in breast cancer. Proc Natl Acad Sci U S A 2006;103(20):7795–800.

97. Arpino G, Weiss H, Lee AV, et al. Estrogen receptor-positive, progesterone receptor-negative breast cancer: association with growth factor receptor expression and tamoxifen resistance. J Natl Cancer Inst 2005;97(17):1254–61.

98. Polychronis A, Sinnett HD, Hadjiminas D, et al. Preoperative gefitinib versus gefitinib and anastrozole in postmenopausal patients with oestrogen-receptor positive and epidermal-growth-factor-receptor-positive primary breast cancer: a double-blind placebo-controlled phase II randomised trial. Lancet Oncol 2005;6(6):383–91.

99. Smith IE, Walsh G, Skene A, et al. A phase II placebo-controlled trial of neoadjuvant anastrozole alone or with gefitinib in early breast cancer. J Clin Oncol 2007;25(25):3816–22.

100. Mita M, de Bono J, Patnaik A, et al. A phase II and biologic correlative study investigating anastrozole in combination with gefitinib in post menopausal patients with estrogen receptor positive metastatic breast carcinoma who have previously failed hormonal therapy. Breast Cancer Res Treat 2005;94 (Suppl 1):Abstract 1117.

101. Cristofanilli M, Valero V, Mangalik A, et al. A phase II multicenter, double-blind, randomized trial to compare anastrozole plus gefinitib with anastrozole plus placebo in postmenopausal women with hormone receptor-positive (HR) metastatic breast cancer (MBC). J Clin Oncol 2008;26:abstr 1012.

102. Osborne K, Neven P, Dirix L, et al. Randomized Phase II study of gefitinib (IRESSA) or placebo in combination with tamoxifen in patients with hormone receptor positive metastatic breast cancer. San Antonio Breast Cancer Symposium 2007:Abstr 2067.

103. Mayer I, Ganja N, Shyr Y, Muldowney N, Arteaga C. A phase II trial of letrozole plus erlotinib in post-menopausal women with hormone-sensitive metastatic breast cancer: preliminary results of toxicities and correlative studies. Breast Cancer Res Treat 2006;100(Suppl 1):Abstr. 4052.

104. Marcom PK, Isaacs C, Harris L, et al. A phase II trial of letrozole and trastuzumab for ER and/or PgR and HER2 positive metastatic breast cancer: Final results. J Clin Oncol (Meeting Abstracts) 2005;23(16_suppl):596.

Chapter 11 / Signal Transduction Inhibitors in the Treatment of Breast Cancer 201

105. Mackey JR, Kaufman B, Clemens M, et al. Trastuzumab prolongs progression-free survival in hormone-dependent and HER2-positive metastatic breast cancer. Breast Cancer Res Treat 2006;100(Suppl 1):Abstr. 3.
106. Boulay A, Rudloff J, Ye J, et al. Dual inhibition of mTOR and estrogen receptor signaling in vitro induces cell death in models of breast cancer. Clin Cancer Res 2005;11(14):5319–28.
107. Johnston SR, Semiglazov VF, Manikhas GM, et al. A phase II, randomized, blinded study of the farnesyltransferase inhibitor tipifarnib combined with letrozole in the treatment of advanced breast cancer after antiestrogen therapy. Breast Cancer Res Treat 2008;110(2):327–35.
108. Baselga J, Roche H, Fumoleau P, et al. Treatment of postmenopausal women with locally advanced or metastatic breast cancer with letrozole alone or in combination with temsirolimus: a randomized, 3-arm, phase 2 study. Breast Cancer Res Treat 2005;94(Suppl 1):Abstr. 1068.
109. Chow LWC, Sun Y, Jassem J, et al. Phase 3 study of temsirolimus with letrozole or letrozole alone in postmenopausal women with locally advanced or metastatic breast cancer. Breast Cancer Res Treat 2006;100(Suppl 1):Abstr. 6091.
110. Traina TA, Dickler MN, Caravelli JF, et al. A phase II trial of letrozole in combination with bevacizumab, and anti-VEGF antibody in patients with hormone receptor positive metastatic breast cancer. Breast Cancer Res Treat 2005;94(Suppl 1):Abstr. 2030.
111. Fan M, Yan PS, Hartman-Frey C, et al. Diverse Gene Expression and DNA Methylation Profiles Correlate with Differential Adaptation of Breast Cancer Cells to the Antiestrogens Tamoxifen and Fulvestrant. Cancer Res 2006;66(24):11954–66.

12

Integration of Target-Based Agents in Current Protocols of Breast Cancer Therapy

Maria Carmela Piccirillo, Fabiano Falasconi, Antonia Del Giudice, Gianfranco De Feo, Jane Bryce, Mario Iaccarino, Francesco Perrone, and Alessandro Morabito

SUMMARY

Breast cancer is a heterogeneous disease sustained by the dysregulation of numerous molecular pathways, such as cell cycle progression, angiogenesis, and apoptosis. Recent progress in molecular technology has allowed better characterization of the transformed phenotype, identifying molecular features that distinguish tumor from normal tissue and represent rational targets for more selective therapeutic approaches. In this chapter, we focus on the molecular target-based agents in the most advanced state of clinical development in breast cancer. Trastuzumab, a monoclonal antibody with high specificity for the HER2 protein, is the first targeted agent approved for the treatment of metastatic and early breast cancer. Bevacizumab, a monoclonal antibody directed against the VEGF-A ligand, with antiangiogenetic properties, and lapatinib, a dual tyrosine-kinase inhibitor of both EGFR and HER2, have been recently approved for use in the treatment of metastatic breast cancer. Several other compounds directed against different targets have also entered clinical evaluation. Key issues in the clinical development of targeted therapy include the proper selection of patients, the identification of the optimal combinations with conventional treatments, predictive markers of activity and toxicity, and the most appropriate therapeutic strategies.

Key Words: Breast cancer; Targeted therapy; Trastuzumab; Pertuzumab; Lapatinib; Bevacizumab; Sunitinib; Temsirolimus; Everolimus

From: *Current Clinical Oncology: Breast Cancer in the Post-Genomic Era,*
Edited by: A. Giordano and N. Normanno, DOI: 10.1007/978-1-60327-945-1_12,
© Humana Press, a part of Springer Science + Business Media, LLC 2009

1. INTRODUCTION

Worldwide, breast cancer is the most common female tumor and it is the leading cause of cancer deaths. In 2000 alone, more than one million women were diagnosed (22% of all female cancer diagnoses) and 373,000 women died (14% of all cancer deaths among women) of breast cancer *(1)*. Mortality rates have begun to fall in the last 20 years, with a substantial reduction both in middle age (approximately 25%) and, to a lesser extent, in old age. This decrease is due to improvements in awareness and screening as well as in multidisciplinary cancer treatment. Both chemotherapy and hormone therapy have significantly impacted survival of these patients, although therapy for metastatic disease still remains palliative. Recent progress of molecular technology has allowed for a better understanding of the mechanisms sustaining breast cancer transformation and progression, which are characterized by a dysregulation of numerous molecular pathways, such as cell cycle progression, angiogenesis, and apoptosis, each representing rational targets for more selective therapeutic approaches. Target-based agents include antibodies that form complexes with antigens on the surface of cancer cells and small molecules that have been engineered to block key enzymatic reactions. Since these agents are specific for a target that is usually amplified or overexpressed in cancer cells, they generally have fewer side effects than most conventional chemotherapeutic agents and can be combined with conventional chemotherapeutic agents to improve the response to treatment without a major increase in side effects.

In this chapter, we will discuss the target-based agents in the most advanced state of clinical development in breast cancer (Table 1), while the agents that are in preclinical development or in the initial phases of clinical study will be the topic of a separate chapter of this book.

Table 1
Target-based agents in phase III clinical development in breast cancer

Target	Agent	Class and mechanism of action	Setting of development
ErbB receptors	Trastuzumab	Monoclonal antibody against HER2	Advanced, adjuvant, neoadjuvant
	Lapatinib	TK inhibitor of HER2 and EGFR	Advanced, adjuvant, neoadjuvant
	Pertuzumab	Monoclonal antibody against HER2	Advanced
Angiogenesis	Bevacizumab	Monoclonal antibody against VEGF	Advanced, adjuvant
	Sunitinib	TK inhibitor of VEGFRs, PDGFR, c-Kit	Advanced
mTOR	Temsirolimus	Rapamycin analogue inhibitor of mTOR	Advanced
	Everolimus	Rapamycin analogue inhibitor of mTOR	Neoadjuvant

2. TARGETING ERBB RECEPTORS

The human epidermal growth factor receptor (HER) family of receptor tyrosine kinases comprises four members: epidermal growth factor receptor (EGFR; also named HER1 or ErbB1), HER2 (also named ErbB2 or neu), HER3 (ErbB3), and HER4 (ErbB4). Collectively, these are also referred to as the ErbB receptors. ErbB receptors are composed of an extracellular ligand binding domain, a single transmembrane domain, and an intracellular domain with tyrosine kinase activity. Evidence from experimental systems and from primary human breast tumors indicate that ErbB signaling network is involved in the pathogenesis of breast cancer. In particular, EGFR and HER2/neu are overexpressed in approximately 50% and 25% of breast cancers, respectively *(2)*. Their overexpression is associated with an aggressive tumor phenotype, which is characterized by increased cell proliferation, tumor cell motility and invasiveness, angiogenesis, and inhibition of apoptosis *(2)*. In particular, overexpression of HER2/neu identifies a subgroup of patients with aggressive disease, frequently hormone receptor negative and with poor prognosis *(3,4)*. Furthermore, tumor amplification of the HER2 gene has been associated with resistance to a variety of cytotoxic agents and tamoxifen *(5,6)*.

There are two major classes of ErbB receptors inhibitors in advanced clinical evaluation: ectodomain-binding antibodies or monoclonal antibodies (mAbs), such as trastuzumab and pertuzumab, and small molecule tyrosine kinase inhibitors (TKIs) competing with ATP for the tyrosine kinase domain, such as gefitinib, erlotinib, and lapatinib.

2.1. Trastuzumab

Trastuzumab is a humanized monoclonal antibody with high specificity for the HER2 protein. It showed activity as single agent in first- or second-line treatment of HER2 positive metastatic breast cancer *(7–9)*. In a pivotal randomized prospective controlled trial of first-line therapy, 469 HER2 positive metastatic breast cancer patients, who had not received previous treatment for advanced disease, were randomized to receive chemotherapy or chemotherapy plus weekly trastuzumab *(10)*. Patients who had received anthracyclines in the adjuvant setting or who were not suitable to receive anthracyclines ($n = 188$), received 3-weekly paclitaxel. All other patients received an anthracycline plus cyclophosphamide. The addition of trastuzumab to chemotherapy significantly improved all clinical outcomes. Median time to progression was 7.4 months in the combination group, whereas in the group treated with chemotherapy alone it was 4.6 months ($p < 0.001$). Compared with chemotherapy alone, combination treatment was associated with a significantly higher response rate (50% vs. 32%, $p < 0.001$), a longer duration of response (median 9.1 vs. 6.1 months, $p < 0.001$), and a longer time to treatment failure (median 6.9 vs. 4.5 months, $p < 0.001$). The improvement was significant in both the chemotherapy subgroups (either paclitaxel or anthracycline based). Median survival was 25.1 months in the combination group and 20.3 months in the group that received chemotherapy alone ($p = 0.046$). The risk of death was reduced by 18–20% in the arms with trastuzumab, but the result might be diluted as it included patients given chemotherapy alone who received open-label trastuzumab after the occurrence of disease progression. Trastuzumab given in combination with chemotherapy resulted in an increased incidence of anemia, leukopenia, diarrhea, and infections. These events were not severe and might be due to the longer duration of chemotherapy in trastuzumab arms. There was an unacceptable high rate of cardiotoxicity in the subgroup of patients treated concurrently with anthracyclines (27% of patients exhibited a cardiac toxicity that was severe in 16% of cases), which limited the use of such a combination in clinical practice.

The combination of trastuzumab with paclitaxel was well tolerated, also considering cardiac toxicity, which was severe in only 2% of cases. The benefit of combination treatment was supported by a successive analysis of health-related quality of life that revealed a significant improvement in global quality of life for patients receiving trastuzumab and chemotherapy *(11)*.

Several clinical studies have since assessed the efficacy and safety of two-drug combinations of trastuzumab with paclitaxel *(12–16)*, docetaxel *(17–19)*, vinorelbine *(20–25)*, platinum salts *(26)*, gemcitabine *(27)*, capecitabine *(28,29)*, or of three-drug combinations with taxanes and platinum salts as front-line therapy *(30–33)* (Table 2).

The combination of trastuzumab and taxanes is supported by preclinical data demonstrating a synergistic cytotoxicity in breast cancer cell lines. Combinations of trastuzumab and taxanes induce a response rate of 40–75% as first-line therapy *(10,12,16,19)* and a high percentage of objective responses also in pretreated patients *(13–15,17,18)*. Moreover, taking into account the low systemic toxicity and the good tolerability of weekly schedules, weekly taxanes seem to exhibit, at the moment, one of the best therapeutic indexes when associated with trastuzumab. The weekly schedule of administration of both paclitaxel or docetaxel and trastuzumab has been successfully evaluated in several clinical trials *(12,13,15–19)* and offers the potential of improving certain toxicities associated with tri-weekly administration. Weekly schedules of taxanes are characterized by moderate hematological toxicity, allowing their administration for prolonged period of time, and by several non-hematological toxicities, mainly consisting of fatigue, myalgia, and neurotoxicity. Although only combinations with taxanes have been approved, there is interest in developing alternative trastuzumab-based treatment options, because of the increasing use of taxanes in the adjuvant setting. Trastuzumab plus vinorelbine showed one of the most interesting tolerability and activity profiles, with response rates ranging from 50% to 70% in phase II clinical trials of first- or second-line therapy *(20–25)*. The most common toxicity was manageable neutropenia, while few non-hematological toxicities were reported and the incidence of neuropathy was limited. Two clinical trials with the combination of trastuzumab and capecitabine have been published, reporting a response rate of almost 50% in first- or second-line and no overlapping toxicities *(26,27)*. The combinations of trastuzumab and cisplatin or gemcitabine have been evaluated in patients with extensively pretreated metastatic breast cancer only, resulting in a response rate of 24% and 38%, respectively, with a favorable toxicity profile *(28,29)*.

The favorable safety profile exhibited by the combinations of trastuzumab plus single agent chemotherapy prompted researchers to evaluate the addition of the antibody to polychemotherapy. Most of the studies investigated combinations with a taxane and a platinum salt *(30–33)*. This triple combination showed a high response rate, ranging from 65% to 85% in first-line therapy and being more than 50% in second line also. Nevertheless, these regimens induced severe nonhematologic toxicities, including fatigue, nausea, vomiting, and neurotoxicity, which limit the use of such combinations in clinical practice. A randomized study of trastuzumab and paclitaxel versus the same regimen in combination with carboplatin demonstrated an improvement in response rate and time to progression with the triplet association *(33)*. An attractive triplet for taxanes-pretreated patients with HER2 positive tumors is the combination of trastuzumab with gemcitabine and vinorelbine, that has shown, as second-line therapy, a response rate of 50%, increasing to 73.3% in patients with HercepTest 3+ *(34)*. However, further prospective clinical trials need to establish the relative benefit of three-drug versus two-drug combinations.

Another debated question is the opportunity of continuing trastuzumab in combination with a non-cross resistant chemotherapeutic regimen in patients with progressive disease on trastuzumab. Preclinical observations provide some evidence to support the concept of

Table 2
Main phase II–III clinical studies of trastuzumab plus chemotherapy in metastatic breast cancer

Author; reference	Study phase	Trastuzumab	Chemotherapy	Line	# Pts	Median age (mean)	RR (%)	TTP (months)	OS (months)	Cardiotoxicity (%) Any	Severe
Slamon D [10]	Phase III	Weekly	Paclitaxel	1	92	(51)	41[b]	6.9[b]	22.1	13	2
		None	Paclitaxel	1	96	(51)	17	3	18.4	1	1
		Weekly	Doxorubicin (Epirubicin) + Cyclophosphamide	1	143	(54)	56[b]	7.8[a]	26.8	27	16
		None	Doxorubicin (Epirubicin) + Cyclophosphamide	1	138	(54)	42	6.1	21.4	8	3
Fountzilas G [12]	Phase II	Weekly	Paclitaxel weekly	1	34	48	62	9	n.r.	3	–
Seidman AD [13]	Phase II	Weekly	Paclitaxel weekly	1–2	95	51	56.8			10	3
Leyland-Jones B [14]	Phase II	3-weekly	Paclitaxel	1–2	32	53	59	12.2		31	3
Gori S [15]	Phase II	Weekly	Paclitaxel weekly	1–2	25	43	56	8.6	n.r.	8	8
Gasparini G [16] Rand. Phase II		Weekly	Paclitaxel weekly	1	63	56	75	9.9[a]	n.r.	1.7	–
		None	Paclitaxel weekly	1	60	54.3	56.9	6.6[a]	n.r.	1.7	–
Esteva FJ [17]	Phase II	Weekly	Docetaxel weekly	1–2	30	43	63	9		29	3
Tedesco KL [18]	Phase II	Weekly	Docetaxel weekly	1–2	26	53	50	12.4	22.1	8	4
Marty M [19] Rand. Phase II		Weekly	Docetaxel	1	92	53	61	11.7	31.2	17	2.2
		None	Docetaxel	1	94	55	34	6.1	22.7	8	–

(continued)

Table 2
(continued)

Author, reference	Study phase	Trastuzumab	Chemotherapy	Line	# Pts	Median age (mean)	RR (%)	TTP (months)	OS (months)	Cardiotoxicity (%) Any	Cardiotoxicity (%) Severe
Burstein HJ (20)	Phase II	Weekly	Vinorelbine weekly	1–2	40	50	75	n.r.	n.r.	26	–
Jahanzeb M (21)	Phase II	Weekly	Vinorelbine weekly	1	40	51	78	16.6	n.r.	2.5	–
Burstein HJ (22)	Phase II	Weekly	Vinorelbine weekly	1	54	54.5	68			15	2
Chan A (23)	Phase II	Weekly	Vinorelbine weekly	1	69	53	62.9	9.9[a]	23.7	6	1.4
Papaldo P (24)	Phase II	Weekly	Vinorelbine weekly	2–3	35	53	51.4	9	27	20	3
De Maio E (25)	Phase II	3-weekly	Vinorelbine	1–2	50	54	50	9.6[a]	22.7	6	–
Yamamoto D (26)	Phase II		Capecitabine	1–3	59		50			1.7	–
Schaller G (27)	Phase II	Weekly	Capecitabine	1–3	27	54	45	6.7[a]	28	n.r.	4
Pegram MD (28)	Phase II	Weekly	Cisplatin	2–4	39	50	24.3			n.r.	2.6
O'Shaughnessy JA (29)	Phase II	Weekly	Gemcitabine	2–3	64	55	38	5.8	14.7	4/38	–
Burris H (30)	Phase II	Weekly	Paclitaxel Carboplatin (weekly)	1	32	51	84	14.2	32.2	16	3
Pegram MD (31)	Phase II	Weekly	Docetaxel Cisplatin	1–2	62	52	79	9.9	n.r.	12	2
	Phase II	Weekly	Docetaxel Carboplatin	1–2	62	54	58	12.7	n.r.	8	2
Perez EA (32)	Phase II	3-weekly	Paclitaxel Carboplatin	1	43	56	65	9.9	27.6	4.6	–
	Phase II	3-weekly	Paclitaxel Carboplatin (weekly)	1	48	55	81	13.8	38.4	–	–
Robert N (33)	Phase III	Weekly	Paclitaxel Carboplatin	1	98	56	52	10.7[a,b]	35.7	2	2
		Weekly	Paclitaxel	1	98	55	36	7.1[a]	32.2	–	–
Morabito A (34)	Phase II	Weekly	Gemcitabine Vinorelbine	2	30	58	50	7[a]	15	–	–

aPFS; n.r. not reached; bstatistically significative difference

Chapter 12 / Integration of Target-Based Agents in Current Protocols 209

trastuzumab treatment beyond progression (35). However, retrospective analyses of case series have shown conflicting results (36–40). Two recently published phase II clinical trials have evaluated safety and activity of the combination of trastuzumab with capecitabine or gemcitabine, respectively, as salvage therapy in heavily pretreated patients with metastatic breast cancer after earlier trastuzumab exposure (41,42). Both studies showed a moderate activity of the combinations, with a response rate of 20% and a median time to progression of 3 months for gemcitabine and 8 months for capecitabine combinations, respectively. To date, the opportunity of continuing trastuzumab beyond progression remains unknown and needs to be defined with prospective randomized clinical trials.

The evidence that a molecular cross-talk exists between estrogen receptors and HER2 pathway and that HER2 overexpression is associated with preclinical and clinical resistance to hormonal therapy suggested that combining treatments that target both pathways may provide additional benefits for patients with breast cancer (43). A randomized, controlled, open-label phase III trial investigated the efficacy and safety of the combination of trastuzumab and anastrozole versus anastrozole alone as first-line therapy in postmenopausal patients with estrogen receptor (ER) and/or HER2 positive metastatic breast cancer (44). Patients on combination arm achieved significant improvements in progression-free survival (4.8 vs. 2.4 months; $p = 0.0016$), time to progression (4.8 vs. 2.4 months; $p = 0.0007$), and response rate (20.3% vs. 6.8%; $p = 0.018$). It is worth noting that a median time to progression of 2.4 months in the anastrozole-alone arm does not fit with what is expected for a first-line treatment in hormone responsive patients, even for HER2 positive disease. No significantly longer overall survival was reported in the combination arm (28.5 vs. 23.9 months; $p = 0.325$). However, this result includes the crossover of more than half of the patients in the monotherapy arm to receive trastuzumab after progression of disease. The combination of trastuzumab and letrozole, as first- or second-line therapy, has been evaluated in a phase II trial (45) including ER/HER2 positive patients with metastatic breast cancer. An overall response rate of 26% was reported, with a median time to progression of 5.8 months. Responding patients had long remission, lasting longer than 1 year. However, half of the patients experienced early progressive disease. A phase III trial of letrozole with or without trastuzumab as first-line therapy in postmenopausal ER/HER2 positive patients with locally advanced or metastatic breast cancer is ongoing, with time to progression as the primary end point. A phase II trial of trastuzumab and exemestane in the same population has recently been completed. The combination of trastuzumab and fulvestrant is also being studied in a randomized phase II study, while a randomized, open-label phase III trial is comparing trastuzumab plus tamoxifen to tamoxifen alone. Therefore, in the next few years we should know more about the efficacy of the strategy of combining biologic and endocrine therapy in breast cancer.

The proven benefits of trastuzumab therapy in metastatic breast cancer provided the rationale for its use in the adjuvant setting. Four large international randomized phase III clinical studies evaluated the efficacy of adjuvant trastuzumab in women with HER2 positive early breast cancer (Table 3): the Herceptin® Adjuvant (HERA) trial (46), the National Surgical Adjuvant Breast and Bowel Project (NSABP) B-31 trial and the North Central Cancer Treatment Group (NCCTG) N9831 trial, whose results are available as a pooled analysis (47), and the Breast Cancer International Research Group (BCIRG) 006 trial (48). Data from a subgroup in a smaller Finnish study, FinHer, were also available on adjuvant trastuzumab therapy (49). Despite differences in the patient population and design of these studies, all showed similar results, namely, a significant reduction of risk of first event, with an hazard ratio (HR) of 0.46–0.67 for women receiving trastuzumab. Furthermore, the HERA and BCIRG 006 trials and the American joint-analysis also showed improvements in

Table 3

Phase III clinical trials of trastuzumab as adjuvant treatment of early breast cancer patients

Trial	Patients	N	Treatments	DFS HR (95% CI) p	OS HR (95% CI) p
HERA [Piccart-Gebhart MJ (46)]	5,090	N–/N+	Any accepted chemotherapy followed by observation vs. H for 1 year vs. H for 2 years	0.64 (0.54–0.76) p < 0.0001	0.66 (0.47–0.91) p = 0.0115
NSABP B-31 NCCTG N9831 [Romond EH (47)]	3,351	N+ N–/N+	AC → P vs. AC → P + H AC → wP vs. AC → wP + H	0.48 (0.39–0.59) p < 0.0001	0.67 (0.48–0.93) p = 0.015
BCIRG 006 [Slamon D (48)]	3,222	N–/N+	AC → D vs. AC → D + H vs. DCbH	0.61 (0.37–0.65) p < 0.0001 0.67 (0.47–0.79) p = 0.0002	0.59 (0.40–0.85) p = 0.004 0.66 (0.47–0.93) p = 0.0017
FINHER [Joensuu H (49)]	232	N–/N+	D or V ± H → FEC	0.42 (0.21–0.83) p = 0.001	0.41 (0.16–1.08) p = 0.07

N: nodal status; DFS: disease-free survival; H: trastuzumab; AC: adriamycin + cyclophosphamide; P: paclitaxel; wP: weekly paclitaxel; D: docetaxel; V: vinorelbine; FEC: 5-fluorouracil, epirubicin, cyclophosphamide; DCbH: docetaxel + carboplatin + trastuzumab overall survival (reported HR range 0.59–0.67). These results have led to the approval of the use of adjuvant trastuzumab for 1 year.

The HERA trial is a three arm study with more than 5,000 women, who were randomized to 1 year or 2 years of 3-weekly trastuzumab or observation, after completion of adjuvant chemotherapy and radiotherapy. A minimum of four cycles of any standard adjuvant or neoadjuvant chemotherapy were accepted, warranting with this heterogeneity general relevance for clinical results regarding both efficacy and safety of combining trastuzumab with chemotherapy. To date, results of 1 year of trastuzumab versus observation are available *(46)*. After 2 years of follow up, trastuzumab showed a significant benefit in disease-free (HR 0.64, 95% CI 0.54–0.76; $p < 0.0001$) and overall survival (HR 0.66, 95% CI 0.47–0.91; $p = 0.0115$). Results of 1 versus 2 years comparison are awaited, as the optimal duration of trastuzumab adjuvant treatment remains unknown. Nevertheless, the smaller FinHer trial showed, in the subset of HER2 positive patients, that 9 weeks of trastuzumab given concurrently with three cycles of docetaxel or vinorelbine and followed by three cycles of fluorouracil, epirubicin, and cyclophosphamide significantly improve disease-free survival (HR 0.42, 95% CI 0.21–0.83; $p = 0.01$) *(49)*. However, considering the small sample size (232 patients), the wide confidence interval, and the absence of overall survival benefit, confirmatory data are required.

The American NSABP B-31 and NCCTG N9831 trials investigated the addition of 1 year of trastuzumab treatment to the standard adjuvant chemotherapy regimen of doxorubicin plus cyclophosphamide (AC) followed by paclitaxel. The joint-analysis plan compared the two arms that provided trastuzumab beginning on the first cycle of paclitaxel with the two arms without trastuzumab *(47)*. The N9831 had a third arm providing trastuzumab following chemotherapy, which was not included in this analysis. At 2 years of median follow up, patients receiving trastuzumab experienced a significative benefit in terms of both disease-free (HR 0.48, 95% CI 0.39–0.59; $p < 0.0001$) and overall survival (HR 0.67, 95% CI 0.48–0.93; $p = 0.015$). An unplanned analysis, comparing the two trastuzumab arms in the N9831 trial, showed a better disease-free survival for those patients receiving concurrent versus sequential trastuzumab. However, the analysis was not sufficiently powered to draw definite conclusions. A longer follow up will clarify the relative benefit of adding trastuzumab concurrently or sequentially to paclitaxel. Finally, the BCIRG 006 study evaluated the addition of trastuzumab to two different chemotherapy regimens, with and without anthracyclines. The trial had a three-arm design, comparing AC followed by docetaxel with the same chemotherapy plus trastuzumab (AC-DH) and with a regimen of docetaxel and carboplatin plus trastuzumab (DCbH). At a median follow up of 36 months, both trastuzumab arms showed significant longer disease-free survival (HR 0.61, CI 95% 0.37–0.65; $p < 0.0001$ in the AC-DH arm and HR 0.67, CI 95% 0.47–0.79; $p = 0.0002$ in the DCbH arm, respectively) and overall survival (HR 0.59, CI 95% 0.4–0.85; $p = 0.004$ in the AC-DH arm and HR 0.66, CI 95% 0.47–0.93; $p = 0.0017$ in the DCbH arm, respectively) *(48)*. A longer follow up is needed to demonstrate whether efficacy differs between the two trastuzumab arms. Therefore this study, besides demonstrating that trastuzumab is effective when combined with a regimen of AC followed by docetaxel, also showed the efficacy and safety of adding trastuzumab to a non-anthracycline regimen and provided an alternative adjuvant treatment for those women who are unsuitable for receiving anthracyclines. The BCIRG protocol also included a subgroup analysis comparing the efficacy of anthracycline and non-anthracycline regimens according to topoisomerase IIa amplification. The topoisomerase-IIa gene is on the same chromosomal region of HER2 gene (17q21) and it has been suggested that its amplification is a positive marker for efficacy of anthracycline-based chemotherapy *(50)*. Patients whose tumors showed coamplification of HER2 and topoisomerase-IIa genes had a better outcome than those whose did not, when treated with an anthracycline containing regimen. Unfortunately, although two interim analyses were reported at San Antonio Breast Cancer Symposium with contrasting results about the comparison of AC-DH and DCbH arms, quality of life analysis and molecular analysis, no definitive results of the BCIRG 006 study have been published to date. Therefore, caution has to be taken to interpret reported data.

In conclusion, trastuzumab has become a milestone in the adjuvant treatment of HER2 positive early breast cancer but several clinical issues remain to be solved: (1) the optimal duration of trastuzumab treatment; (2) the use of trastuzumab as sequential or concurrent to chemotherapy; (3) the optimal combination regimen in terms of efficacy and safety. Moreover, as the cited adjuvant clinical trials did not enroll women with tumor size less than 1 cm and with low grade of malignancy, trastuzumab treatment advisability remains uncertain for HER2 positive tumor with these favorable prognostic factors. Finally, HER2 positive patients who are not candidates for chemotherapy are still not candidates for trastuzumab, since to date there is no evidence for the addition of the antibody to hormonal adjuvant treatment or for an exclusive trastuzumab adjuvant treatment.

2.2. Pertuzumab

Pertuzumab is a humanized recombinant monoclonal antibody directed against the extracellular dimerization domain of the HER2 receptor. This antibody directly inhibits the dimerization of the HER2 protein with other HER family receptors thus preventing the activation of HER signaling pathways and resulting in tumor cell apoptosis. The different and potentially complementary mechanism of action is the rationale for associating pertuzumab with trastuzumab *(51)*. These two monoclonal antibodies have been combined in a phase II study as treatment of locally advanced or metastatic heavily pretreated patients with HER2 positive breast cancer, whose disease had progressed during trastuzumab therapy. Early results have shown activity of this combination *(52)*. Out of 33 enrolled patients, 1 had a complete response, 5 had partial responses (response rate of 18.2%), and further 7 patients achieved a stabilization of disease lasting 6 months or more (21.2%). On the basis of the encouraging phase II data, phase III trials are evaluating the effectiveness of pertuzumab in combination with trastuzumab and chemotherapy as first-line therapy in metastatic disease.

2.3. Lapatinib

Lapatinib is an oral, dual tyrosine-kinase inhibitor of both EGFR and HER2. In preclinical studies lapatinib determined growth inhibition, in vitro and in vivo, in a variety of human tumor cell lines overexpressing either EGFR or HER2, including breast cancer *(53)*. Early clinical trials provided evidence that lapatinib is active against EGFR expressing and/or HER2 overexpressing heavily pretreated breast cancer *(54,55)*. Two phase II trials of lapatinib as single agent were conducted in patients with refractory metastatic breast cancer *(56,57)*. The first trial enrolled HER2 positive breast cancer patients with progressive disease after prior trastuzumab. In the second trial, patients who had received prior anthracyclines, taxanes, and capecitabine were distributed in two cohorts according to their positivity or negativity for HER2. Both studies showed activity of lapatinib in this unfavorable setting, with a disease control rate of 22% and 15.7%, respectively. A combined biomarker analysis was conducted for these studies to determine clinical or biological factors that would predict response to lapainib. Initial data showed that estrogen and progesterone receptors (PgR) negativity and EGFR overexpression may be predictive markers of response to lapatinib in

Chapter 12 / Integration of Target-Based Agents in Current Protocols 213

trastuzumab pretreated patients. Moreover, a decline in serum HER2 extracellular domain after 4 and 8 weeks of lapatinib therapy could be related to clinical response.

A phase I study demonstrated the activity of lapatinib in combination with capecitabine in HER2 positive trastuzumab pretreated patients *(58)*. The combination showed no overlapping toxicities and no relevant pharmacokinetic interactions at the recommended dose and schedule of the combination therapy (lapatinib at 1,250 mg daily and capecitabine at 2,000 mg/m^2 daily, on days 1 through 14 of a 21-day cycle). A phase III randomized study demonstrated the efficacy of lapatinib plus capecitabine over capecitabine alone in women with advanced, progressive HER2 positive breast cancer, who had received multiple previous treatments *(59)*. A planned interim analysis of time to progression met specified criteria for early reporting on the basis of superiority in the combination-therapy group. Patients receiving lapatinib plus capecitabine had a significantly longer median time to progression than patients treated with capecitabine alone (37 vs. 20 weeks, $p = 0.00016$), corresponding to a 51% reduction in the risk of disease progression. Treatment was well tolerated and the rate of adverse events was similar in the two arms, the main difference being an increase of grade 1 and 2 diarrhea in the combination arm (45% vs. 28%). Unfortunately, the cross-over offered to women in the monotherapy group after the report of these results invalidated the overall survival analysis.

Lapatinib has been evaluated in combination with paclitaxel in a randomized phase III study, as first-line therapy of a heterogeneous population of HER2 negative/untested advanced breast cancer. Patients were assigned to receive paclitaxel alone or paclitaxel plus lapatinib *(60)*. Overall, the addition of lapatinib to paclitaxel did not lead to significant improvement in time to progression, which was the primary end point for the study. However, a planned subgroup analysis according to HER2 status showed that among the 12% of all cases that had HER2 positive tumors (71 patients), adding lapatinib to chemotherapy improved the time to progression and response rate, suggesting that the spectrum of major activity for lapatinib is in the group of HER2 positive tumors.

Data from phase I and II clinical trials indicated that lapatinib may have an important role in the treatment of inflammatory breast cancer. This disease has a higher prevalence of HER2 overexpression than non-inflammatory locally advanced breast cancer, thus the use of HER2 antagonists would have a great rationale. In a phase II study of relapsed or refractory inflammatory HER2 positive breast cancer, lapatinib showed a response rate of 62%, with an added 21% of stabilization of disease, while only 8.3% of HER2 negative tumors achieved a partial response *(61)*. A phase II study of neoadjuvant therapy of lapatinib and paclitaxel is ongoing to better evaluate the activity of lapatinib in this setting.

An interesting issue is the combination of lapatinib with endocrine agents. Preclinical studies showed promising results and demonstrated that combining lapatinib with antiestrogens delays or prevents the development of lapatinib resistance in HER2-overexpressing/ER positive breast cancer cells and may overcome also endocrine resistance *(62,63)*. A phase I study identified the optimal combination dose of lapatinib and letrozole in advanced ER positive breast cancer and showed preliminary signs of clinical activity in terms of long-lasting stable disease *(64)*. A phase II study is planned with lapatinib plus tamoxifen in endocrine resistant breast cancer patients, while two phase III studies are underway with lapatinib plus letrozole as first-line treatment in ER positive metastatic breast cancer regardless of HER2 status (EGF30008 trial), and lapatinib plus fulvestrant (CALGB40302 trial) in advanced ER positive HER2 overexpressing breast cancer.

Because of the unexpected cardiac toxicity evidenced in trastuzumab trials, great attention has been given to cardiac safety of lapatinib. A review of cardiotoxicity data of nearly 3,000 patients enrolled in 18 phase I-III clinical trials, including 1,674 breast cancer patients, treated with lapatinib alone or in combination with other agents, reported an incidence of symptomatic or asymptomatic decline in left ventricular ejection fraction (LVEF) of 1.3% *(65)*. Cardiotoxicity was severe in 0.1% of cases and generally reversible or non-progressive. It is worth noting that a substantial number of the non-breast cancer patients had not received prior anthracycline or trastuzumab treatment, which could have partially influenced the low incidence of cardiac failure. Lapatinib does not appear to increase the risk of cardiomyopathy, even when combined with trastuzumab. Data from four trials in which patients received both lapatinib and trastuzumab were pooled to analyze cardiotoxicity *(66)*. Among nearly 400 patients who received the combination treatment, the incidence of asymptomatic declines in left ventricular ejection fraction (LVEF) was approximately 2% and 2 patients developed heart failure. However, also in this analysis, the incidence of cardiotoxicity could have been lowered by patients' selection, as the majority of them had received prior trastuzumab exposure without reporting significant cardiotoxicity, which may have reduced the chances of subsequent development of congestive heart failure or change in LVEF.

3. TARGETING ANGIOGENESIS

Angiogenesis, the process of formation of a new network of capillary vessels from pre-existing vessels, is necessary for tumor growth and metastasis. The initiation of the angiogenic process, the angiogenic switch, requires the acquisition of the angiogenic phenotype through a series of molecular events leading to increased expression of angiogenic factors and/or down-regulation of naturally occurring inhibitors *(67)*. Vascular endothelial growth factor (VEGF) is the most specific and powerful angiogenic factor. It is an endothelial cell-specific mitogen and survival factor and also stimulates vascular permeability and recruits progenitor endothelial cells from bone marrow. Other major angiogenic factors are angiopoietin-2, transforming growth factor-b1 (TGF-b1), basic fibroblast growth factor (bFGF), and matrix metalloproteinases (MMPs). The biologic effects of VEGF are mediated through the binding to three specific endothelial surface cell receptors VEGF-R1 (flt-1), VEGF-R2 (flk-1/kdr), and VEGF-R3. VEGF-R1 promotes differentiation and vascular maintenance, VEGF-R2 induces endothelial cell mitogenesis and vascular permeability, whilst VEGF-R3 stimulates lymphangiogenesis *(68)*. VEGF gene expression may be upregulated by a number of stimuli, including hypoxia, nitric oxide, various growth factors, estrogens, progestins, loss of p53, activation of ras, v-src, and HER2/neu *(67)*. In breast cancer, initiation of the angiogenic phenotype is correlated with progression from DCIS to invasive carcinoma *(69)*. In premalignant lesions, VEGF-R1 is absent and VEGF-R2 is minimally expressed. Expression of VEGFR is enhanced in invasive cancer and endothelial cells. VEGF and HER2 signaling pathways are connected at molecular level and cooperate to promote cell proliferation. Many studies indicated VEGF as an independent prognostic marker *(70)*. Indeed, intratumor VEGF levels are predictive of the resistance to various treatments, including radiotherapy, chemotherapy, and hormonal therapy *(69)*. VEGF-targeting treatments include large molecules such as neutralizing antibodies against VEGF (bevacizumab) and VEGFRs and the soluble form of VEGFR-1, and small molecules, such as signal transduction inhibitors. Moreover, a number of other antiangiogenic agents are being tested in Phase I/II clinical trials for the treatment of breast cancer, either alone or in combination with other therapies, including carboxyamidotriazole, interleukin-12, thalidomide, celecoxib, soy isoflavone, anti avb3 integrin monoclonal antibody, and MMPs inhibitors.

3.1. Bevacizumab

Bevacizumab, a humanized monoclonal antibody directed against the vascular endothelial growth factor (VEGF)-A ligand, is the most mature target-based agent with anti-angiogenetic activity. Two phase I clinical studies demonstrated that bevacizumab can be administered safely, without dose-limiting toxicities, up to the dose of 10 mg/kg every 2 weeks, and that it could be combined with chemotherapy without apparent synergistic toxicity *(71,72)*. A phase II study of bevacizumab monotherapy was conducted in 75 patients with previously treated metastatic breast cancer *(73)*. A 9.3% objective response rate with 17% of patients responding or stable at 22 weeks was reported; four (7%) patients continued therapy without progression for over 12 months with good tolerability. Several phase II trials tested bevacizumab in combination with chemotherapy in metastatic breast cancer patients. The safety and activity of bevacizumab (10 mg/kg every 2 weeks) and vinorelbine (25 mg/mq/week) combination were evaluated in 55 metastatic pretreated patients, showing a response rate of 31% with one complete response. Treatment was well tolerated, with only minor occurrence of hypertension, proteinuria, and epistaxis. No major bleeding or thrombotic events were registered *(74)*. Another trial evaluated the combination of bevacizumab with weekly docetaxel as first or second line of treatment of 27 metastatic patients *(75)*. A response rate of 52% was reported, showing a good activity of this combination. The only severe adverse events attributable to bevacizumab were grade 3 hypertension in one patient and venous thromboembolism in two patients, being most toxicity consistent with the safety profile of weekly docetaxel.

A phase III clinical trial was conducted on 462 anthracycline and taxane-refractory metastatic breast cancer patients, who were randomly assigned to receive capecitabine alone or capecitabine plus bevacizumab *(76)*. Despite reporting a significant twofold increase in response rate in the combination arm (19.8% vs. 9.1%; $p = 0.001$), the study failed to show an improvement in progression-free survival, which was the primary end point, and in overall survival. As expected, hypertension requiring treatment (17.9% vs. 0.5%), proteinuria (22.3% vs. 7.4%), and thromboembolic events (7.4% vs. 5.6%) were more frequent in patients receiving bevacizumab. Subsequently, a large international phase III trial of the Eastern Cooperative Oncology Group (E2100) tested the addition of bevacizumab to first-line weekly paclitaxel in 722 metastatic breast cancer patients *(77)*. The combination of paclitaxel plus bevacizumab significantly prolonged progression-free survival, which was the primary end point, as compared with paclitaxel alone (median, 11.8 vs. 5.9 months) with HR of progression of 0.60 (95% CI 0.51–0.70; $p < 0.001$). The addition of bevacizumab to paclitaxel significantly improved also the objective response rate (36.9% vs. 21.2%, $p < 0.001$). Combined therapy increased the 1-year survival rate (81.2% vs. 73.4%, $p = 0.01$), although median overall survival was similar in the two arms (26.7 vs. 25.2 months, respectively; HR 0.88; $p = 0.16$). More neuropathy was seen in women receiving the combination therapy than in those receiving paclitaxel alone (20.5% vs. 14.2%, $p = 0.01$), but this finding might be due to longer exposition to paclitaxel in the combination arm. Almost all of the enrolled patients had tumors that did not overexpress HER2; thus, on the basis of the results of E2100, the combination of bevacizumab plus paclitaxel is a reasonable first-line treatment for women with HER2 negative metastatic disease, while further studies are needed to assess the efficacy of bevacizumab in patients with HER2 positive breast cancer. The E2100 trial demonstrated the efficacy of an early treatment with bevacizumab in the course of metastatic breast cancer, when angiogenic pathways are likely less redundant. Moreover, preclinical studies have shown that initial events in the development of metastasis are VEGF-dependent *(78)*, suggesting that the most successful clinical application of angiogenesis inhibitors is likely to be in patients with micrometastatic disease in the adjuvant setting. Trials evaluating the feasibility and efficacy of bevacizumab treatment in patients with early breast cancer are ongoing. In the neoadjuvant setting, bevacizumab has been tested in combination with docetaxel. Locally unresectable breast cancer patients, with or without metastasis, were randomly assigned to receive bevacizumab and weekly docetaxel or docetaxel alone. Patients whose disease responded underwent definitive surgery followed by adjuvant chemotherapy. Only preliminary safety results are available, showing a good tolerability of the combination therapy *(79)*. Bevacizumab was also tested in combination with doxorubicin and docetaxel as neoadjuvant treatment of women with inflammatory breast cancer *(80)*. Fourteen of 21 enrolled patients experienced a clinical partial response and a decrease in vascular permeability on dynamic contrast-enhanced magnetic resonance imaging was evidence that was consistent with reduced angiogenesis. Moreover, this study also indicated a direct antitumor effect of bevacizumab, suggested by a decrease in phosphorylated VEGF-R2 in tumor cells, and a median increase in tumor apoptosis.

Several questions are open regarding use of bevacizumab. The optimum therapeutic combinations and duration of therapy, the continuance after disease progression, and even the optimum setting of use remain undefined.

3.2. Receptor Tyrosine Kinase Inhibitors Targeting the VEGF Pathway

The small molecules that inhibit tyrosine kinase activity of VEGF receptors represent another opportunity of treatment targeting the VEGF pathway. Sunitinib, targeting the VEGFRs, PDGFR-b, and c-Kit, has been evaluated in a phase II study enrolling 64 metastatic breast cancer patients resistant to anthracyclines and taxanes *(81)*. Seven patients achieved a partial response, giving an overall response rate of 11%. Three additional patients (5%) maintained stable disease for more than 6 months. Of note, responses occurred in triple negative tumors (15%) and HER2 positive, trastuzumab-treated patients (25%), thus a population for which limited treatment options are currently available. Severe transient neutropenia was experienced by 34% of patients, that is higher than reported in sunitinib trials of renal cell or gastrointestinal stromal tumors. This may be due to heavy pretreatment of the study population. Several phase III trials are evaluating the efficacy of the addition of sunitinib to docetaxel, trastuzumab, capecitabine and comparing sunitinib versus chemotherapy or sunitinib and paclitaxel versus paclitaxel and bevacizumab. Moreover, phase I–II studies are ongoing with vatalanib, a potent inhibitor of all known VEGFR tyrosine kinases, and sorafenib, a dual inhibitor of Raf kinase and VEGFRs *(82)*.

4. TARGETING MTOR

Mammalian target of rapamycin (mTOR) is a serine/threonine kinase, belonging to the phosphoinositide kinase-related kinase family. Through the formation of multimolecular complexes, the mTOR pathway controls several fundamental cell functions, playing a central role in the regulation of cell growth, proliferation, and survival. Upstream activators include, but are not limited to, the phosphatidylinositol 3-kinase (PI3K)/AKT signaling pathway. AKT is a serine/threonine kinase that promotes cell survival and is activated in response to many different growth factors, including EGF, heregulin, VEGF, insulin, insulin-like growth factor I, and basic fibroblast growth factor. Activation of mTOR results in the phosphorylation and activation of the ribosomal protein S6 kinase (pS6K) and the eukaryotic initiation factor 4E-binding protein-1 (4E-BP1) that play a key role in translation of mRNAs regulating

Chapter 12 / Integration of Target-Based Agents in Current Protocols 217

cell cycle progression. Although neither mTOR mutations nor overexpression have been reported in human tumors, signaling pathways that are upstream or downstream of mTOR are frequently deregulated in human cancers, including breast cancer. Rapamycin, the prototype of mTOR inhibitors, inhibited tumor growth in a wide range of experimental malignancies *(83)*. Temsirolimus and everolimus are rapamycin analogues currently selected for clinical development.

4.1. Temsirolimus

Temsirolimus (CCI-779) is a water-soluble ester of rapamycin which demonstrated antitumor activity in a variety of cancer models, including breast cancer *(84)*. The growth inhibitory properties of temsirolimus were studied in eight human breast cancer lines. Sensitive lines were estrogen dependent (MCF-7, BT-474, T47D), or lacked expression of the tumor suppressor gene PTEN (MDA-MB-468, BT-549) and/or overexpressed HER2 (SKBR-3, BT-474), while resistant lines (MDA-MB-435, MDA-MB-231) shared none of these properties *(84)*. In vivo, temsirolimus inhibited growth of MDA-MB-468 but not of MDA-MB-435 tumors. AKT resulted highly activated in sensitive but only minimally in resistant cell lines. These results suggested that temsirolimus might be a useful treatment for breast cancer with specific phenotypes, in which AKT activation results from either growth factor dependency or loss of PTEN function. Moreover, a synergistic effect of the combination of temsirolimus with endocrine therapy has been shown *(85)*. MCF7 breast cancer cell lines, expressing a constitutively active AKT, were able to proliferate, in vitro and in vivo, under reduced estrogen conditions and resulted resistant to tamoxifen inhibitory effect. In xenograft models, temsirolimus treatment inhibited mTOR activity and restored sensibility to tamoxifen, with a synergistic interaction. Preclinical findings also revealed the antiangiogenetic potential of temsirolimus *(86)*. In the HER2 overexpressing breast cancer cell line BT474, temsirolimus inhibited VEGF production in vitro under both normoxic and hypoxic conditions through inhibition of hypoxia-stimulated hypoxia-inducible factor (HIF)-1a expression and transcriptional activation. Temsirolimus also directly inhibited endothelial cell proliferation and morphogenesis in vitro and vessel formation in a Matrigel assay in vivo.

Temsirolimus was studied in a phase I trial, as a weekly 30-min intravenous infusion, at doses ranging from 7.5 to 220 mg/m^2 *(87)*. The most frequent drug-related toxicities were skin rash and stomatitis, observed at all doses. All toxicities were reversible on treatment discontinuation. Unexpectedly, the dose of 220 mg/m^2 induced a maniac-depressive syndrome, preventing further dose escalation, although the formal definition of MTD was not met. Evidence of activity was observed over the entire dose range, with no apparent relationship between exposure and clinical benefit, suggesting that target inhibition may be achieved at doses well below those that result in DLT. A translational study of temsirolimus was conducted to develop a pharmacodynamic biomarker, focusing on pS6K activity, a direct downstream substrate of mTOR *(88)*. Pharmacodynamic measurements were done on peripheral blood mononuclear cells (PBMCs), in which pS6K is constitutively activated. Temsirolimus inhibited pS6K activity in PBMCs and tumor tissue in vivo in a parallel fashion, indicating that the PBMCs could be an appropriate surrogate tissue. Moreover, there was a linear association between inhibition of pS6K and time to tumor progression, showing the potential predictive value of this biomarker.

Temsirolimus antitumor activity has been explored in a randomized phase II study with two dose levels (75 and 250 mg/week as a 30-min intravenous infusion), in heavily pretreated patients with locally advanced/metastatic breast cancer *(89)*. A response rate of 9% and a median time to progression of 12 weeks were reported for all patients in the intent-to-treat population. A tolerable safety profile was reported at the 75-mg dose, mucositis, maculopapular rash, and nausea being the most common toxicities. Preliminary data from a randomized phase II trial of letrozole with or without oral temsirolimus as first or second line of treatment have been also reported *(90)*. Locally advanced or metastatic breast cancer patients were randomized to letrozole alone, letrozole plus continuous oral temsirolimus, or letrozole plus intermittent temsirolimus. Clinical activity has been observed in all arms, and the combination treatment resulted well tolerated at the dose of temsirolimus 10 mg daily or 30 mg for 5 days every 2 weeks. However, a large randomized, placebo controlled, double-blind phase III trial exploring the efficacy of the combination of letrozole plus temsirolimus as first-line hormonal therapy was recently closed on the basis of data from a planned interim analysis, reporting the trial was unlikely to achieve the targeted level of efficacy for the combination therapy compared to letrozole alone *(91)*.

4.2. Everolimus

Everolimus (RAD-001) is an orally bioavailable mTOR inhibitor under clinical evaluation in different types of cancer, including breast cancer. Everolimus binds with high affinity to intracellular receptor FKBP12, forming a complex that interacts with mTOR to inhibit downstream signaling events *(92)*. In preclinical models everolimus alone at nanomolar concentrations decreased the growth of BT-474.m1 cells, a subline of BT-474 breast cancer cells that overexpress HER2, and of BT-474.m1 cells transfected with PTEN antisense oligonucleotides *(93)*. Moreover, this drug enhanced, in vitro and in vivo, growth inhibition by trastuzumab in PTEN-deficient cells, overcoming resistance to trastuzumab *(93)*. Everolimus was also active against EGFR-resistant cancer cell lines and partially restored the ability of gefitinib to inhibit growth and survival. In MDA-MB-468, a breast cancer cell line with low sensitivity to gefitinib, everolimus reduced the expression of EGFR-related signaling effectors and VEGF production, inhibiting proliferation and capillary tube formation of endothelial cells, both alone and in combination with gefitinib *(94)*. Everolimus inhibited estrogen-driven proliferation in MCF7 estrogen-dependent breast cancer cells, with specific modulation of mTOR downstream elements *(95)*. In the same breast cancer model, the combination of everolimus with letrozole significantly enhanced the antiproliferative activity as compared with either agent alone, with a synergistic interaction.

A pharmacodynamic phase I study has been conducted to identify the optimal dose and schedule of everolimus in cancer treatment *(96)*. Nineteen of 55 enrolled patients had breast cancer. Everolimus was administered as a single weekly oral dose of 20, 50, and 70 mg, or as a continuous daily oral dose of 5 and 10 mg. Pharmacodynamic effects on mTOR pathways were determined in sequential tumor and skin biopsies. Toxicity profiles were similar in the two schedules. The most frequent toxicities were skin rash, stomatitis, headache, and fatigue. Inhibition of mTOR signaling was observed at all dose levels and schedules, being almost complete at 10 mg daily and 50 mg weekly.

In a phase II preoperative trial, 30 patients with early breast cancer received everolimus 5 mg daily for 14 days, prior to surgery *(97)*. Everolimus produced a significant decrease of Ki67 labeling index. Phospho-AKT (pAKT) levels were reduced in tumors with high pretreatment cytoplasmic staining for pAKT. Moreover, higher pre-treatment pAKT correlated significantly with greater reductions in proliferation, suggesting that AKT activation could be a predictive marker of mTOR activation and, therefore, of everolimus efficacy.

Everolimus is currently undergoing evaluation in combination with docetaxel, paclitaxel, trastuzumab, fulvestrant, erlotinib in patients with metastatic breast cancer. A phase II double-blind, randomized, placebo-controlled trial is ongoing to assess the value of adding

Chapter 12 / Integration of Target-Based Agents in Current Protocols 219

everolimus to letrozole as preoperative therapy of primary breast cancer in postmenopausal women *(98)*. Primary objective is the overall response rate, based on the palpation of the breast tumor and lymph nodes. Preliminary results evidence a higher response rate by palpation in the combination arm (68.1% vs. 59.1%) that was also confirmed by ultrasound (58% vs. 47%). A biomarker analysis has been conducted to identify subpopulations deriving the greatest benefit from the addition of everolimus *(99)*. Results indicate significant changes between baseline and day 15 tumor biopsies for mTOR pathway relevant markers, including PgR, pS6K, pAKT, and cyclinD1. More extensive analysis, after unblinding, will reveal the predictive power of the baseline biomarkers in selecting responding populations. A phase III trial program is exploring the integration of everolimus, bevacizumab, and lapatinib into current neoadjuvant chemotherapy regimens for primary breast cancer.

5. CONCLUSIONS

A large number of molecular-targeted drugs are in clinical development in breast cancer. However, several key issues in the design and conduction of clinical trials with molecular-targeted agents need to be defined *(100)*. First of all, the lack of valid, predictive preclinical models: the doses and schedules tested for some agents may not be appropriate and bulky disease may not be the optimal setting for the evaluation of these drugs. Second, unanswered questions remain regarding the optimal trial design and choice of adequate end-points. Response rate remains the preferred end-point in the early evaluation of new drugs. However, this approach might lead to rejection of potentially useful drugs when significant tumor shrinkage cannot be demonstrated. Therefore, a number of alternative end-points have been proposed for agents which are not expected to cause a major tumor regression: time to progression, progression-free survival, overall survival, early progression rate. Third, the final efficacy of these agents should be validated in appropriately designed phase III trials that must include tissue or circulating surrogate biomarkers of efficacy, biologically driven criteria of patient selection, well-defined schedules of treatment, and predictive markers of activity and toxicity. A tight collaboration between laboratory and clinical researchers is required in order to avoid missing activity and to define relevant biological end-points.

REFERENCES

1. Parkin DM, Bray FI, Devesa SS. Cancer burden in the year 2000 The global picture. Eur J Cancer 2001;37:S4–S66.
2. Salomon DS, Brandt R, Ciardiello F, Normanno N. Epidermal growth factor-related peptides and their receptors in human malignancies. Critical Rev Oncol Hematol 1995;19:183–232.
3. Slamon DJ, Clark GM, Wong SG, Levin WJ, Ullrich A, McGuire WL. Human breast cancer: correlation of relapse and survival with amplification of the HER-2/neu oncogene. Science 1987;235:177–182.
4. Querrel N, Wafflart J, Borrichon F, et al. The prognostic value of c-erbB2 in primary breast carcinomas: a study of 942 cases. Breast Cancer Res Treat 1995;35:283–291.
5. Pegram MD, Finn RS, Arzoo K, et al. The effect of her-2/neu overexpression on chemotherapeutic drug sensitivity in human breast and ovarian cancer cells. Oncogene 1997;15:537–547.
6. Carlomagno C, Perrone F, Gallo C, et al. c-ErbB2 overexpression decreases the benefit of adjuvant tamoxifen in early breast cancer without axillary lymph node metastases. J Clin Oncol 1996;14:2702–2708.
7. Cobleigh M, Vogel C, Tripathy D, et al. Multinational study of the efficacy and safety of humanized anti-HER2 monoclonal antibody in women who have HER2-overexpressing metastatic breast cancer that has progressed after chemotherapy for metastatic disease. J Clin Oncol 1999;17:2639–2648.

8. Baselga J, Tripathy D, Mendelsohn J, et al. Phase II study of weekly intravenous trastuzumab (Herceptin) in patients with HER2/neu-overexpressing metastatic breast cancer. Semin Oncol 1999;26:78–83.
9. Vogel C, Cobleigh M, Tripathy D, et al. Efficacy and safety of trastuzumab as a single agent in first-line treatment of HER2-overexpressing metastatic breast cancer. J Clin Oncol 2002;20:719–726.
10. Slamon D, Leyland-Jones B, Shak S, et al. Use of chemotherapy plus a monoclonal antibody against HER2 for metastatic breast cancer that overexpresses HER2. N Engl J Med 2001;344:783–792.
11. Osoba D, Slamon DJ, Burhmore M, et al. 2002 Effects on quality of life of combined trastuzumab and chemotherapy in women with metastatic breast cancer. J Clin Oncol 2002;20:3106–3113.
12. Fountzilas G, Tsavdaridis D, Kalogera-Fountzila A, et al. Weekly paclitaxel as first-line chemotherapy and trastuzumab in patients with advanced breast cancer A Hellenic Cooperative Oncology Group phase II study. Ann Oncol 2001;12:1545–1551.
13. Seidman AD, Fornire MN, Esteva FJ, et al. Weekly trastuzumab and paclitaxel therapy for metastatic breast cancer with analysis of efficacy by HER2 immunophenotype and gene amplification. J Clin Oncol 2001;19:2587–2525.
14. Leyland-Jones B, Gelmon K, Ayoub JP, et al. Pharmacokinetics, safety, and efficacy of trastuzumab administered every three weeks in combination with paclitaxel. J Clin Oncol 2003;21:3965–3971.
15. Gori S, Colozza M, Mosconi AM, et al. Phase II study of weekly paclitaxel and trastuzumab in anthracycline- and taxane-pretreated patients with HER2- overexpressing metastatic breast cancer. Br J Cancer 2004;90:36–40.
16. Gasparini G, Gion G, Mariani L, et al. Randomized Phase II Trial of weekly paclitaxel alone versus trastuzumab plus weekly paclitaxel as first-line therapy of patients with Her-2 positive advanced breast cancer. Breast Cancer Res Treat 2007;101:355–365.
17. Esteva FJ, Valero V, Booser D, et al. Phase II study of weekly docetaxel and trastuzumab for patients with HER-2–overexpressing metastatic breast cancer. J Clin Oncol 2002;20:1800–1808.
18. Tedesco KL, Thor AD, Johnson DH, et al. Docetaxel combined with trastuzumab is an active regimen in HER-2 3+ overexpressing and fluorescent in situ hybridization–positive metastatic breast cancer: a multi-institutional phase II trial. J Clin Oncol 2004;22:1071–1077.
19. Marty M, Cognetti F, Maraninchi D, et al. Randomized phase II trial of the efficacy and safety of trastuzumab combined with docetaxel in patients with human epidermal growth factor receptor 2–positive metastatic breast cancer administered as first-line treatment: the M77001 Study Group. J Clin Oncol 2005;23:4265–4274.
20. Burstein HJ, Kuter I, Campos SM, et al. Clinical activity of trastuzumab and vinorelbine in women with HER2-overexpressing metastatic breast cancer. J Clin Oncol 2001;19:2722–2730.
21. Jahanezeb M, Joanne E, Mortimer JE, et al. Phase II trial of weekly vinorelbine and trastuzumab as first-line therapy in patients with HER2+ metastatic breast cancer. Oncologist 2002;7:410–417.
22. Burstein HJ, Harris LN, Marcom PK, et al. Trastuzumab and vinorelbine as first-line therapy for HER2-overexpressing metastatic breast cancer: multicenter phase II trial with clinical outcomes, analysis of serum tumor markers as predictive factors, and cardiac surveillance algorithm. J Clin Oncol 2003;21:2889–2895.
23. Chan A, Martin M, Untch M, et al. Vinorelbine plus trastuzumab combination as first-line therapy for HER 2-positive metastatic breast cancer patients: an international phase II trial. Br J Cancer 2006;95:788–793.
24. Papaldo P, Fabi A, Ferretti G, et al. A phase II study on metastatic breast cancer patients treated with weekly vinorelbine with or without trastuzumab according to HER2 expression: changing the natural history of HER2-positive disease. Ann Oncol 2006;17:630–636.
25. De Maio E, Pacilio C, Gravina A, et al. Vinorelbine plus 3-weekly trastuzumab in metastatic breast cancer A single-centre phase 2 trial. BMC Cancer 2007;7:50.
26. Yamamoto D, Iwase S, Kitamura K, et al. A phase II study of trastuzumab and capecitabine for patients with HER2-overexpressing metastatic breast cancer: Japan Breast Cancer Research Network (JBCRN) 00 Trial. Cancer Chemother Pharmacol 2008;61:509–514.
27. Schaller G, Fuchs I, Gonsch T, et al. Phase II study of capecitabine plus trastuzumab in human epidermal growth factor receptor 2 overexpressing metastatic breast cancer pretreated with anthracyclines or taxanes. J Clin Oncol 2007;25:3246–3250.

Chapter 12 / Integration of Target-Based Agents in Current Protocols

28. Pegram MD, Lipton A, Hayes DF, et al. Phase II study of receptor-enhanced chemosensitivity using recombinant humanized anti-p185HER2/neu monoclonal antibody plus cisplatin in patients with HER2/neu-overexpressing metastatic breast cancer refractory to chemotherapy treatment. J Clin Oncol 1998;16:2659–2671.

29. O'Shaughnessy JA, Vukelja S, Marsland T, et al. Phase II study of trastuzumab plus gemcitabine in chemotherapy-pretreated patients with metastatic breast cancer. Clin Breast Cancer 2004;5:142–147.

30. Burris H, Yardley D, Jones S, Phase II trial of trastuzumab followed by weekly paclitaxel/carboplatin as first-line treatment for patients with metastatic breast cancer. J Clin Oncol 2004;22:1621–1629.

31. Pegram MD, Pienkowski T, Northfelt DW, et al. Results of two open-label, multicenter phase II studies of docetaxel, platinum salts, and trastuzumab in HER2-positive advanced breast cancer. J Natl Cancer Inst 2004;96:759–769.

32. Perez EA, Suman VJ, Rowland KM, et al. Two concurrent phase II trials of paclitaxel/carboplatin/ trastuzumab (weekly or every-3-week schedule) as first-line therapy in women with HER2-overexpressing metastatic breast cancer: NCCTG study 983252. Clin Breast Cancer 2005;6:425–432.

33. Robert N, Leyland-Jones B, Asmar L, et al. Randomized phase III study of trastuzumab, paclitaxel, and carboplatin compared with trastuzumab and paclitaxel in women with HER-2–overexpressing metastatic breast cancer. J Clin Oncol 2006;24:2786–2792.

34. Morabito A, Longo R, Gattuso D, et al. Trastuzumab in combination with gemcitabine and vinorelbine as second-line therapy for HER-2/neu overexpressing metastatic breast cancer. Oncol Rep 2006;16:393–398.

35. Fujimoto-Ouchi K, Sekiguchi F, Kazushige M. Preclinical study of continuous administration of trastuzumab as combination therapy after disease progression with trastuzumab monotherapy. Proc Am Assoc Cancer Res 2005;46:5062a.

36. Fountzilas G, Razis E, Tsavdaridis D, et al. Continuation of trastuzumab beyond disease progression is feasible and safe in patients with metastatic breast cancer: A retrospective analysis of 80 cases by the Hellenic Cooperative Oncology Group. Clin Breast Cancer 2003;4:120–125.

37. Gelmon KA, Mackey J, Verma S, et al. Use of trastuzumab beyond disease progression: Observations from a retrospective review of case histories. Clin Breast Cancer 2004;5:52–58; discussion 59–62.

38. Tripathy D, Slamon DJ, Cobleigh M, et al. Safety of treatment of metastatic breast cancer with trastuzumab beyond disease progression. J Clin Oncol 2004;22:1063–1070.

39. Montemurro F, Donadio M, Clavarezza M, et al. Outcome of patients with HER2-positive advanced breast cancer progressing during trastuzumab-based therapy. The Oncologist 2006;11:318–324.

40. Bartsch R, Wenzel C, Hussian D, Analysis of trastuzumab and chemotherapy in advanced breast cancer after the failure of at least one earlier combination: An observational study. BMC Cancer 2006;6:63.

41. Bartsch R, Wenzel C, Altorjai G, et al. Capecitabine and trastuzumab in heavily pretreated metastatic breast cancer. J Clin Oncol 2007;25:3853–3858.

42. Bartsch R, Wenzel C, Gampenrieder SP, et al. Trastuzumab and gemcitabine as salvage therapy in heavily pre-treated patients with metastatic breast cancer. Cancer Chemother Pharmacol 2008 Feb 7 [Epub ahead of print].

43. Jones A. Combining trastuzumab (Herceptin®) with hormonal therapy in breast cancer: what can be expected and why? Ann Oncol 2003;14:1697–1704.

44. Mackey JR, Kaufman B, Clemens M, Trastuzumab prolongs progression-free survival in hormone-dependent and HER2-positive metastatic breast cancer. Breast Cancer Res Treat 2006;100 (suppl 1):S5. abst 3.

45. Marcom PK, Isaacs C, Harris L, et al. The combination of letrozole and trastuzumab as first- or second-line biological therapy produces durable responses in a subset of HER2 positive and ER positive advanced breast cancers. Breast Cancer Res Treat 2007;102:43–49.

46. Piccart-Gebhart MJ, Procter M, Leyland-Jones B, et al. Trastuzumab after adjuvant chemotherapy in HER2-positive breast cancer. N Engl J Med 2005;353:1659–1672.

47. Romond EH, Perez EA, Bryant J, et al. Trastuzumab plus adjuvant chemotherapy for operable HER2-positive breast cancer. N Engl J Med 2005;353:1673–1684.

48. Slamon D, Eiermann W, Robert N, et al. BCIRG 006: 2nd interim analysis phase III randomized trial comparing doxorubicin and cyclophosphamide followed by docetaxel (AC T) with doxorubicin and cyclophosphamide followed by docetaxel and trastuzumab (AC TH) with docetaxel, carboplatin and trastuzumab (TCH) in Her2neu positive early breast cancer patients. 29th Annual San Antonio Breast Cancer Symposium Proc; December 14–17, 2006; San Antonio, TX. abst 52.
49. Joensuu H, Kellokumpu-Lehtinen P-L, Bono P, et al. Adjuvant docetaxel or vinorelbine with or without trastuzumab for breast cancer. N Engl J Med 2006;354:809–820.
50. Coon JS, Marcus E, Gupta-Burt S, et al. Amplification and overexpression of topoisomerase II alpha predict response to anthracycline-based therapy in locally advanced breast cancer. Clin Cancer Res 2002;8:1061–1067.
51. Nahta R, Hung MC, Esteval FJ. The HER-2-targeting antibodies trastuzumab and pertuzumab synergistically inhibit the survival of breast cancer cells. Cancer Res 2004;64:2343–2346.
52. Baselga J, Cameron D, Miles D, et al. Objective response rate in a phase II multicenter trial of pertuzumab (P), a HER2 dimerization inhibiting monoclonal antibody, in combination with trastuzumab (T) in patients (pts) with HER2-positive metastatic breast cancer (MBC) which has progressed during treatment with T. J Clin Oncol 2007 ASCO Annual Meeting Proceedings; 25(18S):abst 1004.
53. Rusnak DW, Affleck K, Cockerill SG, et al. The characterization of novel, dual ErbB-2/EGFR, tyrosine kinase inhibitors: potential therapy for cancer. Cancer Res 2001;61:7196–7203.
54. Spector NL, Xia W, Burris H III, et al. Study of the Biologic Effects of Lapatinib, a Reversible Inhibitor of ErbB1 and ErbB2 Tyrosine Kinases, on Tumor Growth and Survival Pathways in Patients With Advanced Malignancies. J Clin Oncol 2005;23:2502–2512.
55. Burris HA III, Hurwitz HI, Dees EC, et al. Phase I Safety, Pharmacokinetics, and Clinical Activity Study of Lapatinib (GW572016), a Reversible Dual Inhibitor of Epidermal Growth Factor Receptor Tyrosine Kinases, in Heavily Pretreated Patients With Metastatic Carcinomas. J Clin Oncol 2005;23:5305–5313.
56. Blackwell KL, Burstein H, Pegram M, et al. Determining relevant biomarkers from tissue and serum that may predict response to single agent lapatinib in trastuzumab refractory metastatic breast cancer. J Clin Oncol 2005;23(16 suppl).
57. Burstein H, Storniolo AM, Franco S, et al. A phase II of lapatinib monotherapy in chemotherapy refractory HER2-positive and HER2-negative advanced or metastatic breast cancer. Ann Oncol 2008 in press.
58. Chu QS, Schwartz G, de Bono J, et al. Phase I and pharmacokinetic study of lapatinib in combination with capecitabine in patients with advanced solid malignancies. J Clin Oncol 2007;25:3753–3758.
59. Geyer CE, Forster J, Lindquist D, et al. Lapatinib plus capecitabine for HER2-positive advanced breast cancer. N Engl J Med 2006;355:2733–2743.
60. Di Leo A, Gomez H, Aziz Z, et al. Lapatinib with paclitaxel compared to paclitaxel as first-line treatment for patients with metastatic breast cancer: a phase III randomized, double-blind study of 580 patients. J Clin Oncol 2007;25:abst 1011.
61. Spector NL, Blackwell K, Hurley J, et al. EGF103009, a phase II trial of lapatinib monotherapy in patients with relapsed/refractory inflammatory breast cancer (IBC): clinical activity and biologic predictors of response. J Clin Oncol 2006;24(18 suppl).
62. Xia W, Bacus S, Hegde P, et al. A model of acquired autoresistance to a potent ErbB2 tyrosine kinase inhibitor and a therapeutic strategy to prevent its onset in breast cancer. PNAS 2006;103:7795–7800.
63. Chu I, Blackwell K, Chen S, et al. The dual ErbB1/ErbB2 inhibitor, lapatinib, cooperates with tamoxifen to inhibit both cell proliferation and estrogen-dependent gene expression in antiestrogen-resistant breast cancer. Cancer Res 2005;65:18–25.
64. Chu Q, Goldstein L, Murray N, et al. A phase I, open-label study of the safety, tolerability and pharmacokinetics of lapatinib (GW572016) in combination with letrozole in cancer patients. J Clin Oncol 2005;23:abst 3001.
65. Perez EA, Byrne JA, Hammond IW, et al. Results of an analysis of cardiac function in 2812 patients treated with lapatinib. Proc Am Soc Clin Oncol 2006;24:abst 583.
66. Storniolo AM, Koehler M, Preston A, et al. Cardiac safety in patients with metastatic breast cancer treated with lapatinib and trastuzumab. Proc Am Soc Clin Oncol 2007;25:abst 514.

Chapter 12 / Integration of Target-Based Agents in Current Protocols 223

67. Hanahan D, Folkman J. patterns and emerging mechanisms of the angiogenic switch during tumorigenesis. Cell 1996;86:353–364.
68. Kim KJ, Li B, Winer J, et al. Inhibition of vascular endothelial growth factor-induced angiogenesis suppresses tumor growth in vivo. Nature 1993;362:841–844.
69. Fox SB, Gasparini G, Harris AL. Angiogenesis: pathological, prognostic and growth factor pathways and their link to trial design and anticancer drugs. Lancet Oncol 2001;2:278–289.
70. Toi M, Matsumoto T, Bando H, Vascular endothelial growth factor: its prognostic, predictive, and therapeutic implications. Lancet Oncol 2001;2:667–673.
71. Gordon MS, Margolin K, Talpaz M, et al. Phase I safety and pharmacokinetic study of recombinant human anti-vascular endothelial growth factor in patients with advanced cancer. J Clin Oncol 2001;19:843–850.
72. Margolin K, Gordon MS, Holmgren E, et al. Phase Ib trial of intravenous recombinant humanized monoclonal antibody to vascular endothelial growth factor in combination with chemotherapy in patients with advanced cancer: pharmacologic and long-term safety data. J Clin Oncol 2001;19:851–856.
73. Cobleigh MA, Langmuir VK, Sledge GW, et al. A phase II dose-escalation trial of bevacizumab in previously treated metastatic breast cancer. Semin Oncol 2003;30:117–124.
74. Burstein HJ, Parker LM, Savoie J, et al. Phase II trial of the anti-VEGF antibody bevacizumab in combination with vinorelbine for refractory advanced breast cancer. Breast Cancer Res Treat 2002;79: (S115)abst 446.
75. Ramaswamy B, Elias AD, Kelbick NT, et al. Phase II trial of bevacizumab in combination with weekly docetaxel in metastatic breast cancer patients. Clin Cancer Res 2006;12:3124–3129.
76. Miller KD, Chap LI, Holmes FA, et al. Randomized phase III trial of capecitabine compared with bevacizumab plus capecitabine in patients with previously treated metastatic breast cancer. J Clin Oncol 2005;23:792–799.
77. Miller K, Wang M, Gralow J, et al. Paclitaxel plus bevacizumab versus paclitaxel alone for metastatic breast cancer. N Engl J Med 2007;357:2666–2676.
78. Steeg PS. Tumor metastasis: mechanistic insights and clinical challenges. Nat Med 2006;12:895–904.
79. Lyons JA, Silverman P, Remick S, et al. Toxicity results and early outcome data on a randomized phase II study of docetaxel ± bevacizumab for locally advanced, unresectable breast cancer. J Clin Oncol 2006, ASCO Annual Meeting Proceedings; 24 (18S): abst 3049.
80. Wedam SB, Law JA, Yang SX, et al. Antiangiogenic and antitumor effects of bevacizumab in patients with inflammatory and locally advanced breast cancer. J Clin Oncol 2006;24:769–777.
81. Burstein HJ, Elias AD, Rugo HS, et al. Phase II study of sunitinib malate, an oral multitargeted tyrosine kinase inhibitor, in patients with metastatic breast cancer previously treated with an anthracycline and a taxane. J Clin Oncol 2008;26:1810–1816.
82. Morabito A, De Maio E, Di Maio M, et al. Tyrosine kinase inhibitors of vascular endothelial growth factor receptors in clinical trials: current status and future directions. The Oncologist 2006;11:753–764.
83. Bjornsti MA, Houghton PJ. The TOR pathway: a target for cancer therapy. Nat Rev Cancer 2004;4:335–348.
84. Yu K, Toral-Barza L, Discafani C, et al: mTOR, a novel target in breast cancer: The effect of CCI-779, an mTOR inhibitor, in preclinical models of breast cancer. Endocr Relat Cancer 2001;8:249–258.
85. DeGraffenried LA, Friedrichs WE, Russel DH, et al. Inhibition of mTOR activity restores tamoxifen response in breast cancer cells with aberrant Akt activity. Clin Cancer Res 2004;10: 8059–8067.
86. Del Bufalo D, Ciuffreda L, Trisciuoglio D, et al. Antiangiogenic potential of the mammalian target of rapamycin inhibitor temsirolimus. Cancer Res 2006;66:5549–5554.
87. Raymond E, Alexandre J, Faivre S, et al. Safety and pharmacokinetics of escalated doses of weekly intravenous infusion of CCI-779, a novel mTOR inhibitor, in patients with cancer. Clin Oncol 2004;22:2336–2347.
88. Peralba JM, deGraffenried L, Friedrichs W, et al. Pharmacodynamic evaluation of CCI-779, an inhibitor of mTOR, in cancer patients. Clin Cancer Res 2003;9:2887–2892.

89. Chan S, Scheulen ME, Johnston S, et al. Phase II study of temsirolimus (CCI-779), a novel inhibitor of mTOR, in heavily pretreated patients with locally advanced or metastatic breast cancer. J Clin Oncol 2005;23:5314–5322.
90. Carpenter JT, Roché H, Campone M, et al. Randomized 3-arm, phase 2 study of temsirolimus (CCI-779) in combination with letrozole in postmenopausal women with locally advanced or metastatic breast cancer J Clin Oncol 2005 ASCO Annual Meeting Proceedings; 23 (16S): abst 564.
91. Chow LWC, Sun Y, Jassem J, et al. Phase 3 study of temsirolimus with letrozole or letrozole alone in postmenopausal women with locally advanced or metastatic breast cancer. SABCS 2006 Proceedings; abst 6091.
92. Beuvink I, O'Reilly T, Zumstein S, et al: Antitumor activity of RAD001, an orally active rapamycin derivative. Proc Am Assoc Cancer Res 2001; 42:366 (suppl, abstr 1972).
93. Lu CH, Wyszomierski SL, Tseng LM, et al. Preclinical testing of clinically applicable strategies for overcoming trastuzumab resistance caused by PTEN deficiency. Clin Cancer Res 2007;13:5883–5888.
94. Bianco R, Garofalo S, Rosa R, et al. Inhibition of mTOR pathway by everolimus cooperates with EGFR inhibitors in human tumours sensitive and resistant to anti-EGFR drugs. Br J Cancer 2008;98:923–30.
95. Boulay A, Rudloff J, Ye J, et al. Dual inhibition of mTOR pathway and estrogen signaling in vitro induces cell death in models of breast cancer. Clin Cancer Res 2005;11:5319–5328.
96. Tabernero J, Rojo F, Calvo E, et al. Dose- and schedule-dependent inhibition of the mammalian target of rapamycin pathway with everolimus: a phase I tumor pharmacodynamic study in patients with advanced solid tumors. J Clin Oncol 2008;26:1603–1610.
97. Macaskill EJ, Bartlett JMS, White S, et al. The mammalian target of rapamycin inhibitor RAD001 (everolimus) in postmenopausal women with early breast cancer: results of a phase II pre-operative trial. SABCS 2006 Proceedings; abst 6092.
98. Baselga J, Semiglazov V, van Dam P, et al. Phase II double-blind randomized trial of daily oral RAD001 (everolimus) plus letrozole (LET) or placebo (P) plus LET as neoadjuvant therapy for ER+ breast cancer. SABCS 2007 Proceedings; abst 2066.
99. Gardner H, Bandaru R, Barrett C, et al. Biomarker analysis of a phase II double-blind randomized trial of daily oral RAD001 (everolimus) plus letrozole or placebo plus letrozole as neoadjuvant therapy for patients with estrogen receptor positive breast cancer. SABCS 2007 Proceedings; abst 4006.
100. Morabito A, Di Maio M, De Maio E, et al. Methodology of clinical trials with new molecular-targeted agents: where do we stand? Ann Oncol 2006;17(suppl 7):vii128–vii131.

Index

A

Activin type II, 91
Adjuvant trastuzumab, 209–212
Amplified in breast cancer 1 (AIB1), 111–112
Angiogenesis, 140–141
  bevacizumab
    clinical trial, phase III, 215
    docetaxel and paclitaxel, 215–216
    safety and activity, 215
    VEGF role, 214
Ankyrin repeat domain 17 (ANKRD17), 7
Anti-EGFR drugs
  erlotinib, 184–185
  gefitinib, 181–184
Antigen presenting cells (APCs), 141
Antisense (AS) oligonucleotides, 96
Apoptosis, 140
Aromatase, 112
Arylamine N-acetyltransferase. *See*
        N-acetyltransferase 2 (NAT2)
A-type cyclins, 58
5-Aza-deoxy-cytidine, 162

B

BAG1 protein, 6
Basal-like tumors, BRCA1
    immunohistochemical surrogate, 41–42
    vs. triple negative tumors, 42–43
BCL2 associate X protein (BAX), 5
Bosutinib, 189
BRCA1. *See also* Basal-like tumors
  double-strand breaks (DSB), 45
  founder mutations, 46
  germline mutations, 48
BRCA2 protein, 45
Breast development
  architecture, 1–2
  cancer susceptibility, 2–3
  cell proliferation, 2
  genomic approaches
    DNA repair genes, 6–7

    epithelial apoptosis, 5–6
    immunosurveillance and detoxification,
      7–9
    transcription factors, 9–12
  pathogenesis, 3–4
Bromodomain PHD finger transcription factor
    (BPTF), 9–10

C

Cancer stem cells, 28–30
Caspase-2, 6
β-Catenin, 93–94. *See also* Wnt signaling
    pathways
CDK inhibitors (CDKIs)
  pathway alterations
    Cip/Kip proteins, 71
    p21 cytoplasmic localization, 73
    p27 cytoplasmic mislocalization, 72
    p21Cip1/Waf1, 61–62
    p27 expression, 63
    p16INK4a and p15INK4b, 61
Cell cycle
  breast cancer pathogenesis
    Cdk inhibitors pathway alterations,
      71–73
    cyclin D1 role, 67–69
    cyclin E role, 69–70
    Rb direct and indirect role, 70–71
  CDK inhibitors (CDKIs)
    pathway alterations, 71–73
    p21Cip1/Waf1, 61–62
    p27 expression, 63
    p16INK4a and p15INK4b, 61
  cell fate, 56
  cyclin-dependent kinases (CDKs), 58–59
  DNA damage checkpoints, 57–58
CellSearch™, 128–129
Cip/Kip family, 61
Circulating tumor cells (CTCs), 128–129
c-*myc* transcription factor, 110–111
Colony stimulating factor (CSF-1), 107–108

Index

Cre recombinase, 22
Cripto-1 (CR-1/Cr-1)
  chemistry and composition, 88
  EGF-CFC protein family, 89–90
  Glypican-1/c-src/MAPK/Akt signaling
    pathway, 92
  human breast carcinomas, 95–96
  mammary epithelium tumorigenesis,
    94–95
  Nodal/Alk4/Alk7/Smad-2 signaling
    pathways, 91–92
  O-linked fucosylation, 88–89
  signaling pathways, 90
  Wnt signaling pathway and activin
    proteins, 92–93
Custom-made microarray assay. *See*
    Mammaprint assay
Cyclin B, 58–59
Cyclin D1
  estrogen-induced breast cancer, 68
  mammary tumorigenesis, 67
  overexpression, 68–69
Cyclin-dependent kinases (CDKs)–cyclins
  cell cycle machinery, 59
  definition and types, 58
Cyclin E
  low molecular weight (LMW) isoforms, 70
  overexpression, 69
cyclops (cyc) gene, 93

D

Dasatinib, 188
Deleterious mutations, 47
Differentiation therapy, 29
DNA damage checkpoints, 57–58
DNA methylation
  aberrations, 161
  bilateral relationship, 160
  chromatin modifications and cancer
    EZH2, 153
    histone acetylation, 152
    nucleosome, 151–152
    NurD complex, 153
  demethylation enzymes
    deamination and excision repair, 159
    DNA methyltransferases, 155
    equilibrium, 157
    isoforms, 156
    MBD2, 158–159
    reversible and irreversible reaction, 157
    targeting events, 155–156
  gene expression silencing, 154–155
  hypermethylation, tumor suppressor genes
    5-aza-deoxy-cytidine, 162–163

p16 gene, 162
  therapeutic implications, 163–164
hypomethylation
  demethylation inhibition, 166
  DNMT, 165–166
  global hypomethylation, 164
  and hypermethylation, 164–165
  MBD2, 166
  p16 gene, 165
  SAM, 166–167
  therapeutic implications, 164–167
pattern of, 153–154
prometastatic genes, 157, 161
DNA methyltransferases (DNMT), 155
D-type cyclins, 110
  description, 58–59
  G1/S transition modulator, 59–60

E

E-cadherin, 94
E2F transcription factors
  composition, 65
  molecular functions, 66
Ephrin B3 molecule, 12
Epidermal growth factor (EGF) family
  EGF-CFC protein
    activins, 91–92
    embryonic development, 93
    mammary gland development, 93–94
    related genes, 88
  protein destination and intranuclear
    localisation, 80
  receptors and ligands, 79
Epidermal growth factor receptor (EGFR), 107
Epithelial-mesenchymal transition (EMT), 143
Epoxide hydrolase (EPHX1), 8–9
ErbB2 growth factor receptor, 106–107
ErbB receptors
  lapatinib
    capecitabine, 213
    EGFR and HER2, 212
    endocrine agents and cardiac toxicity,
      213–214
    paclitaxel, 213
  pertuzumab, 212
  trastuzumab
    chemotherapy, 205, 207–208
    estrogen receptors and HER2 pathway,
      209–212
    polychemotherapy, 206
Erlotinib, 184–185
Estrogen receptor alpha (ERα), 2, 111
E-type cyclins, 58
Everolimus, 218–219

Index

F

Farnesyl transferase inhibitors (FTIs), 187
Fibroblast growth factors (FGFs), 105–106

G

G1 checkpoint, 57
Gefitinib
  bone metastasis and bone pain, 184
  phase II clinical trials, 181–182
  PI3K/AKT pathway, 182–183
Gene expression profiling technique
  diagnosis and prognosis
    CellSearch™, 128–129
    diagnostic test (VDX2), 129
    70-gene prognosis signature, 128
    Mammostrat®, 129
    Oncotype DX™ assay, 128
    recurrence, 129
  microarrays
    expression profile, 124
    integrated data analysis, 131
  molecular classification
    ER-positive tumors, 126
    hormone receptor negative breast
      cancers, 127
    normal breast-like subtype, 127
    prognosis, 127
    subtypes, 126
  therapeutic response
    docetaxel and topoisomerases, 130
    ER status, 130
    tamoxifen, 130–131
Genomic profiling technique, 43.
    See also Gene expression
    profiling technique
Genomic signature, 3, 5
Glutathione S-transferase (GST) theta 1
    (GSTT1), 8–9
Glypican-1/c-src/MAPK/Akt signaling
    pathways, 92
GRP78 protein, 92
G1/S transition regulation. *See* CDK inhibitors
    (CDKIs)
GTB2B, 11

H

HDAC inhibitors (HDACi), 152
Hereditary breast cancer (HBC)
  clinical and histopathological
    features, 48
  clinical management, 48–49
  founder mutations, 46
  genetics, 44
  lifetime risk, 45

oncogenetic counseling
    genetic test, 47–48
    mathematical models, 46–47
  susceptibility genes
    BRCA1, 44–45
    BRCA2, 45
HER4/ErbB4 receptor, 80–81
Histone acetyl transferase (HAT), 152
Histone, chromatin modifications, 152–153
Histone deacetylase inhibitors (HDACi), 152
Histone methyltransferase (HMETase), 153
Homeobox (HOX) genes, 11
Human breast cancer, transgenic mice model
  c-myc protooncogene, 110–111
  D-type cyclins, 110
  growth factor receptor
    CSF-1, 107–108
    EGFR10, 107
    ErbB2, 106–107
    met receptor tyrosine kinase family,
      108–109
    Wnt family, 109
  growth factors
    FGFs, 105–106
    TGFα, 104–105
  hormones
    AIB1, 111–112
    aromatase, 112
    estrogen receptor α, 111
  promoters, 104
  signal transduction, 109
  stromal components, 113
Human breast carcinomas, cripto-1
    (CR-1/Cr-1)
  enzyme-linked immunosorbent assay
    (ELISA), 95
  therapeutic intervention, 96
Human epidermal growth factor receptor
    (HER), 205

I

Immunohistochemical staining technique,
    81–82
Inhibitor of DNA binding 4 (ID4), 11
INK4/ARF locus, 73
INK4 gene family, 61
Intracellular signal transduction pathways
    AZD0530, 188–189
    AZD3409, 188
    AZD6244, 189–190
    bosutinib, 189
    dasatinib, 188
    tipifarnib, 187
Intranucleoplasmic localisation, 83

228 Index

L
β-Lactoglobulin (BLG) promoter, 104
Lapatinib, 212–214
Lob 1 (TDLU), 3
Lonafarnib, 187–188
Long-label retaining epithelial cells
  (LREC), 26

M
Mammalian target of rapamycin (mTOR)
  everolimus
    phase II trial, 218–219
    phase I study, 218
  temsirolimus
    antitumor activity, 217
    phase II study, 217–218
    phase I trial, 217
MammaPrint®, 128, 132
Mammaprint assay, 43
Mammary gland, stem cells
  human fibroblasts transplant, 26–27
  mammosphere culture system, 27–28
  niches
    autonomous phenotype, 34
    co-localization, 33
    ex vivo culture, 33–34
    homeostasis, 30–31
    Sca-1 marker, 32
    systemic hormonal stimuli, 31–32
    terminal end buds (TEBs), 32
  progenitor cells, 27
  tumorigenesis
    cancer stem cells, 21
    characterization, 28–29
    MMTV transformation, 19–20
    pregnancy and MMTV-neu induced
      tumors, 29–30
    xenotransplatation and mammosphere, 29
Mammary tumor virus model, 19–20
Mammosphere culture system, 27
Mammostrat®, 129
Matrix-associated proteins, 83
Metallothionein (MT) promoter, 104, 105
Metastasis associated proteins (MTA), 153
Methylated DNA binding proteins (MBDs),
  154, 160
Met receptor tyrosine kinase family
  hepatocyte growth factor, 108
  Ron receptor, 108–109
  tpr-met fusion gene, 108
MicroRNA (miRNA) expression, 44
Missense mutations, 47
Mitogen-activated protein kinase (MAPK), 180
Mitosis promoting factor (MPF), 58

Mitotic catastrophe, 58
MMTV-CR-1 transgenic mice, 94
Molecular target based agents
  angiogenesis
    bevacizumab, 215–216
    VEGF role, 214
  ErbB receptors
    lapatinib, 212–214
    pertuzumab, 212
    trastuzumab, 205–212
  mammalian target of rapamycin (mTOR)
    everolimus, 218–219
    temsirolimus, 217–218
Morphogenesis checkpoint, 58
Mouse mammary tumour virus long
      terminal repeat (MMTV-LTR)
      promoter, 104
Multilineage progenitor cells, 27
Multiple ligation-dependent probe
      amplification techniques
      (MLPA), 48

N
N-acetyltransferase 2 (NAT2), 8–9
Neoadjuvant chemotherapy, 43
Neuregulins (NRGs)
  biological functions, 80–81
  immunohistochemical staining technique,
    81–82
  nuclear functions
    coimmunoprecipitation, 84
    EGF receptors, 82–83
    HER4/ErbB4 receptor, 84
    protein localisation, 83
NRG1β3, 81
Nuclear membrane associated ribosomes, 83
Nuclear protein Ki67, 2

O
Oep mutant phenotype, 93
O-linked fucosylation, 88–89
Oncogenes
  growth factor receptors
    CSF-1, 107–108
    EGFR, 107
    ErbB2, 106–107
    met receptor tyrosine kinase family,
      108–109
    Wnt family, 109
  growth factors
    FGFs, 105–106
    TGFβ, 104–105
Oncotype DxTM assay, 43, 128
Open reading frames (ORF), 7

Index

P

Parity-induced mammary epithelial cells
  (PI-MECs)
  LacZ expression, 22
  long-label retaining epithelial cells
    (LREC), 25–26
  mammary tumorigenesis, 25
  pregnancy-induced changes, 21
  self renewal capacity and pluripotency
    LacZ-positive cells role, 23
    WAP TGF expression, 23–25
Parous *vs.* nulliparous women, 4
p300/CBP-associated factor (PCAF), 11
Pertuzumab, 212
p27 expression, 63
PI3K/AKT pathway, 180
P53-mediated apoptosis, 6
Pocket proteins, 64
Polyomavirus middle T antigen (PyVmT),
  107, 109
p21 protein, 72–73
pRb protein
  breast cancer direct and indirect role,
    70–71
  cell growth regulator, 65–66
  E2F factors, 65
  functional significance, 64
  phosphorylation, 64–65
  retinoblastoma tumor suppressor, 64
Progesterone receptor (PgR), 2
Protein phosphatases, 6

R

RAD51-like 3 gene, 7
Restriction point (R point), 56–57
Retinoblastoma gene product. *See* pRb protein
Reverse transcriptase polymerase chain
  reaction (RT-PCR), 125
RNA-induced silencing complex (RISC). *See*
  MicroRNA expression
Ron receptor tyrosine kinase, 108–109

S

S-adenosyl methionine (SAM), 152
Serial transplantation, 27–28
Signal transducer and activator of
  transcription-1 (STAT-1), 11
Signal transduction inhibitors
  anti-EGFR drugs
    erlotinib, 184–185
    gefitinib, 181–184
  endocrine therapy
    EGFR-TKIs clinical trials, 191
    gefitinib and anastrozole, 190, 192

letrozole, 193
tamoxifen, 192–193
intracellular signal transduction pathways
  AZD0530, 188–189
  AZD3409, 188
  AZD6244, 189–190
  bosutinib, 189
  dasatinib, 188
  Lonafarnib, 187–188
  Ras proteins, 187
  tipifarnib, 187
molecular targets
  EGFR and ErbB receptors, 178–179
  PI3K/AKT pathway, 180
  ras/raf/MEK/MAPK pathway, 180
  RPS6KB1 gene, 180
  src protein, 180–181
  vascular endothelial growth factor
    (VEGF), 181
VEGFR signalling
  sorafenib, 185–186
  sunitinib, 186
  vandetanib, 186
Sorafenib, 185–186
SOX-2 factor, 10
Spindle checkpoint, 57–58
Spliceosome localisation, 81–82
Split hand/foot malformation (ectrodactyly)
  type 1, 6
Sporadic breast cancer
  genomic profiling, 43
  immunohistochemical panel, 42
  MicroRNA expression identification, 44
  molecular portrait, 40–42
  pathological factors, 40
  triple-negative and basal-like tumors
    BRCA1 protein, 42
    characterization, 42
    trial tests and therapies, 43
squint (sqt) gene, 93
Src protein, 180–181
Sub-nuclear localisation, 84
Sunitinib, 186
Suppressor of hairy wing homolog 4, 12

T

T-cells, 141
Terminal ductal lobular unit, 4
Terminal end buds (TEBs), 32
The American Society of Clinical Oncology
  (ASCO), 46
Thioredoxin reductase 1 (TR1), 8–9
Tipifarnib, 187
Tissue microarrays (TMAs), 124

Toll-like receptors (TLRs), 7
Tomoregulin-1, 91
Transforming growth factor-α (TGF-α), 104–105
Transforming growth factor-beta (TGF-β)
  alterations, evidence for, 141–142
  angiogenesis, 140–141
  apoptosis, 140
  dichotomy of, 142
    epithelia, 143
    mesenchymal cells, 143–144
  immune system, 141
  migration and invasion, 140
  proliferation, 139–140
  signaling cascade, 138
  therapeutic strategy
    antibody, 145
    immune system, 145–146
    increased expression, 144
    small molecule inhibitors, 145
Trastuzumab
  adjuvant therapy
    clinical issue, 212
    Herceptin® Adjuvant (HERA) trial, 209
    National Surgical Adjuvant Breast and Bowel Project (NSABP) B-31 trial, 209, 211
    North Central Cancer Treatment Group (NCCTG) N9831 trial, 209
  chemotherapy, 205, 207–208
  estrogen receptors and HER2, 209–212
  polychemotherapy, 206
  taxanes, 206
Trichostatin A (TSA), 160
Triple-negative tumors. *See* Basal-like tumors
Tsg101 gene, 25

Tumor necrosis factor receptor 1 (TNFR1), 6
Tumor suppressor genes, hypermethylation, 162–163
Tyrosine kinase inhibitors (TKIs), 181

U
Unknown variants (UV), 47

V
Vandetanib, 186
Vascular endothelial growth factor receptor (VEGFR) signaling inhibitors
  sorafenib, 185–186
  sunitinib, 186
  vandetanib, 186
Vascular endothelial growth factor (VEGF), 181
  angiogenesis, 214
  receptor tyrosine kinase inhibitors, 216

W
Whey acidic promoter (WAP)
  gene promoter
    Cre transgenic expression, 22–23
    TGF-β1 expression, 23–25
  mammary-specific gene expression, 104
  pregnancy-associated tumorigenesis, 29–30
  transgene expression, 94
Wnt signaling pathways
  β-catenin translocation, 95
  colon carcinoma, 92–93
  growth factor receptors, 109

X
X ray repair complementing defective repair I (XRCC4), 7